Respiratory Syncytial Virus

PERSPECTIVES IN MEDICAL VIROLOGY

Volume 14

Series Editors

A.J. Zuckerman

Royal Free and University College Medical School
University College London
London, UK

I.K. Mushahwar

Abbott Laboratories
Viral Discovery Group
Abbott Park, IL, USA

Respiratory Syncytial Virus

Editor

Patricia Cane

Health Protection Agency
Salisbury, Wiltshire, UK

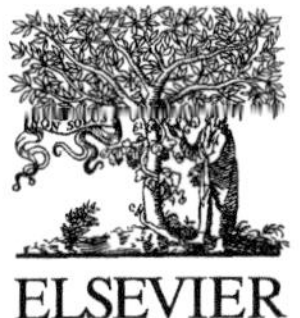

Amsterdam – Boston – Heidelberg – London – New York – Oxford – Paris
San Diego – San Francisco – Singapore – Sydney – Tokyo

Elsevier
Radarweg 29, PO Box 211, 1000 AE Amsterdam, The Netherlands
The Boulevard, Langford Lane, Kidlington, Oxford OX5 1GB, UK

First edition 2007

Library of Congress Cataloguing-in-Publication Data
A catalog record for this book is available from the Library of Congress

British Library Cataloguing in Publication Data
A catalogue record for this book is available from the British Library

ISBN-13: 978-0-444-52030-2
ISBN-10: 0-444-52030-9
ISSN: 0168-7069

For information on all Elsevier publications
visit our website at books.elsevier.com

Transferred to digital print 2007
Printed and bound by CPI Antony Rowe, Eastbourne

Contents

Contents

Preface

Respiratory syncytial virus (RSV) was first identified half a century ago in 1956. Following its discovery, the virus soon became recognised as a major viral pathogen causing extensive outbreaks of respiratory tract infections in both the very young and in vulnerable adults. It is an unusual virus in that it can cause repeated re-infections throughout life. Our understanding of the molecular biology and immunology of the virus is now very extensive. However, some aspects of its pathology, biology within the community setting, and interactions with other microorganisms remain elusive and a clear understanding of these factors will be necessary for effective control. Vast effort has been devoted over the years by both academia and industry towards the development of an effective and safe vaccine. It seems that goal may finally be almost within reach and it is to be hoped that a vaccine will be available to reduce the burden of disease due to the virus within the next few years.

The topics covered within this volume are wide ranging in scope from the most basic molecular biology of the virus to the clinical picture of RSV in the developing world. The first two chapters provide the background of the molecular biology and immunology of the virus, the next looks at the molecular epidemiology followed by the influence of host genetics. Chapters by Brearey and Smyth, Murata and Falsey, and Nokes examine the clinical picture of RSV in children, the elderly, and in the developing world, respectively. The next two chapters that follow review the current status of interventions against RSV, covering vaccine development and antiviral drugs. Recently, work has resumed on a much neglected surrogate virus, namely pneumonia virus of mice, and the final chapter describes progress with that model.

This volume of Perspectives in Medical Virology has enlisted many of the internationally recognised experts in their particular field of RSV research. The writers were invited not only to review the present state of knowledge, but also to give their perspective on the current situation and to identify the gaps and future requirements for research. It is to be hoped that the views expressed will stimulate new cross-cutting approaches to tackle this major viral pathogen.

Patricia Cane
Health Protection Agency,
UK

Respiratory Syncytial Virus
Patricia Cane (Editor)

DOI 10.1016/S0168-7069(06)14001-X

Molecular Biology of Human Respiratory Syncytial Virus

José A. Melero
Centro Nacional de Microbiología, Instituto de Salud Carlos III, Majadahonda, 28220 Madrid, Spain

Introduction

Human respiratory syncytial virus (HRSV) is the prototype of the *Pneumovirus* genus, which also includes the closely related bovine, ovine and caprine RSV and a more distantly related virus, the pneumonia virus of mice (PVM). The *Pneumovirus* genus is classified within the subfamily *Pneumovirinae* of the family *Paramyxoviridae*. Viruses of this family are grouped, together with those of the *Rhabdoviridae and Filoviridae* families, in the *Mononegavirales* order, which is characterized by having a linear, negative-sense, single-stranded RNA molecule as the genome (Mononegavirales, 2003). Viruses of this order share certain structural and functional features, including: (i) their genomes are tightly associated with the nucleoprotein (N) to form RNase-resistant nucleocapsids, which are the templates for all RNA synthesis, (ii) transcription proceeds in a sequential and polar manner from the 3′-end of the viral RNA (vRNA) by terminating and reinitiating at each of the gene junctions, (iii) replication of the viral genome involves the synthesis of a complementary antigenome (cRNA), (iv) the virus particles are surrounded by a lipid bilayer in which the viral glycoproteins are inserted, and (v) entry of the viral nucleocapsids into the host cells involves membrane fusion. Given these analogies, some details of the HRSV infectious cycle, which have not been addressed directly, are inferred from knowledge acquired from related viruses, particularly paramyxoviruses.

HRSV was first isolated in 1956 from a chimpanzee with coryza (Morris et al., 1956), and a year later from two children with respiratory illness (Chanock et al., 1957). Variability of HRSV isolates was first demonstrated at the antigenic level in a neutralization test performed with hyperimmune serum (Coates et al., 1966). Different panels of monoclonal antibodies were later used to subdivide HRSV isolates into two antigenic groups, A and B (Anderson et al., 1985; Mufson et al., 1985), which correlate with genetically distinct viruses (Cristina et al., 1990). Further variability among viruses of the same antigenic group has been found, particularly in the attachment (G) glycoprotein. This variability is discussed extensively in another chapter of this book.

The virion

HRSV virions are heterogeneous in size and shape. When observed by electron microscopy (EM), two types of viral particles are identified: (i) round- or kidney-shaped particles ranging in diameter from 150 to 250 nm and (ii) filaments up to 10 μm in length (Bächi and Howe, 1973) (Fig. 1A). These two types of particles can be separated, at least partially, by sucrose gradient centrifugation and both are infectious (Gower et al., 2005).

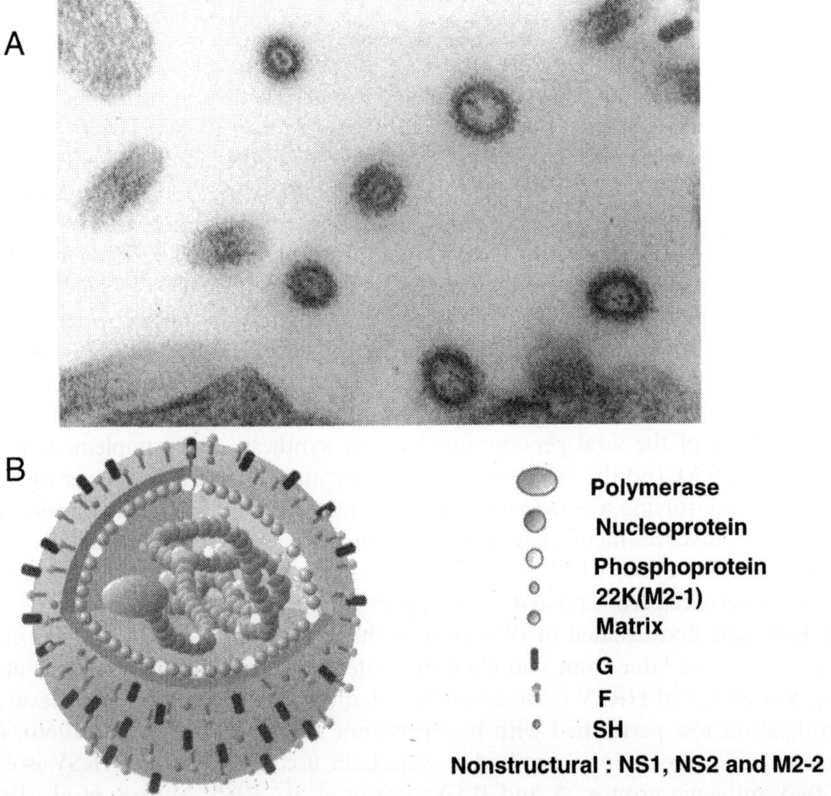

Fig. 1 Electron microscopy (A) and scheme (B) of the HRSV virion. The structural (colour-coded) and non-structural proteins are listed in part B of the figure (for colour version: see colour section on page 323).

Virus particles are surrounded by a lipid bilayer in which the two major surface glycoproteins are inserted (Fig. 1B). These consist of the attachment (G) glycoprotein involved in binding the virus to the cell surface (Levine et al., 1987) and the fusion (F) glycoprotein that mediates fusion of the viral and cell membranes (Walsh and Hruska, 1983). Both G and F form the characteristic spikes of HRSV virions seen by EM. A third small hydrophobic (SH) glycoprotein encoded by HRSV is expressed abundantly at the surface of virus-infected cells but is incorporated only in low amounts in the virus particles (Collins and Mottet, 1993).

The virus nucleocapsid, found inside the virion, consists of the vRNA (the genome) tightly bound to the nucleoprotein (N), forming a helix of "herringbone" morphology when imaged under a transmission electron microscope. The helical nucleocapsids of HRSV are more flexible and appear less well ordered than those of other paramyxoviruses. Pitches range from 68 to 74 Å and the nucleocapsid diameter from 14 to 16 nm, considerably narrower than that of other paramyxoviruses (Bhella et al., 2002). In addition to vRNA and N, other viral proteins are incorporated into the nucleocapsid but they are not observed by EM. These include the RNA-dependent RNA polymerase (or L protein), the phosphoprotein (P) and, probably, the 22k (or M2-1) protein.

HRSV encodes three non-structural proteins (NS1, NS2 and M2-2), which are produced in the infected cell but are not incorporated in the virus particles (Fig. 1B).

The infectious cycle

The different steps of the HRSV infectious cycle are illustrated in Fig. 2. Viral entry into the host cell occurs by the initial binding of virions to cell surface components, followed by activation of the F protein to trigger fusion of the viral and cell membranes. After the internalization of the viral nucleocapsids into the cell cytoplasm, sequential transcription of the viral genome is activated to generate a set of mRNAs that instruct translation of the corresponding gene products by the cell ribosomes. Sometime after infection RNA synthesis changes from transcription to the replication mode, generating a full-length copy of the vRNA of opposite polarity, named cRNA (or antigenome). This antigenome also complexes in nucleocapsids with the N protein, which are the templates for the synthesis of progeny genomes. Eventually, the different HRSV gene products accumulate near the cell membrane where they are assembled into progeny virus particles that are released from the infected cell by budding. The entire infectious cycle of HRSV, which follows the archetype of other paramyxoviruses, can take place in enucleated cells (Follet et al., 1975). However HRSV infection influences the expression of certain nuclear genes, as discussed latter in this chapter and in other chapters of this book.

Experimental systems to study the replicative cycle of HRSV

A wide range of animal species, including mice, cotton rats, mice, ferrets, guinea pigs, marmosets, lams and several non-human primates can be infected by the

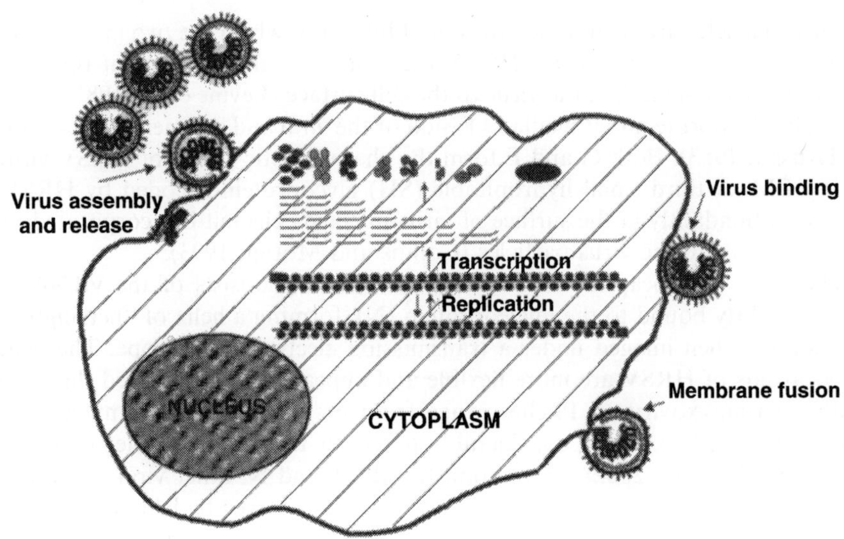

Fig. 2 Diagram of the HRSV infectious cycle (for colour version: see colour section on page 323).

administration of HRSV directly into the respiratory tract (Collins et al., 2001). The chimpanzee alone reproduces faithfully the infection observed in humans. The related bovine RSV infects calves and, perhaps, represents the best model to study RSV infections, since calves are the natural host of this virus (Taylor et al., 2005). However, the high cost of calves and the intensive labour involved in manipulation of calves precludes the routine use of these animals for experimental purposes.

Although animal models are useful to study HRSV infections, the *in vivo* approach is not open to manipulations that allow dissection of the different steps of the replicative cycle. Therefore, infection of established cell lines, or occasionally certain primary cultures, has been employed as the standard system to study the replicative cycle of HRSV. This virus can infect a wide variety of human and animal cells but it should be borne in mind that *in vivo* the epithelial cells of the respiratory tract are the major sites of virus replication.

The reverse genetics approach has revolutionized studies of mononegavirales since the rescue of infectious rabies virus from a full-length cDNA clone was achieved (Schnell et al., 1994). In the case of HRSV, the standard procedure involves cloning of the entire genome in the form of DNA (cDNA), flanked by a promoter of the bacteriophage T7 polymerase and a hammerhead ribozyme followed by T7 terminator(s) (Collins et al., 1995; Jin et al., 1998; Buchholz et al., 1999) (Fig. 3A). When this plasmid is transfected into cells that express the T7 polymerase, transcription by this enzyme generates a positive-stranded copy of the viral RNA (the cRNA or antigenome), which after ribozyme cleavage has the correct ends of the antigenome (although HRSV allows certain flexibility at the RNA ends). If the cells are co-transfected with support plasmids that encode N, P,

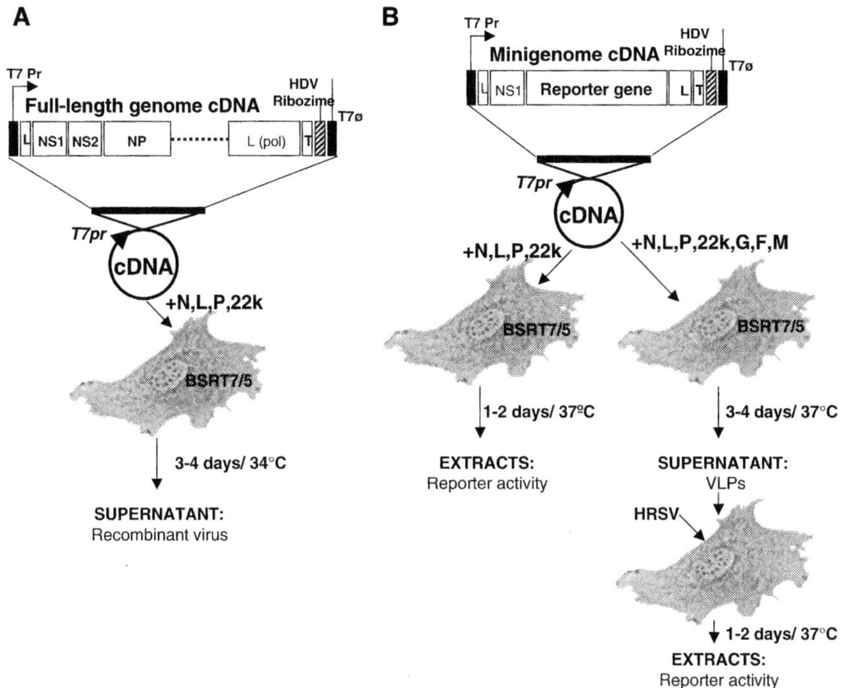

Fig. 3 Reverse genetics systems to study the HRSV replicative cycle. (A) Rescue of recombinant HRSV. BHK cells, expressing constitutively the bacteriophage T7 RNA polymerase (BSR T7/5 cells, Buchholz et al., 1999), are transfected with a plasmid carrying a full-length cDNA copy of the HRSV genome and co-transfected with plasmids encoding N, L, P and 22k proteins under a T7 promoter. Recombinant viruses are generated and released to the culture supernatant from where they can be grown to high titres in new cells. (B) Amplification of minigenomes. BSR T7/5 cells are co-transfected with plasmids carrying a minigenome version of the HRSV vRNA and supporting plasmids encoding N, P, L and 22k proteins under a T7 promoter (left). Extracts are made after 1–2 days in culture to measure reporter activity. If supporting plasmids encoding G, F, and M are also included in the transfection mixture (right), virus like particles (VLPs) carrying the minigenome are generated and released to the culture supernatant. These VLPs are used to infect fresh cultures that are superinfected with helper virus (HRSV). Reporter gene activity, coming from the minigenome encapsidated in the VLPs, is assayed in extracts of the infected cells, made after 1-2 days in culture. See text for details.

L and 22k proteins under the transcriptional control of the T7 promoter, the antigenome is replicated to yield copies of the viral genome that can be transcribed to generate the different gene products thus ensuring virus replication. This system provides the means to introduce predetermined changes into infectious virus via the cDNA intermediate and to test their effects on virus replication and phenotype.

A simplified model system of reverse genetics is based on minireplicons, which are short cDNA versions of the genome or antigenome in which most (or all) of the viral genes have been replaced by a reporter gene (Grosfeld et al., 1995), or shorter RNA analogues (Yu et al., 1995) (Fig. 3B). As with the full-length cDNA clones, transfection of plasmids carrying the minireplicon into cells expressing the T7 polymerase generates minigenomes or antiminigenomes that can be amplified by superinfection with wild-type helper virus (Grosfeld et al., 1995), or by providing the support plasmids encoding N, P, L and 22k proteins under control of a T7 promoter (Grosfeld et al., 1995; Yu et al., 1995). Transcription and amplification of the minireplicon can be assessed by biochemical tests (Yu et al., 1995) or indirectly by measuring the reporter gene activity (Grosfeld et al., 1995).

When cells transfected with the plasmid carrying the minireplicon are provided with plasmids encoding the proteins required for virus maturation (M, F and G), besides the proteins required for transcription and replication (N, P, L and 22k), virus-like particles (VLPs) are formed that are released into the culture supernatant (Teng and Collins, 1998). The presence of VLPs is detected by passage of the transfected cell supernatants into fresh cells which are superinfected with helper virus. The expression of the reporter gene is assayed in these newly infected cells. The minireplicon systems (Fig. 3B) are widely used as rapid methods to identify *cis*-acting sequences that regulate HRSV transcription and/or replication and to study the effect of certain mutations upon the functional properties of specific gene products.

Besides the reverse genetics systems described above, some *in vitro* assays have been developed that reproduce certain steps of the HRSV replicative cycle in the test tube. For instance, synthesis of viral mRNAs has been reproduced, at least to a certain extent, using crude extracts of HRSV-infected cells (Barik, 1992) or partially purified nucleocapsids (Mason et al., 2004). These *in vitro* assays provide an opportunity to set up high throughput systems to search for inhibitors that may have a prophylactic/therapeutic use (Liuzzi et al., 2005).

Finally, the last system to be mentioned here is the expression of individual proteins in tissue culture cells. In this way, their effects on cell metabolism and/or cell behaviour can be assessed independently of other viral gene products. Examples of this approach include the expression of NS1 and NS2 proteins in transfected cells that decreases Stat2 levels and the consequent downstream interferon-α/β response (Lo et al., 2005), or the expression of the F protein which leads to cell–cell fusion and syncytia formation (González-Reyes et al., 2001).

Here, follows a description of the different steps of the HRSV replicative cycle and the viral products that participate in each step.

Virus entry

Virus entry by enveloped viruses has been a topic of intensive investigation in recent years since this step occurs outside the host cell, and consequently is more accessible to inhibition by antiviral candidates than later steps of the infectious cycle that occur inside the infected cell. Two steps are well differentiated in this process: (i) binding of the virus to certain cell surface components and (ii) fusion of the virus and cell membranes at the cell surface. The HRSV G and F glycoproteins mediate these two steps, respectively, although G is not required for infection of certain cell types in tissue culture (see later).

The G glycoprotein

This protein is produced in two different forms in the infected cell: (i) as a type II transmembrane protein (Gm) that is incorporated into virions and (ii) as a soluble protein (Gs) that is secreted by the infected cells (Hendricks et al., 1987, 1988) (Fig. 4). The Gm polypeptide precursor of about 300 amino acids (depending on the strain) contains a single hydrophobic domain (residues 38–63) that acts as a combined signal and a transmembrane anchor domain. This hydrophobic region targets the nascent chain, as it emerges from the ribosome, to the endoplasmic reticulum (ER) and ensures translocation of the polypeptide chain across the membrane, bringing about the stable anchoring of the protein in the lipid bilayer. Gm has neither sequence nor structural homology with the attachment protein of other paramyxoviruses (Wertz et al., 1985).

The Gm polypeptide precursor is extensively modified by the addition of both N- and O-linked oligosaccharides and is also palmitylated, probably at a single cysteine residue located in the N-terminal cytoplasmic tail (Collins and Mottet, 1992). High-mannose N-linked sugar chains are co-translationally added to the G protein precursor to yield intermediate species of 40–50 kDa (Wertz et al., 1989; Collins and Mottet, 1992). This step is followed by the conversion of the N-linked sugars into the complex type and addition of O-linked sugars in the Golgi compartment before reaching the plasma membrane. These modifications convert the 32 kDa precursor into a mature protein of 80–90 kDa, as estimated by SDS–PAGE. Although this technique does not provide a very accurate estimate of the molecular mass of glycoproteins, due to the abnormal interaction of oligosaccharides with SDS, the large difference in the electrophoretic mobility between the precursor and the mature protein highlights the contribution of carbohydrates to the mass of the mature Gm.

The C-terminal Gm ectodomain has a central region (amino acids 164–176) and four cysteines (residues 173, 176, 182 and 186), which are, conserved in all HRSV isolates (Johnson et al., 1987). Disulfide bridges occur between Cys173 and 186, and between Cys176 and 182, resulting in a cystine noose motif which resembles the structure found in the 55 kDa tumour necrosis factor receptor (Doreleijers et al., 1996; Langedijk et al., 1996, 1998). Flanking this region, there are two protein segments that have a high level of sequence variation among HRSV isolates. While the conserved region is essentially devoid of carbohydrates, the variable regions have several potential sites for N-glycosylation and multiple serines and threonines which are predicted to be O-glycosylated by the NetOglyc software (Hansen et al., 1998). Both, N- and O-linked carbohydrates are found in the mature Gm. The variable regions have overall amino acid composition similar to that of the mucins secreted by epithelial cells, which are also extensively modified by the addition of O-linked sugars (Apostopoulos and McKenzie, 1994; García-Beato et al., 1996).

Fig. 4 shows a model for the three-dimensional (3-D) structure of the Gm molecule, modified from the one proposed by Langedijk et al. (1996). Although illustrated as a dimer, native Gm is probably a homotetramer, as inferred from its sedimentation behaviour in sucrose gradients (Escribano-Romero et al., 2004).

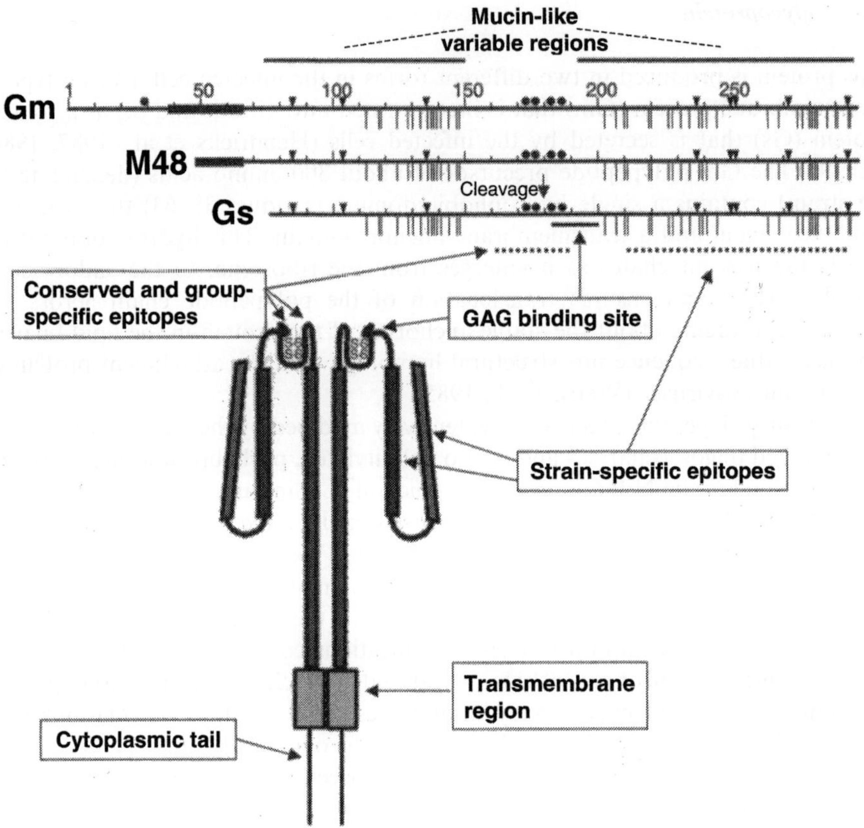

Fig. 4 Scheme of the G protein of HRSV. A straight line of 298 amino acids denotes the Gm polypeptide of the HRSV Long strain. The hydrophobic transmembrane region is indicated by a thick solid line (residues 38–66). The potential N-glycosylation sites (▼), the O-glycosylation sites predicted with the NetOGlyc software (|) (Hansen et al., 1998) and the cysteines (●) are also indicated. Formation of Gs occurs by translation initiation at Met48, and subsequent cleavage after residue 65 (Roberts et al., 1994). A model of the 3-D structure of the mature Gm molecule is depicted in the lower part of the figure. Although Gm is likely a tetramer (Escribano-Romero et al., 2004), it is represented as a homodimer for simplicity. Several structural motifs are denoted in the model and in the primary structure.

Several structural domains can be identified in each protein monomer. The first N-terminal 37 amino acids represent the cytoplasmic tail and the following 26 residues the transmembrane region. The first hypervariable region, preceding the cysteine cluster, probably adopts a rod-like structure due to the presence of multiple, closely spaced, O-linked sugar chains that leads to elongation of the polypeptide backbone (Jentoft, 1990). The cystine noose, made up of the conserved Gm region, including the cluster of four cysteines, follows this region. The 3-D structure of the cystine noose was determined by nuclear magnetic resonance of a 19 amino acid core, within a 32-residue peptide corresponding to amino acids

158–189 (Doreleijers et al., 1996). The cystine noose core structure has a relatively flat surface formed by two short α-helices connected by a type I′ turn. A characteristic hydrophobic pocket, lined by conserved residues, lies at the surface of the cystine noose motif. This hydrophobic pocket was proposed tentatively to act as a receptor-binding site (Johnson et al., 1987), although there is still a lack of experimental evidence to support this hypothesis. However, a short amino acid segment near the cystine noose (residues 184–198) has been implicated in binding of Gm to cell surface glycosaminoglycans (GAGs) (Feldman et al., 1999). This type of structural arrangement places the site of interaction of Gm with cell-surface components (GAGs) at an appropriate distance from the transmembrane region that is inserted in the viral envelope. In agreement with its conserved nature, the central segment of the Gm ectodomain contains epitopes that are either maintained in all HRSV isolates (conserved epitopes) or are shared by viruses of the same antigenic group (group-specific epitopes) (Martínez et al., 1997; Melero et al., 1997).

The second C-terminal hypervariable region of the Gm molecule, which follows the cluster of cysteines, is externally located in the 3-D model of Fig. 4, indicating its accessibility to antibodies that recognize strain-specific epitopes and that map in this region of the molecule. Cell-type specific glycosylations influence the expression of epitopes located in this hypervariable region (Palomo et al., 1991, 2000; García-Beato et al., 1996). Notably, this region, in particular the first half, is partially resistant to protease degradation. In addition, cell-specific glycosylations in the C-terminal half of this region influence the expression of certain epitopes in its N-terminal half, suggesting interactions between the two halves of the C-terminal hypervariable region of Gm (García-Beato et al. 2000), as denoted in Fig. 4.

Interestingly, none of the anti-G monoclonal antibodies described to date are highly neutralizing; however, either polyclonal antiserum raised against purified G protein, pools of anti-G monoclonal antibodies (Martínez and Melero, 1998) or an anti-anti-iditotypic antiserum raised against an anti-G monoclonal antibody (Palomo et al., 1990) exhibit enhanced neutralization. These results suggest that inhibition of HRSV infectivity by anti-G antibodies may be determined by steric hindrance of virus interactions with some component of the cell surface.

The soluble form of the G glycoprotein (Gs) is synthesized by alternative translation initiation by the ribosomes at a second in-frame AUG codon, which lies within the signal/anchor domain of the G protein reading frame (Fig. 4). The N-terminal hydrophobic signal peptide is then proteolytically processed following residue 65 (Roberts et al., 1994). The soluble Gs is transported from the lumen of the ER to the exterior of the cell via the exocytic pathway. Secreted Gs remains monomeric, as assessed by sucrose gradient sedimentation, suggesting that the transmembrane region of Gm is required for oligomerization (Escribano-Romero et al., 2004). Despite the differences between Gs and Gm in the oligomerization state, the former protein is also heavily glycosylated by N- and O-linked oligosaccharides and both forms of G are indistinguishable when tested for reactivity with an extensive panel of monoclonal antibodies. Thus, Gs can be considered the monomeric form of the Gm ectodomain.

As mentioned before, Gm is thought to mediate binding of HRSV particles to the host cell surface (Levine et al., 1987); however it has been reported that viruses lacking the G gene are still capable of replicating in cell culture, although they are attenuated *in vivo* (Karron et al., 1997; Teng et al., 2001). Thus, alternative routes for HRSV binding to cells, independent of Gm, should exist. The actual role of Gs is still not known. Several studies have provided evidence that Gs may act as a decoy for antibodies or it may play some immunomodulatory role *in vivo* (Polack et al., 2005). Interestingly, recombinant viruses expressing only Gs can replicate efficiently in cell culture and are only moderately attenuated *in vivo* (Teng et al., 2001).

The F glycoprotein

The fusion (F) protein of HRSV has low yet significant sequence relatedness and shares some structural motifs with the fusion protein of other paramyxoviruses. It is a type I glycoprotein that is synthesized as an inactive precursor (F0) of 574 amino acids (Johnson and Collins, 1988). This precursor is cleaved by furin-like proteases during maturation to yield two disulfide-linked polypeptides, F2 from the N-terminus and F1 from the C-terminus (Fig. 5). In contrast to other paramyxovirus F proteins that are cleaved only once, the F0 precursor of HRSV (González-Reyes et al., 2001) and that of the related bovine RSV (Zimmer et al., 2001a) are cleaved twice, following residues 109 (site I) and 136 (site II), which are preceded by furin-recognition motifs. Site II is equivalent to the single cleavage site found in other paramyxovirus F proteins. After completion of cleavage at sites I and II, a 27-mer peptide is released from the mature F protein which, in the case of bovine RSV, shares sequence identity with tachykinins, an evolutionary conserved family of peptide hormones (Zimmer et al., 2003). Although tachykinin-like activity was detected in the supernatant of bovine RSV-infected cells, the significance of this finding for the virus life cycle is not known, since HRSV F does not contain a tachykinin motif.

The F protein of all paramyxovirus have three main hydrophobic regions: one at the N-terminus, which acts as the signal peptide for translocation to the ER during synthesis; another near the C-terminus, which is the membrane anchor or transmembrane domain; and a third hydrophobic region at the N-terminus of the F1 chain, called the fusion peptide since it is thought to be inserted into the target membrane during the process of membrane fusion. The F0 precursor is co-translationally translocated to the ER where it is decorated with high-mannose sugar chains. These oligosaccharides are later modified to the complex type while traversing the Golgi compartment (Collins and Mottet, 1991). Before reaching the cell surface the F0 precursor is cleaved at sites I and II by furin; however cleavage is not 100% effective, resulting in cleavage intermediates (cleaved only at site I or site II), which are found in virions in addition to fully processed F molecules (González-Reyes et al., 2001).

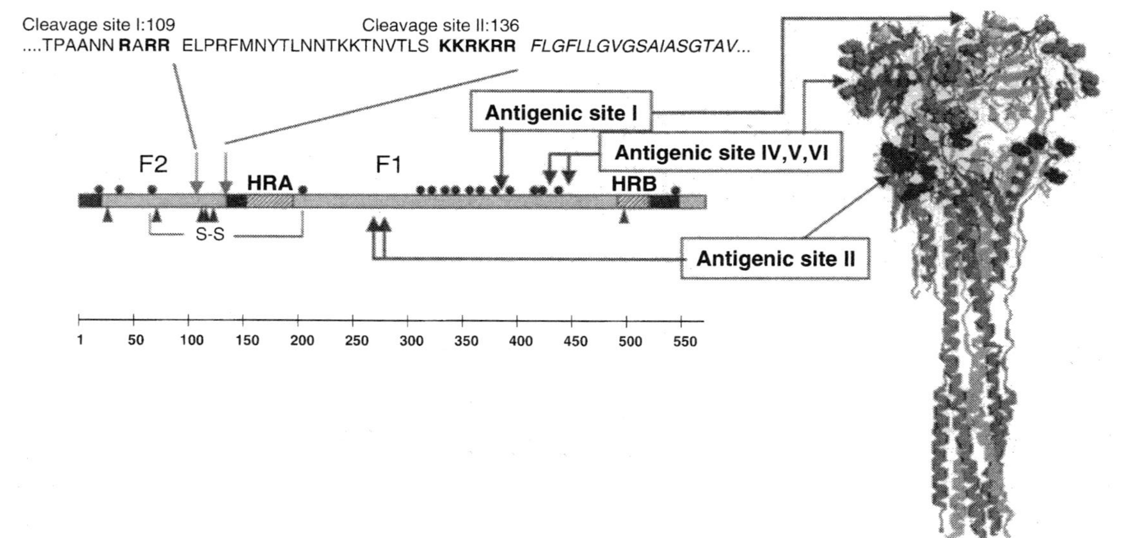

Fig. 5 Scheme of the F protein of HRSV. The F0 precursor is depicted as a grey rectangle of 574 amino acids in length. The hydrophobic regions are shown in black and the heptad repeat sequences (HRA and HRB) in shaded rectangles, respectively. The two cleavage sites that yield the F1 and F2 chains are indicated by vertical arrows (red and blue). A partial amino acid sequence of the F protein, including cleavage sites I and II (with the furin recognition sequences shown in boldface) and the fusion peptide (italics), is shown above the protein diagram. Also shown are the N-glycosylation sites (▲), the cysteine residues (●) and the disulfide bond (–S–S–) between the F2 and F1 chains. A 3-D model of the HRSV F glycoprotein, based on the structure determined for the uncleaved parainfluenza type 3 F ectodomain (Yin et al., 2005), is shown at right. Residues that are changed in escape mutants selected with monoclonal antibodies, whose epitopes map in the different antigenic sites of the F molecule, are indicated in the protein diagram and in the 3-D model (for colour version: see colour section on page 324).

The mature HRSV F protein is a homotrimer in which two heptad-repeat sequences, HRA and HRB (Fig. 5), adjacent to the fusion peptide and to the transmembrane region of each monomer, respectively, serve as important motifs for the formation and stability of the F trimers (Chambers et al., 1992). HRA and HRB peptides form trimeric complexes in solution (Lawless-Delmenico et al., 2000; Matthews et al., 2000) and X-ray crystallography of these complexes has revealed a structure consisting of an internal core of three HRA α-helices bounded by three antiparalell HRB α-helices, packed into the grooves of the HRA coiled-coil trimer (Zhao et al., 2000).

HRSV F protein is palmitylated within the transmembrane region at Cys550 via a thioester bond (Arumugham et al., 1989) and glycosylated by the addition of N-linked glycosylation oligosaccharides at Asn27, Asn70, Asn116, Asn120, Asn126 and Asn500. Elimination of the glycosylation sites on the F2 chain (Asn27 and Asn70) has a minimal effect on membrane fusion, as measured by syncytia formation in transfected cells. In contrast, mutagenesis of Asn500 ablated the fusion activity of bovine RSV F, although did not alter expression at the cell surface (Zimmer et al., 2001b). The effects of the sugar chains bound to Asn116, Asn120 and Asn126 on F fusion activity have not yet been studied. However, these glycosylation sites are located in the intervening segment between cleavage sites I and II and, consequently, the corresponding oligosaccharides are not present in the fully processed mature molecule. In addition, Asn120 is not conserved in all HRSV strains. Whether or not glycosylation of F in the segment between the two cleavage sites influences proteolytic processing of the F0 precursor and/or other property of the F molecule remains to be elucidated.

The 3-D structure of HRSV F has not been solved to date. However, based on a partial atomic structure of the Newcastle Disease Virus (NDV) F protein (Chen et al., 2001), a partial model of HRSV F was proposed (Smith et al., 2002). A more complete model was later constructed by grafting the six-helix core of HRSV F (Zhao et al., 2000) onto the model based on the NDV F structure (Morton et al., 2003). Fig. 5 shows a similar model of the HRSV F 3-D structure, based on the atomic structure of a soluble form of the parainfluenza virus type 3 F protein recently determined by X-ray crystallography (Yin et al., 2005). The 3-D models of HRSV F are in good agreement with EM images of HRSV F molecules (Calder et al., 2000). Furthermore, when the residues altered in monoclonal antibody escape mutants are located in the F protein model, a good correlation is observed between the location of those residues in the 3-D model and the binding sites of the corresponding antibodies, as observed by EM (Calder et al., 2000) (Fig. 5). Although these data lend support to the 3-D model of HRSV F, it is still not known whether the structure presented in Fig. 5 corresponds to the conformation adopted by the F molecule in the pre- or postactive configuration (see later).

Interestingly, highly neutralizing antibodies directed against the F protein bind to epitopes at antigenic sites II or the overlapping sites IV, V and VI, while other antibodies specific to these sites are only weakly neutralizing. Monoclonal antibodies binding at epitopes of site I have all low neutralizing activity (Beeler and van

Wyke Coeling, 1989; García-Barreno et al., 1989; Arbiza et al., 1992; López et al., 1998). Thus, in contrast to the afore-mentioned neutralization by anti-G antibodies based on steric hindrance, the mechanism of HRSV neutralization by anti-F antibodies seems to require specific interactions of antibodies with certain residues of the F protein, perhaps to inhibit conformational changes that occur during the process of membrane fusion. The importance of research into anti-F antibodies is emphasized by the fact that a humanized neutralizing monoclonal antibody (Palivizumab), directed against an epitope of F protein antigenic site II, is the only product available to date for prophylactic treatment of HRSV infections in high-risk infants (Groothuis and Nishida, 2002).

Virus binding and membrane fusion

As mentioned previously, paramyxoviruses enter the cell by fusion of the viral and cell membranes at the cell surface. Preceding this step, the virus is likely to bind to a specific cell surface component. The nature of the viral receptor has been elucidated for certain paramyxovirus (Lamb and Kolakofsky, 2001), and may involve carbohydrates, such as sialic acid in the case of Sendai virus (Markwell et al., 1980, 1985), or protein components of the cell surface, such as CD46 or SLAM (Dhiman et al., 2004), in the case of measles virus. However, it is worth noting that the same virus may use alternative receptors depending on the cell type being infected.

An initial observation indicated that heparin (a soluble proteoglycan) could inhibit HRSV infectivity in cell cultures (Krusat and Streckert, 1997). Subsequently, it was demonstrated that HRSV could bind to the glycosaminoglycan (GAG) moiety of proteoglycans (Hallak et al., 2000a; Martínez and Melero, 2000). Proteoglycans are macromolecules of the cell surface or extracellular matrix in which one or more GAG chains are joined covalently to either membrane or secreted proteins, commonly through Ser residues. The GAG chains are long oligosaccharides of heterogeneous length, which consist of alternating units of *N*-acetylglucosamine and glucuronic or iduronic acid. GAGs normally contain high levels of sulfate groups linked to the sugar hydroxyl groups, which confer a net negative charge to proteoglycans that is at the basis of interactions with positively charged regions of protein ligands.

Preincubation of HRSV with different GAGs or elimination of these components of the cell surface with specific enzymes provided evidence that heparan sulfate is the main GAG involved in binding to HRSV (Hallak et al., 2000a; Martínez and Melero, 2000). Specifically, iduronic acid, sulfate groups and a minimal length of 10 saccharides seem to be critical requirements for interaction of GAGs with HRSV (Hallak et al., 2000b).

The HRSV G glycoprotein was originally proposed as the attachment protein because a specific antiserum blocked virus binding to HeLa cells (Levine et al., 1987). In agreement with this hypothesis, it was found that binding of HRSV to GAGs is mediated mainly by the G glycoprotein (Techaarpornkul et al., 2002). Studies with overlapping peptides derived from consensus sequences of the

G protein ectodomain identified a positively charged region, including residues 184-198 for antigenic group A and 183–197 for antigenic group B viruses, which was involved in binding to heparin (Feldman et al., 1999). However, this heparin binding domain (HBD) may not be the only region of the G protein capable of interacting with GAGs, since recombinant HRSV lacking that segment could still infect cells in a GAG-dependent manner (Teng et al., 2001). In addition, Gs lacking the HBD had a reduced capacity to bind to cells but the remaining activity was still sensitive to heparinase treatment of cells (Escribano-Romero et al., 2004). Furthermore, studies with G protein fragments expressed in bacteria provided evidence of GAG binding outside HBD (Shields et al., 2003). Since the G protein ectodomain is rich in positively charged residues, it is possible that other regions outside HBD may contribute to attachment to proteoglycans.

While the G protein may be the main HRSV component involved in binding to GAGs, a recombinant virus with the F protein as its only viral glycoprotein (rgRSV-F) could still infect certain cell types in tissue culture, in a proteoglycan-dependent manner. Comparison of the attachment and infection activities of wild-type and rgRSV-F virions with CHO cell mutants defective in GAG biosynthesis indicated that approximately 50% of the wild type attachment is due to G protein–GAG binding, 25% to F protein–GAG binding and 25% to an independent pathway (Techaarpornkul et al., 2002). The latter observation is important since HRSV, as observed for other viruses, may use alternative receptors (or co-receptors) in order to infect different cell types. It has been postulated that, owing to the highly glycosylated nature of the G protein, cell surface lectins could serve as HRSV receptors. In support of this hypothesis, HRSV G is able to bind to several lectins (García-Beato et al., 1996), including surfactant proteins—A and D (LeVine et al., 1999, 2004). The latter interaction may facilitate clearance of virus by alveolar macrophages. Furthermore, it has been suggested that HRSV G may bind to the fractalkine receptor by mimicry of the CX3C motif present in the fractalkine chemokine (Tripp et al., 2001). However, the significance of G binding to alternative receptors during natural infection and the identity of cell surface components which interact with rgRSV-F remain to be elucidated.

Following binding of HRSV to the cell surface, membrane fusion is triggered by activation of the F glycoprotein. Fig. 6 illustrates the process of membrane fusion mediated by HRSV F, adapted from a general model of fusion by class I viral fusion proteins, which are characterized by having a fusion peptide at the N-terminus of the membrane-anchored polypeptide (Skehel and Wiley, 2000). Activation of the F protein for membrane fusion must occur in the vicinity of the cell membrane since it involves exposure of the fusion peptide. In the absence of a target membrane, exposure of the highly hydrophobic fusion peptide would lead to its insertion in the viral membrane and consequently inhibition of virus infectivity. However, once the virus particle is bound to the host cell, exposure of the fusion peptide leads to its insertion in the cell membrane (Fig. 6B). In this way, the F1 chain is bound simultaneously to the target cell membrane through its N-terminus and to the viral membrane through the transmembrane region. Refolding of this

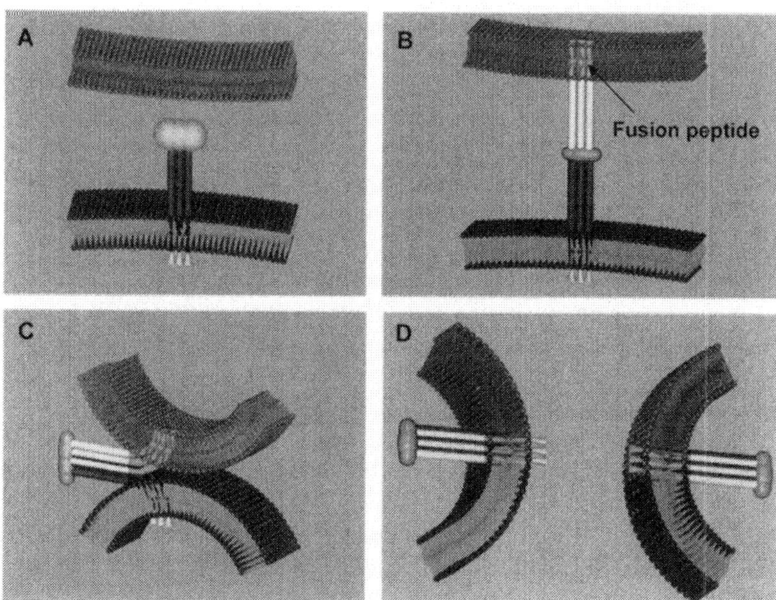

Fig. 6 Model of the viral and cell membrane fusion mediated by the HRSV glycoprotein. (A) Only an F protein trimer is shown inserted into the viral lipid bilayer (green) and in the proximity of the cell membrane (red). (B) After activation of the F protein, the fusion peptide is exposed and consequently it is inserted into the target cell membrane. (C) Refolding of the F protein intermediate brings the viral and cell membranes into close proximity. (D) Lipid mixing of the two membranes forms the fusion pore that probably requires the concerted action of several F molecules (for colour version: see colour section on page 325).

unstable F intermediate brings the viral and cell membranes into close proximity (Fig. 6C). This step probably involves formation of a highly stable structure in which the 6-helix bundle, formed from the two heptad repeats (HRA and HRB) of the F1 polypeptide, plays a crucial role. This step is followed by lipid mixing of the two membranes and formation of the fusion pore that connects the interior of the virus particle with the cell cytoplasm (Fig. 6D).

It has been a matter of some speculation how activation of HRSV F actually occurs. In the case of other paramyxoviruses, it has been postulated that the receptor binding protein (HN or H) interacts with the F protein in the virion maintaining the latter protein in a preactive configuration. After attachment to cells, the HN protein would undergo its own conformational change which, in turn, could trigger a conformational change of the F protein resulting in the release of the fusion peptide (Lamb, 1993; Lamb et al., 2006). In agreement with this hypothesis, induction of syncytia formation in transfected cells expressing the paramyxovirus F protein requires co-expression of the homotypic attachment protein. Co-immunoprecipitation analysis has also indicated that F and HN can form a complex in the cell surface (Stone-Hulslander and Morrison, 1997; Yao et al., 1997) and co-capping of the two proteins has been observed.

In contrast with the situation found in other paramyxoviruses, expression of HRSV F alone in transfected cells leads to syncytia formation (Zimmer et al., 2001b; González-Reyes et al., 2001). Furthermore, both a spontaneous deletion mutant of HRSV lacking SH and G genes (Karron et al., 1997), and a recombinant virus with F as the only viral glycoprotein (Techaarpornkul et al., 2002) can infect certain cell lines in tissue culture and induce syncytia formation, indicating that HRSV F is capable of mediating virus–cell and cell–cell fusion, respectively, in the absence of other viral envelope glycoproteins. Thus, activation of HRSV F does not depend on the interaction of G with a cellular receptor, at least in situations in which F is the only HRSV glycoprotein present.

When purified HRSV F is observed by electron microscopy (EM), after negative staining, it is seen to aggregate into rosettes, consisting of rods formed by the aggregation of F trimers through their transmembrane regions (Calder et al., 2000). In contrast, a soluble anchorless form of HRSV F, lacking the transmembrane and cytoplasmic tail (F_{TM}–), is seen mainly as unaggregated rods. Preparations of both F and F_{TM}– contain, in addition to molecules cleaved to F1 and F2 chains, uncleaved F0 molecules and partially processed intermediates cleaved only at site I or II. When cleavage of the F_{TM}– monomers is completed by controlled trypsin digestion, the F_{TM}– trimers aggregate into rosettes (Ruiz-Argüello et al., 2002). This aggregation requires a functional fusion peptide, indicating that F_{TM}– aggregation may reproduce some of the conformational changes that occur in the F protein during the process of membrane fusion (Martín et al., 2006). Whether or not completion of cleavage at sites I and II is the only activating step for HRSV requires further experimentation.

In summary, during natural viral infection, the G and F proteins mediate HRSV binding to the cell surface GAGs and virus–cell membrane fusion, respectively. However, alternative receptors may mediate binding of G or F to the cell surface. In addition, activation of the F protein does not depend on the presence of G protein. Thus, the mechanisms operating during the initial stages of the HRSV replicative cycle may differ to some extent from the mechanisms that operate for entry of other paramyxoviruses.

Inhibitors of HRSV entry have been the topic of intense research in recent years. Besides the afore-mentioned humanized anti-F monoclonal antibody (Groothuis and Nishida, 2002), small inhibitors of F protein activity have been actively searched. By analogy with synthetic peptides that inhibit human immunodeficiency virus (HIV) replication (Wild et al., 1994), synthetic peptides that reproduce sequences of the heptad repeats (HR) regions of HRSV were synthesized and tested for inhibition of virus infectivity. Peptides containing partial sequences of HRB were found to be highly active inhibitors of HRSV infectivity (Lambert et al., 1996). These peptides presumably bind to the HRA core of an F protein intermediate during the process of virus–cell membrane fusion, blocking latter stages of the fusion process.

Other small molecules obtained by chemical synthesis have been shown to interact with the HRSV F protein and inhibit membrane fusion. One of these molecules (BMS-433771) has been shown to bind to the F1 chain of HRSV, within a hydrophobic pocket formed at the surface of the HRA core. This interaction presumably prevents the formation of the six-helix bundle of HRA and HRB regions during the final stages of the fusion process (Cianci et al., 2004). Other low molecular weight inhibitors of HRSV have also been described that bind to the F protein, although their binding sites have not been identified. Mutants that escape neutralization by these inhibitors accumulate mutations in the F1 chain of the F glycoprotein (Douglas et al., 2003; Morton et al., 2003). A number of these mutations are located in the HRB region, suggesting that these drugs may also block the interactions of HRA and HRB regions that result in the formation of the six-helix-bundle. However, other mutations were found to map outside the heptad repeats and the reason for selection of these mutations is still not known. At any rate, inhibition of F protein activity by synthetic drugs seems a feasible approach for the development of anti-HRSV compounds that may find some future application in the clinic.

Transcription and replication of the viral genome

Transcription of the viral genome is triggered once the viral nucleocapsid has entered into the cell cytoplasm. Transcription requires the coordinated action of at least four viral proteins: N, P, L and 22k (or M2-1). At a certain time after infection RNA synthesis switches from transcription to replication. Replication requires N, P and L proteins but not 22k and involves the synthesis of a complete copy of the vRNA of opposite polarity, dubbed complementary RNA (cRNA) or the antigenome. The switch from transcription to replication seems to require the action of another protein, M2-2. An overview of the HRSV genome and the characteristics of gene products implicated in HRSV transcription and replication is described below.

The HRSV genome

The HRSV genome is a negative-sense, single-stranded RNA molecule of 15,222 nucleotides for the A2 strain (Collins et al., 1995). As shown in Fig. 7A, the genes are arranged in a linear order along the genome, separated by short variable intergenic sequences, with the exception of the last two genes (M2 and L) that overlap by 68 nucleotides. The *Pneumovirus* genome, including HRSV, has additional genes that are not present in other paramyxoviruses (Fig. 7B). Another feature that differentiates the *Paramyxovirinae* from the *Pneumovirinae* subfamily is the coding potential of the P gene. While in the *Paramyxovirinae* subfamily this gene gives rise to several distinct gene products by using overlapping reading frames on a single mRNA or by RNA editing (pseudotemplated addition of nucleotides), the P gene of the *Pneumovirinae* subfamily has a single open reading frame (ORF) (except in

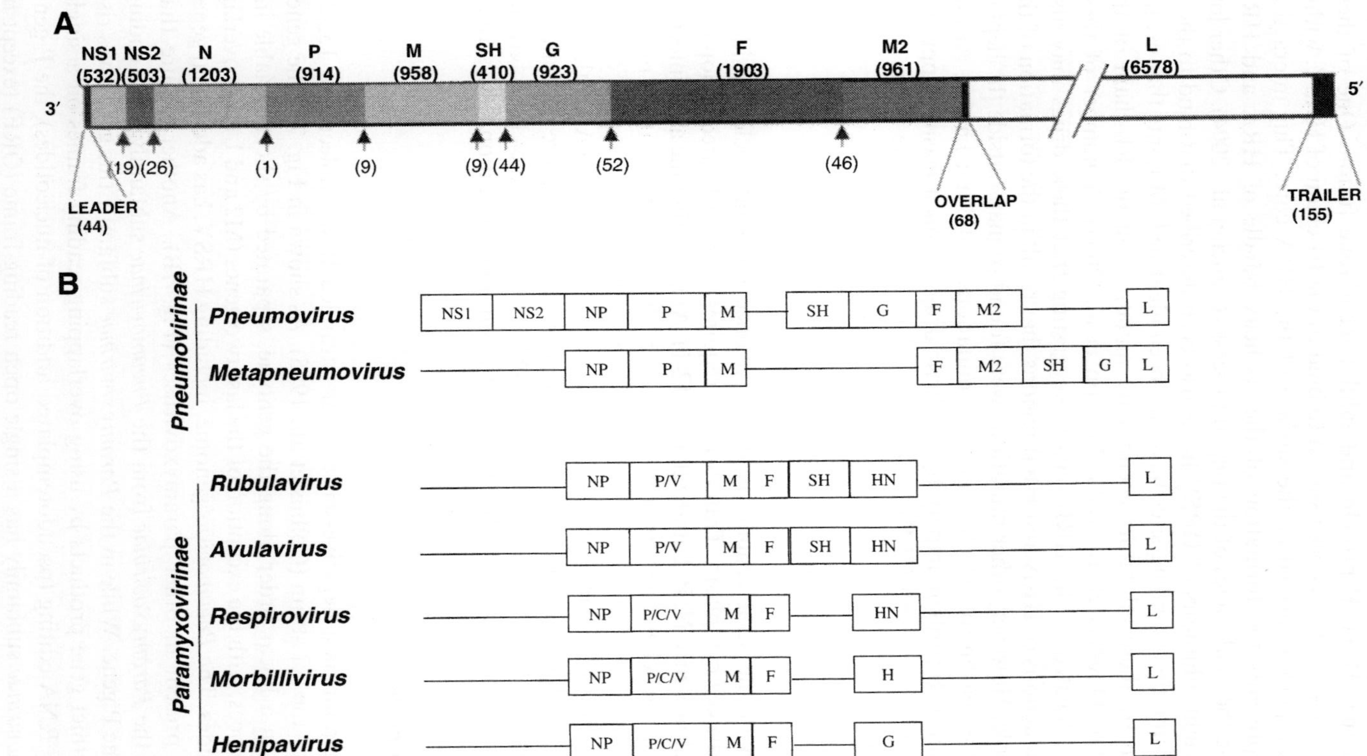

Fig. 7 Scheme of the HRSV genome (A) The different genes of the HRSV A2 strain are shown at scale, except for the L gene that is split into two fragments. The nucleotide lengths of gene and intergenic regions are shown between parentheses above and below the genome diagram, respectively. Also shown are the leader, trailer and overlapping segment between M2 and L genes. (B) Comparison of the gene order in different genus of the *Pneumovirinae* and *Paramyxovirinae* subfamilies.

the case of PVM), and no evidence has been found for an RNA-editing mechanism (Lamb and Kolakofsky, 2001). However, in addition to the full-length P protein, a short 19 kDa polypeptide of unknown function has been found in HRSV-infected cells that is generated by initiation of translation at an internal in-frame AUG codon of P mRNA (Caravokyri et al., 1992).

At the 3′ end of the vRNA (Fig. 7A), there is a leader sequence of 44 nucleotides that contains the promoter sequences for RNA transcription and antigenome synthesis, while the 5′ end is characterized by a 155 nucleotides trailer sequence that contains the antigenome promoter for synthesis of progeny genomes. The 3′ ends of the genome and antigenome are identical in 10 of the first 11 positions, and share 81% identity for the first 24–26 nucleotides, after which sequence identity is insignificant (Mink et al., 1991). While the leader sequence is well conserved, there is a high degree of genetic heterogeneity in the trailer region of HRSV isolates, particularly in the first two-thirds following the L gene. Only the 5′ 40 nucleotides of the trailer (in the genome sense) are required for minigenome rescue (Zambrano, 2000), and most of the variable trailer region is missing from the avian pneumovirus (Randhawa et al., 1997). Thus, it seems that a large segment of the internal trailer sequences do not play a significant role in the infectious cycle.

Each HRSV gene is framed between a gene-start (GS) sequence (3′-CCCCGUUUA(U/C), which is conserved in all genes except in the L gene which is slightly different (3′-CCCUGUUUUA), and a semi-conserved gene-end (GE) sequence (3′-UCA(A/U)UN_{1-4}UUUU_{4-7}). The sequences at each gene-junction differ in length and sequence (as shown in Fig. 7A for the A2 strain) and show also a high degree of genetic variation between HRSV isolates (Moudy et al., 2004).

The nucleoprotein

HRSV encodes a nucleoprotein (N or NP) of 391 amino acids in length (Collins et al., 1985). N is a major component of the virus particle, where it is bound tightly to the genome, forming the helical nucleocapsid. When expressed in insect cells or in bacteria, N binds to RNA in a non-specific manner and forms nucleocapsid-like structures (Murphy et al., 2003). As for other paramyxoviruses (Curran and Kolakofsky, 1999), RNA-binding specificity for the N protein is thought to be provided by interaction with the viral phosphoprotein (P) (Castagné et al., 2004).

N proteins of viruses of the *Paramyxovirinae* subfamily have a modular organization. A large N_{CORE} at the N-terminus, spanning two-thirds of the amino acid sequence, contains all the regions necessary for self-assembly and RNA binding. This is followed by a non-structured N_{TAIL} at the C-terminus that can be released from the nucleocapsids by controlled trypsin digestion and that is required for interaction with the P protein (Karlin et al., 2003). Although HRSV N protein is significantly shorter than its *Paramyxovirinae* counterparts (489–553 amino acids; Barr et al., 1991; Collins et al., 2001), it seems to have a similar organization. Thus, as for other members of the *Paramyxovirinae* subfamily, the N-terminal half of HRSV N is implicated in RNA binding, as suggested by the capacity of deletion mutants to form stable nucleocapsid-like structures (Murphy et al., 2003). Furthermore, monoclonal antibodies binding to the C-terminal half of N or peptides corresponding to this part of the molecule inhibit N–P interaction *in vitro* (Murray et al., 2001). In addition, chimeras of the N proteins of HRSV and PVM (pneumonia virus of mice) have provided evidence that the C-terminal region of HRSV N is required, as in other paramyxoviruses, to interact with the P protein in co-transfected cells (Stokes et al., 2003). Despite these results, deletion mutant analysis indicated that large segments of the N protein are required for efficient interaction with P (García-Barreno et al., 1996), presumably because a large part of the N protein sequence is required for proper folding of the native molecule.

The phosphoprotein

The HRSV P protein is a co-factor of the viral RNA polymerase (L) (Khattar et al., 2001) but also interacts with the N protein (García.Barreno et al., 1996), and possibly with the 22k protein (Mason et al., 2003), playing a central role in the process of RNA synthesis. The P protein is synthesized as a polypeptide of 241 amino acids that self-assembles into oligomers that are eluted as high molecular weight proteins (~500 kDa) from gel-filtration columns (Llorente et al., 2006). However, cross-linking experiments (Asenjo and Villanueva, 2000; Castagné et al., 2004) and analytical centrifugation analysis (Llorente et al., unpublished) support the notion that native P is a tetramer. P is phosphorylated principally at Ser232 (Barik et al., 1995; Sanchez-Seco et al., 1995), although other minor phosphorylation sites have been identified (Navarro et al., 1991; Asenjo et al., 2005). The precise role of phosphorylation for P protein activity remains unclear. Transcription reactions reconstituted *in vitro* in the absence of P or in the presence of phosphate-free P protein produced abortive initiation products but not full-length transcripts (Dupuy et al., 1999), suggesting that P phosphorylation was required to convert the newly initiated polymerase into a stable complex. However, P proteins in which phosphorylation was reduced to 2% by mutation of the major phosphorylation sites retained much of the transcriptase and replicative activity in a minireplicon system (Villanueva et al., 2000). The latter results were confirmed in other minireplicon assays and viruses in which the major phosphorylation sites were eliminated by mutation could be rescued, although they replicated less efficiently than the wild type in certain cell lines and in animal model systems (Lu et al., 2002).

HRSV P protein is much shorter and has no sequence similarity with the P protein of other paramyxoviruses (391–602 amino acids; Collins et al., 2001). Nevertheless, bioinformatic analysis revealed a modular organization of HRSV P, reminiscent of other paramyxovirus P proteins (Llorente et al., 2006), with a central structured domain (amino acids 100–200), flanked by two intrinsically disordered regions (1–99 and 201–241). The structured domain is preceded by a region (amino acids 59–93) that is highly divergent between the P proteins of viruses from antigenic groups A and B (Johnson and Collins, 1990). Within the structured domain, sequences important for self-oligomerization have been identified (Castagné et al., 2004). In addition, a trypsin-resistant fragment (residues 104–163), which represents the oligomerization domain of P, was mapped in the structured domain. This fragment has a high helical content (Llorente et al., 2006) and overlaps with the binding site of the viral polymerase (Khattar et al., 2001), characteristics that are shared with the oligomerization domain of other paramyxovirus P proteins (Tarbouriech et al., 2000). Finally, deletion mutant analysis indicated that the C-terminus of HRSV P, as in other paramyxovirus, is implicated in the interaction with N (García-Barreno et al., 1996; Slack and Easton, 1998). However, point mutations in P protein residues, C-terminal to the oligomerization domain and that conferred a termosensitive (*ts*) phenotype when introduced in recombinant viruses, also affected N–P interactions in a ts manner, suggesting that they affected proper folding of the P protein required for interaction with the N protein (Lu et al., 2002).

The 22k (or M2-1) protein

The first ORF1 of the M2 gene encodes a protein of 194 amino acids in length, named 22k or M2-1 (Huang et al., 1985). This gene is present in all members of the *Pneumovirinae* subfamily but is absent from viruses of the *Paramyxovirinae* subfamily. Based on its solubility properties, the 22k protein was originally proposed as a second matrix protein (Huang et al., 1985) and thus was re-named M2-1. However, the 22k protein associates with characteristic cytoplasmic inclusions found in HRSV-infected cells that also minimally contain the N and P proteins. Moreover, inclusion-like bodies containing 22k were also observed in transfected cells co-expressing N, P and 22k, the first two proteins being sufficient for the formation of the cytoplasmic aggregates (García et al., 1993). In agreement with this subcellular localization, it has been documented that the 22k protein acts as a transcription antiterminator factor, allowing the synthesis of full-length mRNAs (Collins et al., 1996). Thus, the 22k protein is presently considered a component of the HRSV nucleocapsid rather than a second matrix protein.

The 22k protein exists in at least two different isoforms of 24 and 22 kDa, identified by 1-D SDS–PAGE, although further isoforms have been observed by 2-D electrophoresis (Routledge et al., 1987). The slow migrating 24 kDa form is phosphorylated at serine residues 58 and 61 and is the most abundant isoform when expressed in the absence of other HRSV components (Cartee and Wertz, 2001). In contrast, the fast migrating 22 kDa isoform is not phosphorylated and is the most abundantly expressed species in HRSV-infected cells. The reason for the difference in migration and phosphorylation between the two 22k isoforms and their relevance for the HRSV infectious cycle is unknown.

The 22k protein has a Cys_3 His_1 motif ($C–X_7–C–X5—C–X_3–H$) spanning residues 7 to 25, which has been proposed to bind zinc (Hardy and Wertz, 2000), by analogy to a similar motif found in the transcription factor Nup475 (Worthington et al., 1996). Critical residues in this motif are essential for protein function in a minireplicon system (Hardy and Wertz, 2000; Zhou et al., 2003) and for virus infectivity (Tang et al., 2001). Antibody reactivity and deletion mutant analysis provided evidence that the N-terminus of the 22k protein is buried in the native molecule and is important for protein folding (García-Barreno et al., 2005).

The RNA-dependent RNA polymerase (L)

The last gene of the HRSV genome encodes a large (L) protein of 250,226 Da for the A2 strain, which is the viral RNA-dependent RNA polymerase (Stec et al., 1991). The predicted amino acid sequence of the L protein has a high isoleucine and leucine content (21.9% combined) and an estimated net positive charge of +75 at neutral pH. The sequences of L proteins from *Mononegavirales* have been aligned and six relatively conserved sequence regions, I to VI, have been identified (Poch et al., 1990). This conservation is concentrated mainly in the N-terminal half of the L polypeptide (amino acids 422–938), which includes region III. This region contains four polymerase motifs, A–D, present in a wide range of RNA and DNA polymerases from viral and non-viral origin (Poch et al., 1989), including the GDNQ motif, thought to be part of the polymerase active site. In addition to the polymerizing activity, other enzymatic activities have been attributed to the *Mononegavirales* L protein, such as capping, methylation and polyadenylation. Computational analysis identified a 2′-*O*-ribose methyltransferase domain in the C-terminal region of mononegavirales involved in capping of viral mRNAs (Ferron et al., 2002). Interestingly, single amino acid substitutions have been identified in the conserved region IV of the HRSV L polymerase (Cartee et al., 2003), or between regions IV and V (Juhasz et al., 1999), that alter the efficiency of termination at the gene-end sequences (see later).

The M2-2 protein

This protein is encoded by the second ORF of the M2 gene, located towards the 3′ end of the mRNA, partially overlapping the first ORF (Collins and Wertz, 1985). M2-2 is synthesized as a low molecular weight polypeptide (~9–10 kDa), which has been found in the cytoplasm of HRSV-infected cells, with a degree of localization in the inclusion bodies where N, P and 22k are also associated (Ahmadian et al., 1999). A novel process of translational control has been described for the generation of M2-2, whereby initiation of translation of the downstream ORF is coupled to termination of translation of the upstream ORF (Ahmadian et al., 2000). M2-2 modulates the switch of RNA synthesis from transcription to replication (Bermingham and Collins, 1999).

Transcription

UV inactivation experiments provided the first evidence that HRSV transcription proceeds in a sequential manner from the 3′ end of the vRNA (Dickens et al., 1984). Studies with multicistronic minigenomes confirmed that transcription termination of an upstream gene is required to initiate transcription of the downstream gene, ruling out the possibility that the polymerase enters the genome at internal genes to initiate transcription (Fearns and Collins, 1999). Thus, the actual model of HRSV transcription conforms to the start-stop model proposed for other *Mononegavirales* (Lamb and Kolakofsky, 2001).

In this model, the polymerase enters the genome at a single promoter, placed in the 3' end of the vRNA and starts transcription at the gene-start (GS) sequence of the first gene (NS1) in the viral genome. Although nucleotides 1–11 and the 3′ end of the vRNA are sufficient to recruit the viral polymerase to initiate transcription, other sequence elements of the 44 leader (Le) sequence, preceding the NS1 gene, enhance transcription efficiency (McGivern et al., 2005). Therefore, two possibilities exist for the initiation of transcription: (i) that the transcriptase initiates RNA synthesis at the first nucleotide of the vRNA, ending at the Le-NS1 junction to release a leader RNA and reinitiating at the NS1 GS signal to produce the first mRNA and (ii) that the viral polymerase binds to the 3′-end promoter and scans the template to initiate synthesis of the first mRNA at the NS1 GS signal (Cowton and Fearns, 2005).

Transcription initiation occurs by a quasi-templated mechanism at position 1 of each GS sequence (Kuo et al., 1997). Analysis of minireplicons in which the first nucleotide of the GS sequence (C) was changed to U or A indicated that the site of transcription initiation was unchanged. However, the mRNAs were dimorphic at the 5′-terminus: two-thirds contained the predicted mutant substitution but one-third contained the parental assignment. This suggests that the templated mutant assignment at position 1 can sometimes be overridden by an innate preference of the viral polymerase for the parental assignment, in a quasi-templated manner.

Once the polymerase has initiated the transcription process, it travels along the genome until it reaches a gene-end (GE) signal. Polyadenylation occurs by slippage of the viral polymerase on the U tract of the GE signal to generate the poly A tail. At some time during the transcription process, the nascent mRNA is guanylated and methylated by the viral polymerase to produce a cap structure that ensures its translation by the cell ribosomes. The guanylating activity has been located in region V of the L polymerase (Liuzzi et al., 2005), while the methyltransferase activity has been attributed to region VI of the analogous Sendai virus polymerase (Ogino et al., 2005). Inhibition of mRNA guanylation leads to the accumulation of short triphosphorylated transcripts, suggesting that capping is required for transcription to proceed efficiently to the GE sequence (Liuzzi et al., 2005). When the polyadenylation process is completed, the polymerase crosses the intergenic sequence until it reaches the next GS sequence to initiate transcription of the downstream gene. This process of stop-start transcription is repeated at each gene boundary to generate the different mRNA species.

Transcription of the L gene starts within the upstream M2 gene, due to a 68-nucleotide overlap between the two genes. Minigenome analogues provided evidence that transcription initiation at the L gene GS sequence requires that the viral polymerase reaches the M2 GE signal (Fearns and Collins, 1999). Subsequently, the polymerase can presumably scan the nearby sequences to initiate transcription at the L GS signal. This also provides a mechanism whereby the polymerase that prematurely terminates transcription of the L gene at the downstream GE sequence of the M2 gene can recycle back to the L GS signal, thereby accounting for the unexpectedly high level of full-length L mRNA found in infected cells.

Every time that the polymerase ends transcription at a GE sequence there is a chance that it will not start transcription at the downstream GS sequence. This attenuating mechanism reduces the efficiency of transcription 2–3 times at each gene junction and it is a major controlling system of gene expression in HRSV, creating an mRNA gradient such that promoter-proximal genes are transcribed more frequently than downstream genes (Collins and Wertz, 1983). The efficiency of transcriptional stop–start appears to vary among the various gene junctions (which differ in length and nucleotide sequence), providing a second level of regulation of gene expression (Kuo et al., 1996; Hardy et al., 1999). It is still unclear how this differential regulation at each gene junction is determined, however different *cis*-acting elements may contribute to this modulation, including nucleotides outside the consensus GE sequence (Harmon et al., 2001; Harmon and Wertz, 2002). Unexpectedly, neither length nor sequence of a given intergenic junction seems to play a major role in determining the efficiency of stop–start transcription in a dicistronic minigenome (Kuo et al., 1996). However, it has been found that variability in length and sequence of gene junctions among clinical isolates may contribute to differential gene expression (Moudy et al., 2004). As mentioned before, two mutants of the L polymerase have been described with alterations in the efficiency of transcription termination (Juhasz et al., 1999; Cartee et al., 2003), suggesting that termination at the GE signals involves a specific site in the polymerase.

When the polymerase fails to stop transcription at a GE sequence it continues RNA synthesis through the intergenic junction and into the downstream gene, generating polycistronic transcripts that are commonly found in HRSV-infected cells (Dickens et al., 1984). The level of these transcripts is determined by the efficiency of transcription termination at each GE signal. Since only the first gene of a polycistronic transcript is translated by the ribosomes, the level of readthrough transcription may be another factor contributing to regulation of gene expression. Indeed, variability of the GE signals that affects transcription termination has been found in viral isolates (Moudy et al., 2003).

As mentioned before, the following viral proteins are required for transcription: (i) the L polymerase that catalyses the polymerization steps of RNA synthesis and capping and polyadenylation of the mRNAs, (ii) the N protein that is tightly bound to the vRNA, forming the nucleocapsid template recognized by the polymerase, (iii) the P protein that is a co-factor of the L polymerase and (iv) the 22k protein, a transcription antitermination factor that enhances completion of mRNA synthesis.

Based on a model proposed for the P protein of other paramyxoviruses (Curran and Kolakofsky, 1999), it is thought that HRSV P plays a dual role in the process of

RNA synthesis. On the one hand, P binds to newly synthesized N protein (named N°), preventing its illegitimate interaction with non-viral RNA, and facilitating the correct assembly of N molecules into newly formed nucleocapsids. On the other hand, the P protein oligomer binds simultaneously to one molecule of the L polymerase and transiently to the N protein of the viral nucleocapsid, through the C-termini of its monomers. This transient interaction of P with N allows cartwheeling of P along the nucleocapsid template, locally destabilizing the interaction of N with the RNA and facilitating the access of the viral polymerase to the bases of the RNA template.

The mechanism of action of the 22k protein is not totally understood. Originally it was found that the 22k protein co-precipitated with the N protein from extracts of either HRSV-infected cells or cells transfected with the corresponding plasmids (García et al., 1993). However, this interaction seems to occur via RNA, since it is sensitive to RNase treatment (Cartee and Wertz, 2001), and its significance for 22k activity is unclear because 22k–N interaction and 22k activity in a minireplicon system could be separated by mutagenesis (Hardy and Wertz, 2000). It has also been reported that the 22k protein binds to RNA, specifically to leader RNA sequences (Cuesta et al., 2000). However, it was later found that the 22k protein binds to mRNAs generated during infection without specificity (Cartee and Wertz, 2001). Therefore, the RNA-binding capacity of the 22k protein was attributed to the common finding that zinc-binding motifs (such as the Cys3His1 motif of the 22k protein) also bind nucleic acids. Finally, it has been reported that phosphorylation of the 22k protein is required for efficient activity in a minireplicon system (Cartee and Wertz, 2001). However, since mutants in which the two phosphorylated Ser residues were changed to Ala still retained certain activity, it is possible that such mutations altered proper folding of the 22k protein rather than having a direct effect on protein activity. It is worth mentioning here that the major isoform (>90%) of the 22k protein found in HRSV-infected cells is not phosphorylated.

In vitro reconstitution assays of the transcriptase activity have provided evidence that, in addition to viral proteins, other cellular factors are needed for efficient transcription. Cellular factors which have been characterized include actin (Burke et al., 1998), and the actin-modulatory protein, profilin (Burke et al., 2000). The exact role of these cellular proteins in the transcription process of the HRSV genome remains to be elucidated, but these findings suggest that transcription (and perhaps replication) of the viral genome associates with some components of the cytoskeleton.

Replication

As for other paramyxovirus, replication of the HRSV genome involves synthesis of uninterrupted positive-sense complementary copies of the vRNA (the antigenome or cRNA), which are also tightly bound to the N protein in RNase-resistant nucleocapsids. The antigenome is 10–20-fold less abundant in HRSV-infected cells than the genome. The current model of HRSV replication implies that the encapsidated antigenome is the template for the synthesis of progeny genomes that can function as templates for secondary transcription.

It is not yet clear how the polymerase complex alters its activity and switches from the transcription to the replication mode of RNA synthesis during the HRSV replicative cycle. A simple model put forward for other paramyxovirus is based on the availability of N protein. As the amount of N protein builds up in the infected cell, unassembled N may bind to the RNA being synthesized from the 3′ end of the vRNA. Assembly of the nascent RNA into nucleocapsids would force the viral polymerase to continue RNA synthesis, ignoring the gene junction signals, until it reaches the 5′ end of the viral genome (Vidal and Kolakofsky, 1989). However, this model does not seem to apply to HRSV since increased expression of N stimulates genome replication but does not alter the balance between transcription and replication (Fearns et al., 1997).

It has been reported that, while overlapping extensively, the transcription and replication promoters at the 3′end of the genome are not identical (Fearns et al., 2002). It is thus possible that the polymerase complex committed to transcription differs from the replication complex. According to this model, the replicative polymerase would initiate RNA synthesis at the 3′ end of the vRNA to continue uninterrupted until the 5′ end, while the transcriptase also would bind at the 3′ end of the vRNA but initiates RNA synthesis at the GS signal of the NS1 gene. However, an alternative possibility is that the additional promoter residues required for RNA replication may be involved in encapsidation of the nascent RNA chain, and that binding of unassembled N to the nascent RNA chain would determine either transcription or replication of the vRNA template.

In the case of HRSV, contrary to other paramyxovirus, other viral gene products in addition to L, N and P proteins have been implicated in transcription and replication. As mentioned before, the 22k protein is required for efficient transcription of full-length mRNAs and the M2-2 protein has been associated with the switch from transcription to replication (Bermingham and Collins, 1999). Indeed, silencing of M2-2 leads to a 7—18-fold increase in transcription versus replication (Bermingham and Collins, 1999; Cheng et al., 2005). Therefore, the transition from synthesis of mRNAs to synthesis of the antigenome may involve the formation of different polymerase complexes, which recruit different sets of viral, and perhaps non-viral components, to the 3′ end of the vRNA and that utilize overlapping but distinct promoters.

The synthesis of progeny genomes, using the antigenome as template, may require the same replication complex of the viral polymerase. The antigenome promoter is identical to the genome promoter in 10 of the first 11 positions; however, the terminal complementarity of the HRSV genome is not required for its function as template (Peeples and Collins, 2000). Thus, it may be that sequence identity of the genome and antigenome promoters simply reflects recognition by identical (or very similar) polymerase complexes engaged in RNA replication.

Virus assembly

The process of paramyxovirus morphogenesis is poorly understood. It has been postulated that the matrix (M) protein plays a dual role in the assembly and release of new virus particles by: (i) binding to the nucleocapsids to render them transcriptionally inactive before packaging and (ii) mediating association of the nucleocapsid with the nascent viral envelope.

The matrix protein of HRSV is smaller than its paramyxovirus counterparts (256 amino acids versus 335–375). However, as for other matrix proteins, HRSV M has a hydrophobic domain in the C-terminal half of the molecule that is probably responsible for its binding to the cytoplasmic side of the plasma membrane in HRSV-infected cells (Marty et al., 2004). Although M can associate with the plasma membrane in the absence of other HRSV gene products, co-expression of F and/or G glycoproteins is required for its incorporation into lipid rafts (Henderson et al., 2002; Ghyldial et al., 2005), probable sites of HRSV maturation. In the case of the G protein, the site of interaction with M has been mapped within the first six residues of the G polypeptide, lending support to the notion that the M protein is able to interact with the cytoplasmic tail of the HRSV glycoproteins (Ghyldial et al., 2005). In addition, a fraction of the M protein has been shown to co-purify with nucleocapsids and is incorporated, together with other nucleocapsid components, into the inclusion bodies found in HRSV-infected cells (Ghyldial et al., 2002). When M is bound to lipid rafts, it forms structures that can be dissociated with high salt buffers, suggestive of interaction with cytoskeleton components (Henderson et al., 2002). These interactions may be important to drive the budding process that leads to the release of new virions.

Confocal microscopy showed that the M protein is localized in the nucleus of HRSV-infected cells at an early stage following infection (Ghyldial et al., 2003). It was thus proposed that incorporation of M into the cell nucleus might inhibit host cell transcription. Indeed, it was reported that nuclear extracts from HRSV-infected cells were less active in an *in vitro* transcriptional assay than nuclear extracts from mock-infected cells. However, the significance of these findings is unclear since no major inhibition of host gene expression has been found in infected cells. It has also been reported that M can bind to RNA and it has been speculated that this activity may mediate inactivation of viral nucleocapsids for RNA synthesis (Rodríguez et al., 2004). However, this activity has not been confirmed in a minireplicon system where addition of an M protein-encoding plasmid, together with the basic set of plasmids encoding N, P, L and 22k proteins, has no effect either on minigenome rescue or on the RNAs being synthesized (Zambrano, 2000; Rodríguez et al., 2004).

In summary, the results described so far support the notion that the M protein plays a major role in coordinating the assembly of new virions by bridging the interaction between newly synthesized nucleocapsids with the viral glycoproteins at specific sites of the cell membrane (probably lipid rafts). The importance of the M protein for virus assembly is also inferred from its absolute requirement for the formation of virus-like particles in a minireplicon system (Teng and Collins, 1998).

The role of the SH protein in the HRSV infectious cycle is not known, being the only viral gene product that remains without an allocated activity. SH is synthesized as an abundant non-glycosylated polypeptide of 7.5 kDa (SH_0), although a minor non-glycosylated species of 4.5 kDa (SH_t), produced by initiation of translation at a second in-frame AUG is also produced in HRSV-infected cells (Collins and Mottet, 1993). Only a proportion of SH_o molecules are modified by the addition of N-linked oligosaccharides to yield SH_g (13–15 kDa), which are further modified to SH_p by the addition of polylactosaminoglycans (Anderson et al., 1992; Collins and Mottet, 1993). Unexpectedly, SH was also found to be phosphorylated at specific tyrosine residues (Rixon et al., 2005).

The SH protein is inserted into the cell membrane of HRSV-infected cells through a central hydrophobic region, with the C-terminus located extracellularly (Collins and Mottet, 1993). Analysis of the SH protein by sedimentation in sucrose gradients showed that rapidly assembled into homo-oligomers containing all forms of the protein. However, the SH protein is incorporated very inefficiently (or not at all) into virus particles (Collins and Mottet, 1993; Rixon et al., 2004). In addition to the cell membrane, the SH protein also accumulates in the Golgi complex within membrane structures enriched in lipid raft markers (Rixon et al., 2004). Expression of SH in bacteria increased permeability of their membranes to low molecular weight compounds (Pérez et al., 1997). Some of these properties resembled those attributed to the M2 protein of influenza virus, which has an ion channel activity highly specific for H^+ ions (Chizhmakov et al., 1996; Mould et al., 2000). The M2 activity presumably modifies the *trans*-Golgi pH to maintain the influenza hemagglutinin (HA) in a preactive configuration before reaching the cell membrane. However, it is unclear how this activity could benefit HRSV since membrane fusion mediated by the F protein, in contrast to fusion mediated by influenza HA, is not triggered by low pH. In addition, recombinant viruses from which the SH gene was deleted grew efficiently in certain cell lines and formed large syncytia, although they were attenuated *in vivo* (Bukreyev et al., 1997; Whitehead et al., 1999).

Virus–host cell interactions

HRSV infects a large number of cell lines *in vitro*. In most cases, infection leads to virus replication and lysis of the infected cell. However, the actual outcome of HRSV infection is determined, at least partially, by the specific cell-type being infected. For instance, alveolar macrophages are semi-permissive for HRSV infection. Infected macrophages support HRSV replication, with low virus yield, for up to 25 days after infection *in vitro*, without apparent decrease in the number of viable cells (Panuska et al., 1990). HRSV infection of BALB/c mouse fibroblasts led to the establishment more than 20 years ago of a persistently infected cell line (BCH4) that sheds very low amounts of infectious virus to the culture supernatant (Fernie et al., 1981). The virus shed by BCH-4 cells is apparently wild type but its replication is constrained in these cells by the low expression levels of surface glycoproteins (G and F), which limit production of progeny virus (Martínez et al., 2001). Persistent infections of transformed human B lymphocytes (Bangham and McMichael, 1986) and a murine macrophage-like cell line (Guerrero-Plata et al., 2001) have been reported, although the actual mechanisms of persistence were not analysed. Persistent infections have also been reported in *in vivo* models, such as guinea-pigs (Hegele et al., 1994) and BALB/c mice (Schwarze et al., 2004) infected with HRSV or in calves infected with bovine RSV (Valarcher et al., 2001).

HRSV induces a delayed cytopathic effect in permissive cells in comparison with other lytic viruses, and only a moderate shut-off of cellular protein synthesis (García-Barreno et al., 1988). As mentioned before, HRSV can replicate and produce infectious progeny in enucleated cells (Follet et al., 1975), indicating that the different steps of the replicative cycle do not need active nuclear functions. However, HRSV alters the expression of numerous cytokines and chemokines in epithelial cells and in other cell types. It is thought that production of chemokines by HRSV-infected epithelial cells is a major determinant of the inflammatory response that influences severity of the infection (Hoffman et al., 2004) Microarray technology has recently been used to evaluate the impact of HRSV upon expression of cellular genes (Zhang et al., 2001; Martínez et al., unpublished). Besides cytokines and chemokines, enhanced expression of different gene subsets implicated in protein metabolism, regulation of nucleotides and nucleic acid metabolism, transcription and immune response were observed. Thus, it is clear that HRSV infection has a major impact on multiple metabolic processes of the infected cell. Some of them may be induced by the virus to enhance its own replication while others may be part of the host cell defence against the virus attack.

Several viral gene products have been implicated directly in the alteration of gene expression. The best characterized example is the inhibitory effect of the human and bovine RSV NS1 and NS2 proteins on the induction of interferons α, β and λ (Valarcher et al., 2003; Spann et al., 2004) and in blocking expression of genes involved in establishing the antiviral state (Schlender et al., 2000; Bossert et al., 2003; Spann et al., 2005). However, NS1 and NS2 have also been implicated in the induction of RANTES, IL-8 and TNF-α (Spann et al., 2005), supporting the notion that the same viral product may have contrasting effects on the expression of different cellular genes. The attachment (G) glycoprotein, and particularly its soluble form (Gs), has also been implicated in reducing the inflammatory and innate immune responses elicited by HRSV in human epithelial cells (Arnold et al., 2004; Polack et al., 2005). It is thought that reduction of the inflammatory response may enhance virus replication, in agreement with the behaviour of a recombinant virus expressing only Gs that replicates efficiently in cell culture and is only moderately attenuated *in vivo* (Teng et al., 2001).

Although HRSV infects multiple cell lines *in vitro*, the epithelial cells of the respiratory tract are the major sites of virus replication *in vivo*. This should be borne in mind when trying to extrapolate the *in vitro* findings to the *in vivo* situation. Ideally, the *in vitro* system should reproduce the infection *in vivo*; however, most established epithelial cell lines do not maintain the differentiated state. Recently, cultures of human airway epithelium (HAE) cells from nasal, tracheobronchial and bronchiolar origin obtained by surgical procedures (Zhang et al., 2002) or HAE cells removed at adenoidectomy (Wright et al., 2005) have been obtained. HAE cells can be induced to differentiate *in vitro* forming a multilayered, stratified and polarized epithelium that resembles histologically the epithelium of the respiratory tract. Differentiated HAE cell cultures can be infected with HRSV only from the luminal (apical) surface and the infection is restricted to ciliated cells that shed virus from the apical surface, spreading it to neighbouring ciliated cells. HRSV maturation at the apical surface has also been documented in monolayers of polarized epithelial cells (Roberts et al., 1995). Surprisingly, and in contrast to other viruses such as influenza virus, HRSV infection of differentiated HAE cultures did not lead to obvious cytopathology, suggesting that in the absence of an immune response HRSV infection can be tolerated for >3 months in this system (Zhang et al., 2002). Interestingly, the growth of vaccine candidates in HAE cultures parallels their level of attenuation in children (Wright et al., 2005). Further development of the HAE system, to include elements of the immune response, would be of great interest to study HRSV infections in an environment that may faithfully reproduce the infection *in vivo*.

Acknowledgements

I would like to thank Joanna Rawling and Teresa Corral for critical reading of the manuscript and very helpful comments. Research in the author's laboratory is supported in part by grants from the Instituto de Salud Carlos III, the Ministerio de Educación y Ciencia and the European Union.

References

Ahmadian G, Chambers P, Easton AJ. Detection and characterization of proteins encoded by the second ORF of the M2 gene of pneumovirus. J Gen Virol 1999; 80: 2011–2016.

Ahmadian G, Rhandawa JS, Easton AJ. Expression of the ORF-2 protein of the human respiratory syncytial virus M2 gene is initiated by a ribosomal termination-dependent reinitiation mechanism. EMBO J 2000; 19: 2681–2689.

Anderson LJ, Heirholzer JC, Tson C, Hendry RM, Fernie BN, Stone Y, McIntosh K. Antigenic characterization of respiratory syncytial virus strains with monoclonal antibodies. J Infect Dis 1985; 151: 626–633.

Anderson K, King AMQ, Lerch RA, Wertz GW. Polylactosaminoglycan modification of the respiratory syncytial virus small hydrophobic (SH) protein: a conserved feature among human and bovine respiratory syncytial viruses. Virology 1992; 191: 417–430.

Apostopoulos V, McKenzie IFC. Cellular mucins: targets for immunotherapy. Crit Rev Immunol 1994; 14: 293–309.

Arbiza J, Taylor G, López JA, Furze J, Wyld S, Whyte P, Stott EJ, Wertz G, Sullender W, Trudel M, Melero JA. Characterization of two antigenic sites recognized by neutralizing monoclonal antibodies directed against the fusion glycoprotein of human respiratory syncytial virus. J Gen Virol 1992; 73: 2225–2234.

Arnold R, König B, Werchau H, König W. Respiratory syncytial virus deficient in soluble G protein induced an increased proinflammatory response in human lung epithelial cells. Virology 2004; 330: 384–397.

Arumugham RG, Seid Jr. RC, Doyle S, Hildreth SW, Paradiso PR. Fatty acid acylation of the fusion glycoprotein of human respiratory syncytial virus. J Biol Chem 1989; 264: 10339–10342.

Asenjo A, Rodriguez L, Villanueva N. Determination of phosphorylated residues from human respiratory syncytial virus P protein that are dynamically dephosphorylated by cellular phosphatases: a possible role for serine 54. J Gen Virol 2005; 86: 1109–1120.

Asenjo A, Villanueva N. Regulated but not constitutive human respiratory syncytial virus (HRSV) P protein phosphorylation is essential for oligomerization. FEBS Lett 2000; 467: 279–284.

Bächi T, Howe C. Morphogenesis and ultrastructure of respiratory syncytial virus. J Virol 1973; 12: 1173–1180.

Bangham CRM, McMichael AJ. Specific human cytotoxic T cells recognise B cell lines persistently infected with respiratory syncytial virus. Proc Natl Acad Sci USA 1986; 83: 9183–9187.

Barik S. Transcription of human respiratory syncytial virus genome RNA in vitro: requirement of cellular factor(s). J Virol 1992; 66: 6813–6818.

Barik S, McLean Y, Dupuy LC. Phosphorylation of Ser232 directly regulates the transcriptional activity of the P protein of human respiratory syncytial virus: phosphorylation of Ser237 may play an accessory role. Virology 1995; 213: 405–412.

Barr J, Chambers P, Pringle CR, Easton AJ. Sequence of the major nucleocapsid protein gene of pneumonia virus of mice: sequence comparisons suggest structural homology between nucleocapsid proteins of pneumovirus, paramyxoviruses, rhabdoviruses and filoviruses. J Gen Virol 1991; 72: 677–685.

Beeler JA, van Wyke Coelingh K. Neutralization epitopes of the F glycoprotein of respiratory syncytial virus: effect of mutation upon fusion function. J Virol 1989; 63: 2941–2950.

Bermingham A, Collins PL. The M2-2 protein of human respiratory syncytial virus is a regulatory factor involved in the balance between RNA replication and transcription. Proc Natl Acad Sci USA 1999; 96: 11259–11264.

Bhella D, Ralph A, Murphy LB, Yeo RP. Significant differences in nucleocapsid morphology within the Paramyxoviridae. J Gen Virol 2002; 83: 1831–1839.

Bossert B, Marozi S, Conzelmann K-K. Nonstructural proteins NS1 and NS2 of bovine respiratory syncytial virus block activation of interferon regulatory factor 3. J Virol 2003; 77: 8661–8668.

Buchholz UJ, Finke S, Conzelman K-K. Generation of bovine respiratory syncytial virus (BRSV) from cDNA: BRSV NS2 is not essential for virus replication in tissue culture, and the human RSV leader region acts as a functional BRSV genome promoter. J Virol 1999; 73: 251–259.

Bukreyev A, Whitehead SS, Murphy BR, Collins PL. Recombinant respiratory syncytial virus from which the entire SH gene has been deleted grows efficiently in cell culture and exhibits site-specific attenuation in the respiratory tract of the mouse. J Virol 1997; 71: 8973–8982.

Burke E, Dupuy L, Wall C, Barik S. Role of cellular actin in the gene expression and morphogenesis o human respiratory syncytial virus. Virology 1998; 252: 137–148.

Burke E, Mahoney N, Almo SC, Barik S. Profilin is required for optimal actin-dependent transcription of respiratory syncytial virus genome RNA. J Virol 2000; 74: 669–675.

Calder LJ, González-Reyes L, García-Barreno B, Wharton SA, Skehel JJ, Wiley DC, Melero JA. Electron microscopy of the human respiratory syncytial virus fusion protein and complexes that it forms with monoclonal antibodies. Virology 2000; 271: 122–131.

Caravokyri C, Zajac AJ, Pringle CR. Assignment of mutant *ts*N19 (complementation group E) of respiratory syncytial virus to the P protein gene. J Gen Virol 1992; 73: 865–873.

Cartee TL, Megaw AG, Oomens AGP, Wertz GW. Identification of a single amino acid change in the human respiratory syncytial virus L protein that affects transcriptional termination. J Virol 2003; 77: 7352–7360.

Cartee TL, Wertz GW. Respiratory syncytial virus M2-1 protein requires phosphorylation for efficient function and binds viral RNA during infection. J Virol 2001; 75: 12188–12197.

Castagné N, Barbier A, Bernard J, Rezaei H, Huet J-C, Henry C, Da Costa B, Eléouët J-F. Biochemical characterization of the respiratory syncytial virus P–P and P–N protein complexes and localization of the P protein oligomerization domain. J Gen Virol 2004; 85: 1643–1653.

Chambers P, Pringle CR, Easton AJ. Sequence analysis of the gene encoding the fusion glycoprotein of pneumonia virus of mice suggests possible conserved secondary structure elements in paramyxovirus fusion glycoproteins. J Gen Virol 1992; 73: 1717–1724.

Chanock RM, Roizman B, Myers M. Recovery from infants with respiratory illness of a virus related to chimpanzee coryza agent. I. Isolation, properties and characterization. Am J Hyg 1957; 66: 281–290.

Chen L, Gorman JJ, McKimm-Breschkin J, Lawrence LJ, Tulloch PA, Smith BJ, Colman PM, Lawrence MC. The structure of the fusion glycoprotein of Newcastle disease virus suggests a novel paradigm for the molecular mechanism of membrane fusion. Structure 2001; 9: 255–266.

Cheng X, Park H-J, Zhou H, Jing H. Overexpression of the M2-2 protein of respiratory syncytial virus inhibits viral replication. J Virol 2005; 79: 13943–13952.

Chizhmakov IV, Geraghty FM, Ogden DC, Hayhurst A, Antoniou M, Hay AJ. Selective proton permeability and pH regulation of the influenza virus M2 channel expressed in mouse erythroleukaemia cells. J Physiol 1996; 494: 329–336.

Cianci C, Langley DR, Dischino DD, Sun Y, Yu K-L, Stanley A, Roach J, Li Z, Dalterio R, Colonno R, Meanwell NA, Krystal M. Targeting a binding pocket within the trimer-of-hairpins: small-molecule inhibition of viral fusion. Proc Natl Acad Sci USA 2004; 101: 15046–15051.

Coates HV, Alling DW, Chanock RM. An antigenic analysis of respiratory syncytial virus isolates by a plaque reduction neutralization assay. Am J Epidemiol 1966; 83: 299–313.

Collins PL, Anderson K, Langer SJ, Wertz GW. Correct sequence of the major nucleocapsid protein mRNA of respiratory syncytial virus. Virology 1985; 146: 69–77.

Collins PL, Chanock RM, Murphy BR. Respiratory syncytial virus. In: Fields Virology (Knipe DM, Howley PM, editors). 4th ed. Philadelphia: Lippincott Williams & Wilkins; 2001; pp. 1443–1485.

Collins PL, Hill MG, Camargo E, Grosfeld H, Chanock RM, Murphy BR. Production of infectious human respiratory from cloned cDNA confirms an essential role for the transcription elongation factor from the 5′ proximal open reading frame of the M2 mRNA in gene expression and provides a capability for vaccine development. Proc Natl Acad Sci USA 1995; 92: 11563–11567.

Collins PL, Hill MG, Cristina J, Grosfeld H. Transcription elongation factor of respiratory syncytial virus, a nonsegmented negative-strand RNA virus. Proc Natl Acad Sci USA 1996; 93: 81–85.

Collins PL, Mottet G. Post-translational processing and oligomerization of the fusion glycoprotein of human respiratory syncytial virus. J Gen Virol 1991; 72: 3095–3101.

Collins PL, Mottet G. Oligomerization and post-translational processing of glycoprotein G of human respiratory syncytial virus: altered O-glycosylation in the presence of brefeldin A. J Gen Virol 1992; 73: 849–863.

Collins PL, Mottet G. Membrane orientation and oligomerization of the small hydrophobic protein of human respiratory syncytial virus. J Gen Virol 1993; 74: 1445–1450.

Collins PL, Wertz GW. cDNA cloning and transcriptional mapping of nine polyadenylated RNAs encoded by the genome of human respiratory syncytial virus. Proc Natl Acad Sci USA 1983; 80: 3208–3212.

Collins PL, Wertz GW. The envelope-associated 22k protein of human respiratory syncytial virus: nucleotide sequence of the mRNA and a related polytranscript. J Virol 1985; 54: 65–71.

Cowton VM, Fearns R. Evidence that the respiratory syncytial virus polymerase is recruited to nucleotides 1 to 11 at the 3′ end of the nucleocapsid and can scan to access internal signals. J Virol 2005; 79: 11311–11322.

Cristina J, López JA, Albo C, García-Barreno B, García J, Melero JA, Portela A. Analysis of genetic variability in human respiratory syncytial virus by the RNase A mismatch cleavage method: subtype divergence and heterogeneity. Virology 1990; 174: 126–134.

Cuesta I, Geng X, Asenjo A, Villanueva N. Structural phosphoprotein M2-1 of the human respiratory syncytial virus is an RNA binding protein. J Virol 2000; 74: 9858–9867.

Curran J, Kolakofsky D. Replication of paramyxoviruses. Adv Virus Res 1999; 54: 403–422.

Dhiman N, Jacobson RM, Poland GA. Measles virus receptors: SLAM and CD46. Rev Med Virol 2004; 14: 217–229.

Dickens LE, Collins PL, Wertz GW. Transcriptional mapping of human respiratory syncytial virus. J Virol 1984; 52: 364–369.

Doreleijers JF, Langedijk JPM, Hard K, Boelens R, Rullmann JAC, Schaaper WM, van Oirschot JT, Kaptein R. Solution structure of the immunodominant region of protein G of bovine respiratory syncytial virus. Biochemistry 1996; 35: 14684–14688.

Douglas JL, Panis ML, Ho E, Lin KY, Krawczyk SH, Grant DM, Cai R, Swaminathan S, Cihlar T. Inhibition of respiratory syncytial virus fusion by the small molecule VP-14637 via specific interactions with F protein. J Virol 2003; 77: 5054–5064.

Dupuy LC, Dobson S, Bitko V, Barik S. Casein kinase 2-mediated phosphorylation of respiratory syncytial virus phosphoprotein P is essential for the transcription elongation activity of the viral polymerase; phosphorylation by casein kinase 1 occurs mainly at Ser^{215} and is without effect. J Virol 1999; 73: 8384–8392.

Escribano-Romero E, Rawling J, García-Barreno B, Melero JA. The soluble form of human respiratory syncytial virus attachment protein differs from the membrane-bound form in its oligomeric state but is still capable of binding to cell surface proteoglycans. J Virol 2004; 78: 3524–3532.

Fearns R, Collins PL. Model for polymerase access to the overlapped L gene of respiratory syncytial virus. J Virol 1999; 73: 388–397.

Fearns R, Peeples ME, Collins PL. Increased expression of the N protein of respiratory syncytial virus stimulates minigenome replication but does not alter the balance between the synthesis of mRNA and antigenome. Virology 1997; 236: 188–201.

Fearns R, Peeples ME, Collins PL. Mapping the transcription and replication promoters of respiratory syncytial virus. J Virol 2002; 76: 1663–1672.

Feldman SA, Hendry RM, Beeler JA. Identification of a linear heparin binding domain for human respiratory syncytial virus attachment glycoprotein G. J Virol 1999; 73: 6610–6617.

Fernie BC, Ford EC, Gerin JL. The development of Balb/c cells persistently infected with respiratory syncytial virus: presence of ribonucleoprotein on the cell surface. Proc Soc Exp Biol Med 1981; 167: 83–86.

Ferron F, Longhi S, Henrissat B, Canard B. Viral RNA-polymerases –a predicted 2′-O-ribose methyltransferase domain shared by all Mononegavirales. Trends Biochem Sci 2002; 27: 222–224.

Follet EA, Pringle CR, Pennington TH. Virus development in enucleated cells: echovirus, poliovirus, pseudorabies virus, reovirus, respiratory syncytial virus and Semliki Forest virus. J Gen Virol 1975; 26: 183–196.

García J, García-Barreno B, Melero JA. Cytoplasmic inclusions of respiratory syncytial virus-infected cells: formation of inclusion bodies in transfected cells that co-express the nucleoprotein, the phosphoprotein and the 22k proteins. Virology 1993; 195: 243–247.

García-Barreno B, Delgado T, Melero JA. Identification of protein regions involved in the interaction of human respiratory syncytial virus phosphoprotein and nucleoprotein: significance for nucleocapsid assembly and formation of cytoplasmic inclusions. J Virol 1996; 70: 801–808.

García-Barreno B, Jorcano JL, Aukenbauer T, López-Galíndez C, Melero JA. Participation of cytoskeletal intermediate filaments in the infectious cycle of human respiratory syncytial virus (RSV). Virus Res 1988; 9: 307–322.

García-Barreno B, Palomo C, Peñas C, Delgado T, Perez-Breña P, Melero JA. Marked differences in the antigenic structure of human respiratory syncytial virus F and G glycoproteins. J Virol 1989; 63: 925–932.

García-Barreno B, Steel J, Payá M, Martínez-Sobrido L, Delgado T, Yeo RP, Melero JA. Epitope mapping of human respiratory syncytial virus 22k transcription antitermination factor: role of N-terminal sequences in protein holding. J Virol 2005; 86: 1103–1107.

García-Beato R, Martínez I, Francí C, Real FX, García-Barreno B, Melero JA. Host cell effect upon glycosylation and antigenicity of human respiratory syncytial virus G glycoprotein. Virology 1996; 221: 301–309.

García-Beato R, Melero JA. The C-terminal third of human respiratory syncytial virus attachment (G) protein is partially resistant to protease digestion and is glycosylated in a cell-type-specific manner. J Gen Virol 2000; 81: 919–927.

Ghyldial R, Baulch-Brwon C, Mills J, Meanger J. The matrix protein of human respiratory syncytial virus localises to the nucleus of infected cells and inhibits transcription. Arch Virol 2003; 148: 1419–1429.

Ghyldial R, Li D, Peroulis I, Shields B, Bardin PG, Teng MN, Collins PL, Meanger J, Mills J. Interaction between the respiratory syncytial virus G glycoprotein cytoplasmic domain and the matrix protein. J Gen Virol 2005; 86: 1879–1884.

Ghyldial R, Mills J, Murray M, Vardaxis N, Meanger J. Respiratory syncytial virus matrix protein associates with nucleocapsids in infected cells. J Gen Virol 2002; 83: 753–757.

González-Reyes L, Ruiz-Argüello MB, García-Barreno B, Calder L, López JA, Albar JP, Skehel JJ, Wiley DC, Melero JA. Cleavage of the human respiratory syncytial virus fusion protein at two distinct sites is required for activation of membrane fusion. Proc Nat Acad Sci USA 2001; 98: 9859–9864.

Gower TL, Pastey MK, Peeples ME, Collins PL, McCurdy LH, Hart TK, Guth A, Hohnson TR, Graham BS. RhoA signaling is required for respiratory syncytial virus-induced syncytium formation and filamentous virion morphology. J Virol 2005; 79: 5326–5336.

Groothuis JR, Nishida H. Prevention of respiratory syncytial virus infections in high-risk infants by monoclonal antibody (palivizumab). Pediatr Int 2002; 44: 235–241.

Grosfeld H, Hill MG, Collins PL. RNA replication by respiratory syncytial virus (RSV) is directed by the N, P and L proteins: transcription also occurs under these conditions but requires superinfection for efficient synthesis of full-length mRNA. J Virol 1995; 69: 5677–5686.

Guerrero-Plata A, Ortega E, Gomez B. Persistence of respiratory syncytial virus in macrophages alters phagocytosis and pro-inflammatory cytokine production. Viral Immunol 2001; 14: 19–30.

Hallak LK, Collins PL, Knudson W, Peeples ME. Iduronic acid-containing glycosaminoglycans on target cells are required for efficient respiratory syncytial virus infection. Virology 2000a; 271: 264–275.

Hallak LK, Spillmann D, Collins PL, Peeples ME. Glycosaminoglycan sulfation requirements for respiratory syncytial virus infection. J Virol 2000b; 74: 10508–10513.

Hansen JE, Lund O, Tolstrup N, Gooley AA, Williams KL, Brunak S. NetOglyc: prediction of mucin type O-glycosylation sites based on sequence content and surface accesibility. Glycoconj J 1998; 15: 115–130.

Hardy RW, Harmon SB, Wertz GW. Diverse gene junctions of respiratory syncytial virus modulate the efficiency of transcription termination and respond differently to M2-mediated antitermination. J Virol 1999; 73: 170–176.

Hardy RW, Wertz GW. The Cys_3-His_1 motif of the respiratory syncytial virus M2-1 protein is essential for proper function. J Virol 2000; 74: 5880–5885.

Harmon SB, Megaw AG, Wertz GW. RNA sequences involved in transcription termination of respiratory syncytial virus. J Virol 2001; 75: 36–44.

Harmon SB, Wertz GW. Transcription termination modulated by nucleotides outside the characterized gene end sequence of respiratory syncytial virus. Virology 2002; 300: 304–315.

Hegele RG, Hayashi S, Bramley AM, How JC. Persistence of respiratory syncytial virus genome and protein after acute bronchiolitis in guinea pigs. Chest 1994; 105: 1848–1854.

Henderson G, Murray J, Yeo RP. Sorting of the respiratory syncytial virus matrix protein into detergent-resistant structures is dependent on cell-surface expression of the glycoprotein. Virology 2002; 300: 244–254.

Hendricks DA, Baradaran K, McIntosh K, Patterson JL. Appearance of a soluble form of the G protein of respiratory syncytial virus in fluids of infected cells. J Gen Virol 1987; 68: 1705–1714.

Hendricks DA, McIntosh K, Patterson JL. Further characterisation of the soluble form of the G glycoprotein of respiratory syncytial virus. J Virol 1988; 62: 2228–2233.

Hoffman SJ, Laham FR, Polack FP. Mechanisms of illness during respiratory syncytial virus infection: the lungs, the virus and the immune response. Microb Infect 2004; 6: 767–772.

Huang YT, Collins PL, Wertz GW. Characterization of the 10 proteins of human respiratory syncytial virus: identification of a fourth envelope-associated protein. Virus Res 1985; 2: 157–173.

Jentoft N. Why are proteins O-glycosylated? Trends Biochem Sci 1990; 15: 291–294.

Jin H, Clarke D, Zhou HZ, Cheng X, Coelingh K, Bryant M, Li S. Recombinant human respiratory syncytial virus (RSV) from cDNA and construction of subgroup A and B chimeric RSV. Virology 1998; 251: 206–214.

Johnson PR, Collins PL. The fusion glycoprotein of human respiratory syncytial virus of subgroups A and B: sequence conservation provides a structural basis for antigenic relatedness. J Gen Virol 1988; 69: 2623–2628.

Johnson PR, Collins PL. Sequence comparison of the phosphoprotein mRNAs of antigenic subgroups A and B of human respiratory syncytial virus identifies a highly divergent domain in the predicted protein. J Gen Virol 1990; 71: 481–485.

Johnson PR, Spriggs MK, Olmsted RA, Collins PL. The G glycoprotein of human respiratory syncytial viruses of subgroups A and B: extensive sequence divergence between antigenically related proteins. Proc Natl Acad Sci USA 1987; 84: 5625–5629.

Juhasz K, Murphy BR, Collins PL. The major attenuating mutation of respiratory syncytial virus vaccine candidate cpts530/1009 specify temperature-sensitive defects in transcription and replication and a non-temperature-sensitive alteration in mRNA termination. J Virol 1999; 73: 5176–5180.

Karlin D, Ferron F, Canard B, Longhi S. Structural disorder and modular organization in Paramyxovirinae N and P. J Gen Virol 2003; 84: 3239–3252.

Karron RA, Buonagurio DA, Georgiu AF, Whitehead SS, Adamus JE, Clements-Mann ML, Harris DO, Randolph V-B, Udem SA, Murphy BR, Sidhu MS. Respiratory syncytial virus (RSV) SH and G proteins are not essential for viral replication in vitro: clinical evaluation and molecular characterization of a cold-passaged, attenuated RSV subgroup B mutant. Proc Natl Acad Sci USA 1997; 94: 13961–13966.

Khattar SK, Yunus AS, Samal SK. Mapping the domains on the phosphoprotein of bovine respiratory syncytial virus required for N–P and P–L interactions using a minigenome system. J Gen Virol 2001; 82: 775–779.

Krusat T, Streckert HJ. Heparin-dependent attachment of respiratory syncytial virus (RSV) to host cells. Arch Virol 1997; 142: 1247–1254.

Kuo L, Fearns R, Collins PL. Analysis of the gene start and gene end signals of human respiratory syncytial virus: quasi-templated initiation at position 1 of the encoded mRNA. J Virol 1997; 71: 4944–4953.

Kuo L, Grosfeld H, Cristina J, Hill MG, Collins PL. Effects of mutations in the gene-start and gene-end sequence motifs on transcription of monocistronic and dicistronic minigenomes of respiratory syncytial virus. J Virol 1996; 70: 6892–6901.

Lamb RA. Paramyxovirus fusion: a hypothesis for changes. Virology 1993; 197: 1–11.

Lamb RA, Kolakofsky D. *Paramyxoviridae*: the viruses and their replication. In: Fields Virology (Knipe, DM, Howley PM, editors). 4th ed. Philadelphia: Lippincott Williams & Wilkins; 2001; pp.1443–1485.

Lamb RA, Paterson RG, Jardetzky TS. Paramyxovirus membrane fusion: lessons from the F and HN atomic structures. Virology 2006; 344: 30–37.

Lambert DM, Barney S, Lambert AL, Guthrie K, Medinas R, Davis DE, Bucy T, Erickson J, Merutka G, Petteway Jr. SR. Peptides from conserved regions of paramyxovirus fusion (F) proteins are potent inhibitors of viral fusion. Proc Natl Acad Sci USA 1996; 93: 2186–2191.

Langedijk JPM, de Groot BL, Berendsen JC, van Oirschot JT. Structural homology of the central conserved region of the attachment protein G of respiratory syncytial virus with the fourth subdomain of 55-kDa tumor necrosis factor receptor. Virology 1998; 243: 293–302.

Langedijk JPM, Schaaper WMM, Meloen RH, van Oirschot JT. Proposed three-dimensional model for the attachment protein G of respiratory syncytial virus. J Gen Virol 1996; 77: 1249–1257.

Lawless-Delmenico MK, Sista P, Sen R, Moore NC, Antczak JB, White JM, Greene RJ, Leanza KC, Matthews TJ, Lambert DM. Heptad-repeat regions of respiratory syncytial virus F1 protein form a six-membered coiled-coil complex. Biochemistry 2000; 39: 11684–11695.

LeVine AM, Elliott J, Whitsett JA, Srikiatkhachorn A, Crouch E, DeSilva N, Korfhagen T. Surfactant protein-d enhances phagocytosis and pulmonary clearance of respiratory syncytial virus. Am J Respir Cell Mol Biol 2004; 31: 193–199.

LeVine AM, Gwozdz J, Stark J, Bruno M, Whitsett J, Korfhagen T. Surfactant protein-A enhances respiratory syncytial virus clearance *in vivo*. J Clin Invest 1999; 103: 1015–1021.

Levine S, Klaiber-Franco R, Paradiso PR. Demonstration that glycoprotein G is the attachment protein of respiratory syncytial virus. J Gen Virol 1987; 68: 2521–2524.

Liuzzi M, Mason SW, Cartier M, Lawetz C, McCollum RS, Dansereau N, Bolger G, Lapeyre N, Gaudette Y, Lagace L, Massariol MJ, Do F, Whitehead P, Lamarre L, Scouten E, Bordeleau J, Landry S, Rancourt J, Fazal G, Simoneau B. Inhibitors of respiratory syncytial virus replication target cotranscriptional mRNA guanylation by viral RNA-dependent RNA polymerase. J Virol 2005; 79: 13105–13115.

Llorente MT, García-Barreno B, Calero M, Camafeita E, López JA, Longhi S, Ferrón F, Varela PF, Melero JA. Structural analysis of the human respiratory syncytial virus phosphoprotein: characterization of an α-helical domain involved in oligomerization. J Gen Virol 2006; 87: 159–169.

Lo MS, Brazas RM, Holtzman MJ. Respiratory syncytial virus nonstructural proteins NS1 and NS2 mediate inhibition of Stat2 expression and alpha/beta interferon responsiveness. J Virol 2005; 79: 9315–9319.

López JA, Bustos R, Örvell C, Berois M, Arbiza J, García-Barreno B, Melero JA. Antigenic structure of human respiratory syncytial virus fusion glycoprotein. J Virol 1998; 72: 6922–6928.

Lu B, Brazas R, Ma C-H, Kristoff T, Cheng X, Jin H. Identification of temperature-sensitive mutations in the phosphoprotein of respiratory syncytial virus that are likely involved in its interaction with the nucleoprotein. J Virol 2002; 76: 2871–2880.

Markwell MAK, Paulson JC. Sendai virus utilizes specific sialyloligosaccharides as host cell receptor determinants. Proc Natl Acad Sci USA 1980; 77: 5693–5697.

Markwell MAK, Portner A, Schwartz AL. An alternative route of infection for viruses: entry by means of the asialoglycoprotein receptor of a Sendai virus mutant lacking the attachment protein. Proc Natl Acad Sci USA 1985; 82: 978–982.

Martín D, Calder LJ, García-Barreno B, Skehel JJ, Melero JA. Sequence elements of the fusion peptide of human respiratory syncytial virus fusion protein required for activity. J Gen Virol 2006; 87: 1649–1658.

Martínez I, Bustos J, Melero JA. Reduced expression of surface glycoproteins in mouse fibroblasts persistently infected with human respiratory syncytial virus (HRSV) Arch Virol 2001; 146: 669–683.

Martínez I, Dopazo J, Melero JA. Antigenic structure of the human respiratory syncytial virus G glycoprotein and relevance of hypermutation events for the generation of antigenic variants. J Gen Virol 1997; 78: 2419–2429.

Martínez I, Melero JA. Enhanced neutralization of human respiratory syncytial virus by mixtures of monoclonal antibodies to the attachment (G) glycoprotein. J Gen Virol 1998; 79: 2215–2220.

Martínez I, Melero JA. Binding of human respiratory syncytial virus to cells: implication of sulfated cell surface proteoglycans. J Gen Virol 2000; 81: 2715–2722.

Marty A, Meanger J, Mills J, Shields B, Ghyldial R. Association of matrix protein of respiratory syncytial virus with the host cell membrane of infected cells. Arch Virol 2004; 149: 199–210.

Mason SW, Aberg E, Lawetz C, DeLong R, Whitehead P, Liuzzi M. Interaction between human respiratory syncytial virus (RSV) M2-1 and P proteins is required for reconstitution of M2-1 dependent RSV minigenome activity. J Virol 2003; 77: 10670–10676.

Mason SW, Lawetz C, Gaudette Y, Dô F, Scouten E, Lagacé L, Simoneau B, Liuzzi M. Polyadenylation-dependent screening assay for respiratory syncytial virus RNA transcriptase activity and identification of an inhibitor. Nucl Acids Res 2004; 32: 4758–4767.

Matthews JM, Young TF, Tucker SP, Mackay JP. The core of the respiratory syncytial virus fusion protein is a trimeric coiled coil. J Virol 2000; 74: 5911–5920.

McGivern DR, Collins PL, Fearns R. Identification of internal sequences in the 3′ leader region of human respiratory syncytial virus that enhance transcription and confer replication processivity. J Virol 2005; 79: 2449–2460.

Melero JA, García-Barreno B, Martínez I, Pringue CR, Cane PA. Antigenic structure, evolution and immunobiology of human respiratory syncytial virus attachement (G) protein. J Gen Virol 1997; 78: 2411–2418.

Mink MAD, Stec DS, Collins PL. Nucleotide sequence of the 3′ leader and 5′ trailer regions of human respiratory syncytial virus genomic RNA. Virology 1991; 185: 615–624.

Mononegavirales. In: ICTVdB—The Universal Virus Database, version 3 (Büchen-Osmond C, editor). New York, NY, USA: ICTVdB Management, Columbia University; 2003.

Morris JA, Blount RE, Savage RE. Recovery of cytopathic agent from chimpanzees with coryza. Proc Soc Exp Biol Med 1956; 92: 544–550.

Morton CJ, Cameron R, Lawrence LJ, Lin B, Lowe M, Luttick A, Mason A, McKimm-Breschkin J, Parker MW, Ryan J, Smout M, Sullivan J, Tucker SP, Young PR. Structural characterization of respiratory syncytial virus fusion inhibitor escape mutants: homology model of the F protein and a syncytium formation assay. Virology 2003; 311: 275–278.

Moudy RM, Harmon SB, Sullender WM, Wertz GW. Variations in transcription termination signals of human respiratory syncytial virus clinical isolates affect gene expression. Virology 2003; 313: 250–260.

Moudy RM, Sullender WM, Wertz GW. Variations in intergenic region sequences of human respiratory syncytial virus clinical isolates: analysis of effects on transcriptional regulation. Virology 2004; 327: 121–133.

Mould JA, Li HC, Dudlak CS, Lear JD, Pekosz A, Lamb RA, Pinto LH. Mechanism for proton conduction of the M(2) ion channel of influenza A virus. J Biol Chem 2000; 275: 8592–8599.

Mufson MA, Örvell C, Rafnar B, Norrby E. Two distinct subtypes of human respiratory syncytial virus. J Gen Virol 1985; 66: 2111–2124.

Murphy LB, Loney C, Murray J, Bhella D, Ashton P, Yeo RP. Investigation into the amino-terminal domain of the respiratory syncytial virus nucleocapsid protein reveal elements important for nucleocapsid formation and interaction with the phosphoprotein. Virology 2003; 307: 143–153.

Murray J, Loney C, Murphy LB, Graham S, Yeo RP. Characterization of monoclonal antibodies raised against recombinant respiratory syncytial virus nucleocapsid (N) protein: Identification of a region in the carboxy terminus of N involved in the interaction with P protein. Virology 2001; 289: 252–261.

Navarro J, Lopez-Otín C, Villanueva N. Location of phosphorylated residues in human respiratory syncytial virus phosphoprotein. J Gen Virol 1991; 72: 1455–1459.

Ogino T, Kobayashi M, Iwama M, Mizumoto K. Sendai virus RNA-dependent RNA polymerase L protein catalyzes cap methylation of virus-specific mRNA. J Biol Chem 2005; 280: 4429–4435.

Palomo C, Albar JP, García-Barreno B, Melero JA. Induction of a neutralizing immune response to human respiratory syncytial virus with anti-idiotypic antibodies. J Virol 1990; 64: 4199–4206.

Palomo C, Cane PA, Melero JA. Evaluation of antibody specificities of human convalescent-phase sera against the attachment (G) protein of human respiratory syncytial virus: influence of strain variation and carbohydrate side chains. J Med Virol 2000; 60: 468–474.

Palomo C, García-Barreno B, Peñas C, Melero JA. The G protein of human respiratory syncytial virus: significance of carbohydrate side-chains and the C-terminal end to its antigenicity. J Gen Virol 1991; 72: 669–675.

Panuska JR, Cirino NM, Midulla F, Despot JE, McFadden Jr. ER, Huang YT. Productive infection of isolated human alveolar macrophages by respiratory syncytial virus. J Clin Invest 1990; 86: 113–119.

Peeples ME, Collins PL. Mutations in the 5′ trailer region of a respiratory syncytial virus minigenome which limit RNA replication to one step. J Virol 2000; 74: 146–155.

Pérez M, García-Barreno B, Melero JA, Carrasco L, Guinea R. Membrane permeability changes induced in *Escherichia coli* by the SH protein of human respiratory syncytial virus. Virology 1997; 235: 342–351.

Poch O, Blumberg BM, Bougueleret L, Torodo N. Sequence comparison of five polymerases (L proteins) of unsegmented negative-strand RNA viruses: theoretical assignment of functional domains. J Gen Virol 1990; 71: 1153–1162.

Poch O, Sauvaget I, Delarue M, Tordo N. Identification of four conserved motifs among the RNA-dependent polymerase encoding elements. EMBO J 1989; 8: 3867–3874.

Polack FP, Irusta PM, Hoffman SJ, Schiatti MP, Melendi GA, Delgado MF, Laham FR, Thumar BR, Michael Hendry RM, Melero JA, Karron RA, Collins PL, Steven R, Kleeberger SR. The cysteine-rich region of respiratory syncytial virus attachment protein inhibits innate immunity elicited by the virus and endotoxin. Proc Natl Acad Sci USA 2005; 102: 8996–9001.

Randhawa JS, Marriott AC, Pringle CR, Easton AJ. Rescue of synthetic minireplicons establishes the absence of NS1 and NS2 genes from avian pneumovirus. J Virol 1997; 71: 9849–9854.

Rixon HWM, Brown G, Aitken J, McDonald T, Graham S, Sugrue RJ. The small hydrophobic (SH) protein accumulates within lipid-raft structures of the Golgi complex during respiratory syncytial virus infection. J Gen Virol 2004; 85: 1153–1165.

Rixon HWM, Brown G, Murray JT, Sugrue RJ. The respiratory syncytial virus small hydrophobic protein is phosphorylated via a mitogen-activated protein kinase p38-dependent tyrosine kinase activity during virus infection. J Gen Virol 2005; 86: 375–384.

Roberts SR, Compans RW, Wertz GW. Respiratory syncytial virus matures at the apical surfaces of polarized epithelial cells. J Virol 1995; 69: 2667–2673.

Roberts SR, Lichtenstein D, Ball LA, Wertz GW. The membrane-associated and secreted forms of the respiratory syncytial virus attachment glycoprotein are synthesized from alternative initiation codons. J Virol 1994; 68: 4538–4546.

Rodríguez L, Cuesta I, Asenjo A, Villanueva N. Human respiratory syncytial virus matrix protein is an RNA-binding protein: binding properties, location and identity of the RNA contact residues. J Gen Virol 2004; 85: 709–719.

Routledge EG, Willcocks MM, Morgan L, Samson ACR, Scott R, Toms GL. Heterogeneity of the respiratory syncytial virus 22k protein revealed by western blotting with monoclonal antibodies. J Gen Virol 1987; 68: 1209–1215.

Ruiz-Argüello MB, González-Reyes L, Calder LJ, Palomo C, Martín D, Saíz MJ, García-Barreno B, Skehel JJ, Melero JA. Effect of proteolytic processing at two distinct sites on shape and aggregation of an anchorless fusion protein of human respiratory syncytial virus and fate of the intervening segment. Virology 2002; 298: 317–326.

Sanchez-Seco MP, Navarro J, Martínez R, Villanueva N. C-terminal phosphorylation of human respiratory syncytial virus P protein occurs mainly at serine residue 232. J Gen Virol 1995; 76: 425–430.

Schlender J, Bossert B, Buchholz U, Conzelmann K-K. Bovine respiratory syncytial virus non-structural proteins NS1 and NS2 cooperatirely antagonize alpha/beta interferon-induced antiviral response. J Virol 2000; 74: 8234–8242.

Schnell MJ, Mebatsion T, Conzelmann K-K. Infectious rabies viruses from cloned cDNA. EMBO J 1994; 13: 4195–4203.

Schwarze J, O'Donnell DR, Rohwedder A, Openshaw PJ. Latency and persistence of respiratory syncytial virus despite T cell immunity. Am J Respir Crit Care Med 2004; 169: 801–805.

Shields B, Mills J, Ghyldial R, Gooley P, Meanger J. Multiple heparin binding domains of respiratory syncytial virus G mediate binding to mammalian cells. Arch Virol 2003; 148: 1987–2003.

Skehel JJ, Wiley DC. Receptor binding and membrane fusion in virus entry: the influenza hemagglutinin. Annu Rev Biochem 2000; 69: 317–326.

Slack MS, Easton AJ. Characterization of the interaction of the human respiratory syncytial virus phosphoprotein and nucleocapsid protein using the two-hybrid system. Virus Res 1998; 55: 167–176.

Smith BJ, Lawrence MC, Colman PM. Modelling the structure of the fusion protein from human respiratory syncytial virus. Prot Engin 2002; 15: 365–371.

Spann KM, Tran KC, Chi B, Rabin R, Collins PL. Suppression of the induction of alpha, beta and lambda interferons by the NS1 and NS2 proteins of human respiratory syncytial virus in human epithelial cells and macrophages. J Virol 2004; 78: 4363–4369.

Spann KM, Tran KC, Collins PL. Effects of non-structural proteins NS1 and NS2 of human respiratory syncytial virus on interferon regulatory factor 3, NF-κB, and proinflammatory cytokines. J Virol 2005; 79: 5353–5362.

Stec DS, Hill MG, Collins PL. Sequence analysis of the polymerase L gene of human respiratory syncytial virus and predicted phylogeny of nonsegmented negative-strand virus. Virology 1991; 183: 273–287.

Stokes HL, Easton AJ, Marriott AC. Chimeric pneumovirus nucleocapsid (N) proteins allow identification of amino acids essential for the function of the respiratory syncytial virus N protein. J Gen Virol 2003; 84: 2679–2683.

Stone-Hulslander J, Morrison TG. Detection of an interaction between HN and F proteins of Newcastle disease virus. J Virol 1997; 71: 6287–6295.

Tang RS, Nguyen N, Cheng X, Jin H. Requirement of cysteines and length of the human respiratory syncytial virus M2-1 protein for protein function and virus viability. J Virol 2001; 75: 11328–11335.

Tarbouriech N, Curran J, Ruigrok RWH, Burmeister WP. Tetrameric coiled coil domain of Sendai virus phosphoprotein. Nat Struct Biol 2000; 7: 777–781.

Taylor G, Bruce C, Barbet AF, Wyld SG, Thomas LH. DNA vaccination against respiratory syncytial virus in young calves. Vaccine 2005; 23: 1242–1250.

Techaarpornkul S, Collins PL, Peeples ME. Respiratory syncytial virus with the fusion protein as its only viral glycoprotein is less dependent on cellular glycosaminoglycans for attachment than complete virus. Virology 2002; 294: 296–304.

Teng MN, Collins PL. Identification of the respiratory syncytial virus proteins required for formation and passage of helper-dependent infectious particles. J Virol 1998; 72: 5707–5716.

Teng MN, Whitehead SS, Collins PL. Contribution of the respiratory syncytial virus G glycoprotein and its secreted and membrane-bound forms to virus replication *in vitro* and *in vivo*. Virology 2001; 289: 283–296.

Tripp RA, Jones LP, Haynes LM, Zheng H, Murphy PM, Anderson LJ. CX3C chemokine mimicry by respiratory syncytial virus G glycoprotein. Nat Immunol 2001; 2: 732–738.

Valarcher JF, Bourhy H, Lavenu A, Bourges-Abella N, Roth M, Andreoletti O, Ave P, Schelcher F. Persistent infection of B lymphocytes by bovine respiratory syncytial virus. Virology 2001; 291: 55–67.

Valarcher JF, Furze J, Wyld S, Cook R, Conzelmann K-K, Taylor G. Role of alpha/beta interferons in the attenuation and immunogenicity of recombinant bovine respiratory syncytial viruses lacking NS proteins. J Virol 2003; 77: 8426–8439.

Vidal S, Kolakofsky D. Modified model for the switch from Sendai virus transcription to replication. J Virol 1989; 63: 1951–1958.

Villanueva N, Hardy R, Asenjo A, Yu Q, Wertz GW. The bulk of the phosphorylation of human respiratory syncytial virus phosphoprotein is not essential but modulates viral RNA transcription and replication. J Gen Virol 2000; 81: 129–133.

Walsh EE, Hruska J. Monoclonal antibodies to respiratory syncytial virus proteins: identification of the fusion protein. J Virol 1983; 47: 171–177.

Wertz GW, Collins PL, Hang Y, Gruber C, Levine S, Ball LA. Nucleotide sequence of the G protein of human respiratory syncytial virus reveals an unusual type of membrane protein. Proc Natl Acad Sci USA 1985; 82: 4075–4079.

Wertz GW, Krieger M, Ball LA. Structure and cell surface maturation of the attachment glycoprotein of human respiratory syncytial virus in a cell line deficient in O-glycosylation. J Virol 1989; 63: 4767–4776.

Whitehead SS, Bukreyev A, Teng MN, Firestone CY, St Claire M, Elkins WR, Collins PL, Murphy BR. Recombinant respiratory syncytial virus bearing a deletion of either the NS2 or SH gene is attenuated in chimpanzees. J Virol 1999; 73: 3438–3842.

Wild CT, Shugars DC, Greenvell TK, McDanal CB, Matthews TJ. Peptides corresponding to a predictive alpha-helical domain of human immunodeficiency virus type 1 gp41 are potent inhibitors of virus infection. Proc Natl Acad Sci USA 1994; 91: 9770–9774.

Worthington MT, Amann BT, Nathans D, Berg JM. Metal binding properties and secondary structure of the zinc binding domain of Nup475. Proc Natl Acad Sci USA 1996; 93: 13754–13759.

Wright PF, Ikizler MR, Gonzales RA, Carroll KN, Hohnson JE, Werkhaven JA. Growth of respiratory syncytial virus in primary epithelial cells from the human respiratory tract. J Virol 2005; 79: 8651–8654.

Yao Q, Hu X, Compans RW. Association of the parainfluenza virus fusion and hemagglutinineuraminidase glycoproteins on cell surfaces. J Virol 1997; 71: 650–656.

Yin HS, Paterson RG, Wen X, Lamb RA, Jardetzky TS. Structure of the uncleaved ectodomain of the paramyxovirus (hPIV3) fusion protein. Proc Natl Acad Sci USA 2005; 102: 9288–9293.

Yu Q, Ardí RW, Wertz GW. Functional cDNA clones of the human respiratory syncytial virus N, P and L proteins support replication of RS virus genomic RNA analogs and define minimal *trans*-acting requirements for RNA replication. J Virol 1995; 69: 2412–2419.

Zambrano A. Rescate de minigenomas y análisis funcional de la glicoproteína F del virus respiratorio sincitial humano (VRSH). Ph.D. Thesis, Universidad Autónoma de Madrid; 2000.

Zhang Y, Luxon BA, Casola A, Garofalo RP, Jamaluddin M, Brasier AR. Expression of respiratory syncytial virus-induced chemokine gene networks in lower airway epithelial cells revealed by cDNA microarrays. J Virol 2001; 75: 9044–9058.

Zhang L, Peeples ME, Boucher RC, Collins PL, Pickles RJ. Respiratory syncytial virus infection of human airway epithelial cells is polarized, specific to ciliates cells, and without obvious cytopathology. J Virol 2002; 76: 5654–5666.

Zhao X, Singh M, Malshkevich V, Kim PS. Structural characterization of the human respiratory syncytial virus fusion protein core. Proc Natl Acad Sci USA 2000; 97: 14172–14177.

Zhou H, Cheng X, Jin H. Identification of amino acids that are critical to the processivity function of respiratory syncytial virus M2-1 protein. J Virol 2003; 77: 5046–5053.

Zimmer G, Budz L, Herrler G. Proteolytic activation of respiratory syncytial virus fusion protein. Cleavage at two furin consensus sequences. J Biol Chem 2001a; 276: 1642–1650.

Zimmer G, Rohn M, McGregor GP, Shemann M, Conzelamann KK, Herrler G. Virokinin, a bioactive peptide of the tachykinin family, is released from the fusion protein of bovine respiratory syncytial virus. J Biol Chem 2003; 278: 46854–46861.

Zimmer G, Trotz I, Herrler G. N-glycans of F protein differentially affect fusion activity of human respiratory syncytial virus. J Virol 2001b; 75: 4744–4751.

Respiratory Syncytial Virus
Patricia Cane (Editor)

DOI 10.1016/S0168-7069(06)14002-1

Immunology of RSV

Geraldine Taylor
Institute for Animal Health, Compton Laboratory Compton, Newbury RG20 7NN, UK

Human respiratory syncytial virus (HRSV) is the leading cause of severe viral respiratory disease in infants and young children (Glezen and Denny, 1973) and is an important cause of lower respiratory tract (LRT) disease in the elderly (Falsey et al., 1995) and immunocompromised individuals of any age (Fishaut et al., 1980; Milner et al., 1985; Hall et al., 1986). RSV is closely related to bovine (B)RSV, a major cause of pneumonia in young calves and the epidemiology and pathogenesis of infection with these viruses are similar (Stott and Taylor, 1985). Thus, the viruses cause annual winter outbreaks of respiratory disease, with a peak incidence of severe disease in the first 6 months of life, at a time when maternal antibodies are present and severe, or enhanced, respiratory disease has been seen in infant and calf recipients of inactivated vaccines following HRSV or BRSV infection, respectively. For reasons that are not well understood, RSVs are only weakly immunogenic. Reinfection of humans occurs throughout life and there is evidence that cattle can be reinfected experimentally. The poor duration of immunity following natural infection and the observations of vaccine-augmented disease have complicated the search for effective vaccines.

The innate immune response

The airway epithelium serves as the interface between the environment and the host and acts as the first line of defence against invading pathogens. The ability of airway epithelial cells, alveolar macrophages and dendritic cells (DC) to detect and respond to pathogens is critical for the induction of innate immunity and the establishment of the adaptive immune response. RSV infection of airway epithelial cells and alveolar macrophages results in activation of NF-κB which leads to the induction of inflammatory chemokines and cytokines, such as RANTES (CCL5), MIP-1α (CCL3), MCP-1 (CCL2), eotaxin (CCL11), IL-8 (CXCL8), TNF-α, interleukin (IL)-6, IL-1, etc. (Bitko et al., 1997; Harrison et al., 1999; Noah and Becker, 2000; Haeberle et al., 2002, 2004; Miller et al., 2004) that contribute to inflammation by recruiting neutrophils, macrophages and lymphocytes to the airways.

The molecular mechanisms involved in RSV-induced activation of NF-κB and initiation of the innate response are complex.

Toll-like receptors

One of the mechanisms by which the innate immune system senses the invasion of pathogenic microorganisms is through Toll-like receptors (TLRs), which constitute a family of type I transmembrane receptor proteins that recognise specific molecular patterns present in microbial components. Stimulation of different TLRs induces distinct patterns of gene expression, which not only leads to the activation of innate immunity but also instructs the development of antigen-specific acquired immunity (Takeda et al., 2003). TLRs are constitutively as well as inducibly expressed in a variety of different cells and human bronchial epithelial cells have been shown to express several TLRs that are functionally active (Sha et al., 2004).

There is evidence that like lipopolysaccharide (LPS), the RSV F protein interacts with and signals through TLR4 and CD14 in human monocytes (Kurt-Jones et al., 2000). This interaction leads to activation of NF-κB and the production of proinflammatory antimicrobial mediators such as TNF-α, IL-6 and IL-12. TLR4 is expressed at high levels by macrophages and DC but only at very low levels on airway epithelial cells. However, RSV infection increases TLR4 expression on airway epithelial cells and increases their responsiveness to LPS (Monick et al., 2003).

The role of TLR4 in innate immunity to RSV is unclear. A study in TLR4-deficient mice (C57BL/10 ScCr mice) infected with RSV, demonstrated impaired pulmonary natural killer (NK) cell and $CD14^+$ cell trafficking, deficient NK cell function, impaired IL-12 expression, and impaired virus clearance compared to mice expressing TLR4 (Haynes et al., 2001). However, other studies suggest that these effects were due to a defect in the IL-12 receptor in C57BL/10 ScCr mice rather than to the lack of a functional TLR4 (Ehl et al., 2004). Nevertheless, although an important role for TLR4 in resistance of mice to RSV infection could not be demonstrated, an association between TLR4 mutations and severe RSV disease in humans has been reported (Tal et al., 2004).

TLR3, which is expressed in human bronchial epithelial cells, detects double-stranded RNA (dsRNA) (Alexopoulou et al., 2001). RSV infection upregulates TLR3 expression and there is evidence that induction of MyD88-independent chemokines, such as RANTES (CCL5), by RSV replication is mediated by TLR3 signalling pathways (Rudd et al., 2005). Although the replication of RSV in the lungs of TLR3 deficient B6 mice (TLR3-/-) was similar to that of wild-type mice, TLR3(-/-) mice demonstrated significant increases in mucus production in the airways (Rudd et al., 2006). Changes in pulmonary mucus production in RSV-infected TLR3(-/-) mice were accompanied by an increase in Th2-type cytokines, IL-13 and IL-5, and an accumulation of eosinophils in the airways. Taken together, these studies suggest that although TLR3 may not be required for viral clearance, it is necessary to maintain an immune environment in the lungs that avoids the development of Th-2-mediated pulmonary pathology.

While the studies described above demonstrate that RSV activates NF-κB and production of chemokines and cytokines, there is evidence that the cysteine-rich region of the G protein can suppress TLR4-mediated cytokine production by monocytes and macrophages by inhibiting nuclear translocation of NF-κB (Polack et al., 2005). The mechanisms by which the G protein mediates this effect are not known. However, the conserved cysteine-rich region of the G protein has homology with the fourth domain of the TNF receptor (Langedijk et al., 1998) and it has been suggested that the soluble form of the G protein, which is shed from infected cells early after infection before progeny virus is produced (Hendricks et al., 1988) may be mediating the inhibitory effects by binding to TNF-α or an unknown TNF homologue.

Alpha/beta interferons

One of the earliest responses of cells to virus infection is the production of alpha/beta interferons (IFNα/β). Once produced, these secreted proteins induce gene expression in neighbouring cells by binding to cell surface receptors and activating intracellular signalling pathways, resulting in the induction of proteins that impair viral replication. HRSV and BRSV are not only poor inducers of IFN α/β but are resistant to the antiviral effects of IFNα/β (Atreya and Kulkarni, 1999; Schlender et al., 2000a). These properties of HRSV and BRSV are mediated by the non-structural proteins, NS1 and NS2, which function co-operatively both to disrupt the activity and to prevent the induction of IFNα/β in infected cells (Schlender et al., 2000a; Bossert et al., 2003; Valarcher et al., 2003; Spann et al., 2004).

Although most cell types can produce IFNα/β through recognition of cytosolic dsRNA or upon stimulation of TLR3 and TLR4 (Takeda et al., 2003), the major source of IFN upon bacterial or viral infection is plasmacytoid DC (pDC) (Cella et al., 1999). IFN induction in pDC is triggered through TLR7 and TLR9, located in the endosomal membrane, as well as by recognition of cytosolic virus-specific patterns. TLR7 and TLR9 ligands include single-stranded RNA and CpG-rich DNA, respectively. Both TLR-dependent and TLR-independent IFNα/β responses are abolished in human pDC infected with a number of different clinical isolates of RSV or with the A2 strain of RSV (Schlender et al., 2005). In contrast, the Long strain of HRSV is a potent inducer of IFNα/β in human pDC (Hornung et al., 2004), indicating that the Long strain is not representative of clinical isolates of RSV and therefore that care should be taken in extrapolating results obtained with this strain of virus.

The capacity of RSVs to inhibit IFN production in both airway epithelial cells and pDC may have an important influence on the subsequent development of the adaptive immune response. IFNα/β play a major role in DC maturation, the expansion and activation of NK cells and the differentiation, survival and function of T cells. In addition, IFNα/β can enhance primary antibody responses, promote Ig isotype switching, are important in the induction of IgA and enhance priming of IFNγ-secreting CD4$^+$ T cells (Brinkmann et al., 1993; Biron et al., 1998; Le Bon and Tough, 2002; Proietti et al., 2002). The suggestion that the poor IFNα/β response associated with RSV infections may contribute to the rather inadequate adaptive immune response to HRSV and BRSV in their respective natural hosts is supported by the observation that mice lacking the IFNα/β receptor show little increase in pulmonary CD8$^+$ T cells following HRSV infection when compared with wild-type mice (Johnson et al., 2005). Furthermore, although recombinant BRSVs lacking either the NS1 or the NS2 gene were both highly attenuated in young calves, rBRSVΔNS2, which induced higher levels of IFNα/β, *in vitro*, than rBRSVΔNS1 appeared to be more immunogenic (Valarcher et al., 2003).

Surfactant proteins

Surfactant proteins (SP) A and D, which are produced by alveolar and airway epithelial cells, are pattern recognition molecules that form a first line of defence against infection in the lung. During severe RSV infection SP-A and SP-D levels in bronchoalveolar lavage (BAL) fluid are reduced (Kerr and Paton, 1999). SP-A binds to both the F and G proteins, preventing the virus from infecting the target cell (Ghildyal et al., 1999) and enhancing opsonisation and receptor-mediated uptake of RSV by alveolar macrophages and monocytes (Barr et al., 2000). SP-D also binds to the G protein and inhibits RSV infection both *in vitro* and *in vivo* (Hickling et al., 1999). The observations that SP-A-deficient mice have more severe RSV infection than their wild-type littermates (LeVine et al., 1999) and that susceptibility to severe RSV infection in infants has been linked to polymorphisms in both SP-A and SP-D genes (Lahti et al., 2002; Lofgren et al., 2002) suggest that SP-A plays an important role in pulmonary host defence against RSV. Genetic factors in humans that are involved in susceptibility to severe RSV disease are described in detail in Chapter 4 of this volume.

Interaction with antigen-presenting cells

DC are the primary antigen-presenting cells necessary for the activation of antigen-specific naïve T cells. Studies in experimental models of respiratory virus infection suggest that respiratory DCs, which are located both within intra-epithelial sites and underneath the respiratory epithelium, carry viral antigen from the respiratory tract to the draining lymph nodes where they encounter and activate naïve virus-specific T cells. The level of expression of co-stimulatory/inhibitory molecules on the surface of DCs and the cytokines they produce, which are dependent upon innate signals from pathogens, are important in determining whether T cells are tolerised or activated, and whether they are polarised to become Th1, Th2 or regulatory T cells (de Jong et al., 2005). Although there is little or no virus replication in human or bovine DCs infected with RSV or BRSV, *in vitro*, there is expression of viral proteins, an upregulation of co-stimulatory molecules and an increase in DC apoptosis (Werling et al., 2002; Bartz et al., 2003; de Graaff et al., 2005). Cord blood-derived human DCs infected with HRSV, *in vitro*, produced higher levels of IL-10, IL-11 and prostaglandin E_2, and lower levels of IL-12 than DCs infected with influenza virus (Bartz et al., 2002). Similar studies with bovine monocyte-derived DC (MoDC) demonstrated that exposure of these cells to live BRSV induced more IL-10 mRNA and markedly less IL-12p40 and IL-15 mRNA than did heat-inactivated virus (Werling et al., 2002). HRSV infection appears to decrease the capacity of DCs to activate naïve T cells resulting in low levels of T cell proliferation and impaired cytokine production, a characteristic of regulatory T cells (Bartz et al., 2003; de Graaff et al., 2005). Antigen-specific regulatory T cells secrete IL-10 and/or TGFβ, but little or no IFNγ or IL-4, are capable of suppressing Th1 responses and appear to be important in limiting pathogen-induced immunopathology (McGuirk and Mills, 2002). However, although naïve T cells primed by RSV-infected DCs have some of the characteristics of regulatory T cells, there was no evidence that they were able to inhibit the proliferation of freshly isolated $CD4^+$ T cells (de Graaff et al., 2005). The mechanisms responsible for the impaired capacity of RSV-infected DCs to activate $CD4^+$ T cells appear to be due an unidentified soluble factor produced by RSV-infected DCs (de Graaff et al., 2005).

A number of *in vitro* studies have demonstrated that mitogen-induced activation of human T cells is inhibited by RSV. One study suggested that this effect was mediated by IFNα (Preston et al., 1995) and another that inhibition was mediated by IL-1ra (Salkind et al., 1991). However, as described above, RSVs are poor inducers of type I IFNs. Direct contact of lymphocytes with the F protein expressed on the surface of RSV-infected tissue culture cells also inhibits mitogen-induced activation of lymphocytes (Schlender et al., 2000b). This observation has led to the suggestion that expression of the F protein on the surface of RSV-infected DCs could result in suppression of T-cell activation within the draining lymph nodes. However, surface expression of the F protein does not appear to be the major mechanism by which RSV infection of DCs causes the impaired T cell activation described above (de Graaff et al., 2005).

Subsets of DCs have been identified that express distinct surface markers (Belz et al., 2004; Jahnsen et al., 2004), and which may play a role in the differential activation of T cells. Two phenotypically distinct, major populations of bovine afferent lymph-veiled cells (ALVC) have been identified that differ in their ability to present BRSV to resting memory bovine $CD4^+$ T cells (Howard et al., 1997). $CD11a^-$ ALVC are effective at stimulating proliferative responses of allogeneic $CD4^+$ T cells and $CD8^+$ T cells. These cells are able to present ovalbumin (OVA), but not BRSV to resting memory $CD4^+$ T cells. In contrast, $CD11a^-$ ALVC are effective in presenting both BRSV and OVA to resting $CD4^+$ T cells, but are poor at stimulating an allogeneic response (Howard et al., 1997).

The extent to which these studies on the interaction of DCs with RSVs *in vitro* can be extended to RSV infection *in vivo* is not clear. RSVs primarily invade via the lumenal side of ciliated respiratory epithelial cells and bud via the same face of the cell (Roberts et al., 1995; Zhang et al., 2002). This polarised lifestyle of virus entry and budding is controlled by regulatory motifs in virus surface proteins and the F protein is localised on the apical membrane where virus budding occurs. Since infection is usually limited to superficial cells of the respiratory tract, the extent to which DCs become infected with RSV *in vivo* may not be great. The limited tissue tropism of RSV infection, *in vivo*, may therefore represent a more important method of immune evasion than effects on DCs that are detected after a high multiplicity of infection.

NK cells

NK cells are important effectors of the innate immune response and act as a first line of defence against a variety of pathogens. Chemokines such as MIP-1α (CCL3) are critical for recruitment of NK cells to the site of virus infection where they develop cytotoxic activity and produce IFNγ upon recognition of virus-infected cells. NK cell activation and production of IFNγ therefore plays an important role in the subsequent development of the adaptive immune response. Thus, NK cell activation enhances the differentiation of $CD8^+$ T cells into effector cytotoxic memory T lymphocyte (CTL) and influences the differentiation of $CD4^+$ T cells into those with a Th1 phenotype (Romagnani, 1992; Bancroft, 1993; Kos and Engleman, 1996). In the BALB/c mouse model of RSV infection, NK cells are recruited to the lungs early after infection and reach peak levels at about day 3–4 when they represent a major source of IFNγ (Anderson et al., 1989; Hussell and Openshaw, 1998). Following infection of mice with a mutant subgroup B strain of RSV that lacks the G and SH proteins, greater numbers of pulmonary NK cells were observed compared with mice infected with the parental wild-type virus, suggesting that the G and/or SH proteins may downregulate the NK cell response (Tripp et al., 1999). In these studies, the increased numbers of NK cells correlated with greater levels of expression of mRNAs of chemokines that attract NK cells to the lungs in mice infected with the ΔG/SH mutant (Tripp and Anderson, 2000), suggesting that the G and/or SH protein may downregulate the early chemokine response. These observations are in agreement with studies mentioned previously which demonstrated that the G protein can suppress TLR4-mediated cytokine production by monocytes and macrophages (Polack et al., 2005).

Depletion of asiola GM^+ NK cells resulted in prolonged shedding of RSV from infected mice, suggesting a major role for NK cells in clearance of RSV (Harrop et al., 1994). Production of IFNγ by NK cells is dependent upon IL-12 from macrophages or DCs (Biron et al., 1999) and NK cell recruitment to the lungs of RSV-infected mice deficient in IL-12 signalling is impaired compared with wild-type mice (Ehl et al., 2004). However, IL-12 signalling deficiency had only a minor effect on RSV clearance and did not appear to influence either the pulmonary inflammatory response or the development of RSV-specific $CD8^+$ T cells.

NK T cells are a subpopulation of alpha/beta T cells that coexpress receptors of the NK lineage and which have an extremely restricted TCR repertoire (Bendelac et al., 1997). NK T cells recognise glycosphingolipids presented by CD1d, an antigen-presenting molecule distantly related to the peptide-presenting MHC class I and class II molecules. These cells have the potential to secrete large amounts of cytokines, providing early help for effector cells and regulating the Th1 or Th2 differentiation of some immune responses. Studies of RSV infection in CD1d-deficient mice have demonstrated that NK T cells contribute to the efficient induction of RSV-specific $CD8^+$ T cell responses and that in the absence of NK T-cell activation, early IFNγ production may be reduced (Johnson et al., 2002). The mechanism by which RSV activates NK T cells is not known. It is has been suggested that a weak response to CD1d-presented self antigens may be amplified by IL-12 produced by DCs in response to infection (Brigl et al., 2003). However, since RSVs appear to be poor inducers of IL-12 in human or bovine macrophages or DCs (Tsutsumi et al., 1996), the role of NK and NK T cells in RSV infection in the natural host is not clear.

The adaptive immune response

While the innate immune response plays an important role in the pathogenesis of RSV infection and the development of the adaptive immune response, it is the adaptive immune response that mediates recovery from infection and resistance to reinfection. Epidemiological studies have shown that prior RSV infection does not confer complete protection against reinfection (Henderson et al., 1979). However, there is an accumulation of resistance to LRT disease with successive infections. Adults with pre-existing serum antibodies can be infected experimentally with HRSV (Johnson et al., 1961; Kravetz et al., 1961; Mills et al., 1971) and calves can be experimentally reinfected 3 weeks after a primary BRSV infection (Stott et al., 1984). Nevertheless, the duration and quantity of virus shedding in these studies is significantly less than that occurring during the primary infection. A primary RSV infection in cotton rats induced complete resistance to pulmonary infection lasting for at least 18 months, whereas the nasal passages became susceptible to reinfection by 8 months post-infection (Prince et al., 1983). These observations indicate that immunity to RSV infection in the lung may be more durable than that in the upper respiratory tract (URT). The relative importance of the various components of the immune response in resistance to RSV infection has been studied extensively in experimental animal models. Recovery from and resistance to reinfection are mediated by various components of the adaptive immune response and it is becoming increasingly clear that the balance between different types of immune response is crucial in determining the outcome of RSV infection.

Immune recognition of RSV proteins

Studies in BALB/c mice vaccinated with recombinant vaccinia viruses (rVV) expressing individual proteins demonstrated that the F and G proteins were the major determinants of resistance to RSV infection, although transient protection could be induced by the N and M2 proteins (Connors et al., 1991). Serum antibodies were induced by rVV expressing the F, G, N or P proteins, but only the F or G proteins induced neutralising antibodies. Similar studies in calves vaccinated with rVV expressing the BRSV F, G, N or M2 proteins also highlighted the importance of the F and G proteins in mediating protection and indicated that the N protein could also induce some resistance (Taylor et al., 1997). The F, G and N proteins induced serum antibodies, but only the F and G proteins induced neutralising antibodies.

Antibody recognition of RSV proteins

Although RSV infection induces antibodies against a variety of viral proteins only those to the F and G proteins neutralise the virus and confer resistance to RSV infection (see below). The antigenicity and immunogenicity of the F protein is highly dependent upon its folded structure (Gaddum et al., 1996b). Thus, vaccination of mice with rVV expressing an F protein containing a single point mutation in the F1 subunit which blocks its transport to the cell surface induces antibodies which recognise denatured but not native F protein and which are not neutralising. The antigenic structure of the F protein has been analysed using monoclonal antibodies (mAbs), the majority of which are cross-reactive, recognising the F protein from both subgroups of HRSV as well as BRSV (Taylor et al., 1992), antibody-escape mutants and synthetic peptides (Beeler and Van Wyke Coelingh, 1989; Arbiza et al., 1992; Taylor et al., 1992; Lopez et al., 1993; Lopez et al., 1998). These studies identified two regions of the F protein that are recognised by murine neutralising, fusion-inhibiting mAbs that are also recognised by bovine and human neutralising, fusion-inhibiting mAbs (Taylor et al., 1992; Crowe et al., 1998). The neutralising epitopes are located in the F1 subunit and do not involve the fusion peptide (Calder et al., 2000). Analysis of the repertoire of F-specific antibodies induced by RSV infection demonstrated that highly neutralising antibodies recognised the mature F protein on the cell surface and on virions, whereas poorly neutralising antibodies appeared to recognise immature F protein (Sakurai et al., 1999).

Recognition of the G protein by mAbs does not appear to highly dependent upon the folded structure of the G protein (Martinez et al., 1997; Melero et al., 1997). Few mAbs are cross-reactive and recognise the G protein from both antigenic subgroups of HRSV and these do not recognise BRSV (Taylor et al., 1984; Martinez et al., 1997). The majority of G-specific mAbs are either subgroup specific or strain specific. Cross-reactive or subgroup-specific mAbs react with the non-glycosylated central region of the G protein of HRSV or BRSV, containing the cysteine noose (Furze et al., 1994, 1997; Langedijk et al., 1997; Martinez et al., 1997). Although G-specific polyclonal antiserum (Johnson et al., 1987) and mixtures of G-specific mAbs neutralise virus infectivity, individual mAbs exhibit little or no neutralising activity (Martinez and Melero, 1998).

$CD8^+$ T cell recognition of RSV proteins

In adults, HRSV-specific human $CD8^+$ cytotoxic memory T lymphocytes (CTLs) from the majority of individuals studied recognise the N protein, however the SH, F, M, M2 and NS2 proteins are also recognised in some individuals (Cherrie et al.,

1992). There was little or no recognition of the G, P or NS1 protein by human $CD8^+$ T cells. In BALB/c mice, $CD8^+$ CTLs recognise the F, N and M2 proteins (Bangham et al., 1986; Pemberton et al., 1987; Openshaw et al., 1990). The M2 protein contains the immunodominant H-2K^d epitope and immunisation with this epitope induces levels of RSV-specific CTLs comparable to those induced by RSV infection (Kulkarni et al., 1995). BRSV-specific bovine CTLs recognised antigenically distinct strains of BRSV (Gaddum et al., 1996a) and the F, N and M2 proteins appeared to be the major antigens recognised by bovine $CD8^+$ T cells (Gaddum et al., 2003). Whereas there appears to be little or no recognition of the G protein by $CD8^+$ T cells from man or BALB/c mice, strong recognition of the G protein by $CD8^+$ T cells has been observed in cattle that had been vaccinated with rVV expressing this protein and subsequently challenged with BRSV (Gaddum et al., 2003). More recent studies have demonstrated that the BRSV P protein contains epitopes that are recognised by a variety of cattle expressing different MHC class I haplotypes (unpublished observations).

H-2K^d-restricted epitopes recognised by $CD8^+$ T cells from BALB/c mice have been identified in the M2 (Kulkarni et al., 1993b) and F proteins (Chang et al., 2001; Jiang et al., 2002; Johnstone et al., 2004) and an H-2D^b-restricted CTL epitope recognised by $CD8^+$ T cells from C57Bl/6 mice has been identified in the M protein (Rutigliano et al., 2005). HLA class I-restricted CTL epitopes have also been identified in the F protein (Brandenburg et al., 2000a), N protein (Goulder et al., 2000; Venter et al., 2003), M, NS2 and M2 proteins (Heidema et al., 2004). The identification of CTL epitopes has provided the opportunity to detect and accurately quantitate antigen-specific CTLs and to analyse the kinetics of virus-specific CTL responses at the site of infection. Such studies have contributed to the elucidation of the role of $CD8^+$ CTLs in immunity to and the pathogenesis of RSV infection.

$CD4^+$ T cell recognition

Studies in BALB/c mice scarified with rVV expressing different RSV proteins have demonstrated that the F and G proteins prime different $CD4^+$ T-cell subsets (Alwan and Openshaw, 1993; Alwan et al., 1993; Alwan et al., 1994). Thus, scarification of mice with rVVF primed a $CD4^+$ T-cell response that was biased towards Th1, with production of IL-2 and IFNγ, whereas scarification with rVVG primed a $CD4^+$ T-cell response that was biased towards Th2, with production of IL-4, IL-5, IL-13 and IFNγ (Bembridge et al., 1998; Johnson and Graham, 1999). The Th2-biased response induced by the G protein in BALB/c mice is mediated largely by a single immunodominant epitope (aa 183–197) recognised by a $V\beta14^+$ subset of $CD4^+$ T cells producing both Th1 and Th2 cytokines (IFNγ, IL-4, Il-5 and IL-13) after stimulation with RSV *in vitro* (Sparer et al., 1998; Tebbey et al., 1998; Srikiatkhachorn et al., 1999; Varga et al., 2000; Johnson et al., 2004). The consequences of this differential T-cell priming in RSV pathogenesis are discussed below.

The extent to which the findings of differential CD4$^+$ T-cell priming in mice are applicable to the natural host, is not clear. However, there is evidence that the F and G proteins may prime different T-cell subsets in man and in cattle. Thus, F protein-specific, short-term, human CD4$^+$ T-cell lines produced Th1-biased cytokine responses, whereas G protein-specific human CD4$^+$ T-cell lines produced Th2 cytokines (Jackson and Scott, 1996). In cattle, vaccination with rVVF primed CD4$^+$ T cells for a BRSV-specific proliferative response, *in vitro*, and production of IL-2, IFNγ and Il-4 mRNA, whereas CD4$^+$ T cells from cattle vaccinated with rVVG did not proliferate after stimulation with BRSV *in vitro*, but did appear to respond by production of IL-10 mRNA (Fogg, 1999).

Bovine CD4$^+$ T cells recognised epitopes that were distributed predominantly within the F1 subunit of the F protein, some of which were adjacent to previously identified B cell epitopes (Fogg et al., 2001). In contrast, human CD4$^+$ T-cell epitopes are distributed along the entire length of the F protein, with only the region between amino acids 121 and 168 not recognised (van Bleek et al., 2003). Several immunodominant bovine T-cell epitopes within the F protein that were recognised by calves with different MHC class II haplotypes, are also recognised by human T cells (Levely et al., 1991; Fogg et al., 2001). Thus, cattle and humans appear to recognise similar T-cell epitopes on the F protein. In contrast, CD4$^+$ T-cells from BALB/c mice immunised with the FG protein recognised a relatively hydrophobic peptide within the F2 subunit (Levely et al., 1991).

Epitopes within the non-glycosylated ectodomain of the G protein are recognised by CD4$^+$ Th2 cells from a variety of different mouse strains that had been immunised with highly purified native G protein (Hancock et al., 2003b). However out of 43 human volunteers, only 6 recognised the G protein from the A2 strain of HRSV, of which 3 responded to peptide 184–198 (Tebbey et al., 1998). Other studies have demonstrated immunodominant epitopes within the regions 162–179 of the G protein recognised by human CD4$^+$ T cells that produce both Th1 and Th2 cytokines (de Graaff et al., 2004; de Waal et al., 2004). In contrast to humans and mice, bovine CD4$^+$ T-cell epitopes were mainly located within the cytoplasmic tail of the BRSV G protein (Fogg et al., 2001). However, bovine CD4$^+$ T-cell proliferative responses to G protein peptides were poor. The finding that there was little recognition of the extracellular domain of the G protein by bovine T cells has important implications for vaccine design based on the soluble form of this protein.

Role of antibody in recovery from and resistance to RSV infection

Antibody responses to RSV

Both serum and secretory antibodies are produced in response to RSV infection, even by very young infants (McIntosh et al., 1978; Richardson et al., 1978; Watt et al., 1986). However, the frequency and magnitude of the antibody response in young infants are significantly lower than that in older infants and children. Following infection, serum antibodies fall to very low levels within one year

(Welliver et al., 1980). There then emerges a pattern of gradually increasing levels of serum antibody with successive RSV infections, thus producing substantial temporary immunity (Welliver et al., 1980). In contrast, virus-specific IgA antibodies are more short-lived than serum IgG antibodies, and are only detected for a few months following RSV infection. The avidity of the primary serum antibody response to RSV is low in infants, but increases with age (Meurman et al., 1992). Most children of 9–21 months of age develop moderate levels of IgG and IgA antibodies to the F and G proteins, whereas the response of infants less than 8 months of age to the F or G proteins is poor (Murphy et al., 1986a).

The low magnitude and poor durability of RSV antibody responses in infants is most likely due to a combination of immunological immaturity and the suppressive effect of maternally transmitted transplacental antibody (Murphy et al., 1986a). The antibody response to primary RSV infection is inversely related to the titre of maternally derived, serum neutralising antibodies (Parrott et al., 1973) and studies in mice and cotton rats have shown that passively acquired serum antibodies suppress the immune response to RSV (Murphy et al., 1988; Crowe et al., 2001). Although passively acquired serum antibodies are potent in suppressing the systemic antibody response, their effect on priming of a mucosal immune response may be less marked. Thus, whereas passively acquired RSV antibodies suppressed the immune response and the protective efficacy induced by intradermal vaccination of cotton rats with rVV expressing the F or G proteins, the suppressive effects could be partially overcome by administration of the recombinants by the intranasal route (Murphy et al., 1989). Similarly, a serum and mucosal IgA response, but not a serum IgG antibody response could be detected in 1 to 2-month-old infants inoculated intranasally with a live, attenuated RSV vaccine (Wright et al., 2000).

Young infants mount a relatively poor antibody response to immunisation or infection even when they possess low titres of maternally derived specific antibodies. These observations suggest that immunological immaturity also contributes to the poor immune response of infants to RSV. Little is known about the molecular and cellular basis for the immunological immaturity of human infants. However, the observation that virus-specific B cells from infants exhibit a decreased frequency of somatic hypermutations in their antibody genes compared with those of adults (Weitkamp et al., 2005) may explain, at least in part, the poor quality of antibodies in infants. In contrast to the poor antibody response in infants, the RSV-specific antibody response of the elderly, who are at increased risk of severe RSV infection, was as vigorous as that of young adults, suggesting that severe RSV disease in the elderly is not due to a significant defect in humoral immunity (Falsey et al., 1999).

Some studies suggest that age and the titre of maternally derived antibodies influence the development of antibodies to the F and G proteins differently. Thus, in one study, the serum IgA response to the F protein induced by RSV infection, appeared to be primarily influenced by age, whereas the serum IgA response to the G protein was dependent upon the pre-existing serum antibody titre (Murphy et al., 1986a).

However in another study of infants infected with a live attenuated RSV vaccine, the IgA response to the F protein appeared to be dependent upon the level of maternally acquired antibodies rather than age (Wright et al., 2000). In this study, serum IgA responses to the G protein proved to be the most consistent response in young to infection with the live-attenuated RSV vaccine.

The role of serum antibody in protection against RSV

Antibodies play a primary role in protection against RSV and there is a strong correlation between levels of maternal antibodies to RSV and resistance to infection during the first few weeks of life, when titres of passive antibodies are highest. Both the incidence and the severity of RSV LRT disease in infants exhibit an inverse correlation with the level of serum antibodies in previously obtained umbilical cord blood (Parrott et al., 1973; Lamprecht et al., 1976; Hall et al., 1979; Glezen et al., 1981; Ogilvie et al., 1981; Holberg et al., 1991). Similarly in calves, although maternal antibodies do not prevent infection, both the incidence and severity of BRSV respiratory disease are inversely related to the level of BRSV-specific maternally-derived serum antibodies (Kimman et al., 1989). In the elderly, the level of neutralising antibody is also inversely correlated with the risk of hospitalisation during acute RSV infection (Falsey and Walsh, 1998). However, the difference in mean neutralising antibody titre in the elderly hospitalised with RSV infection was only 2–3-fold lower than that in those not requiring hospitalisation (Walsh et al., 2004).

Further evidence for the role of serum antibody in protection against RSV comes from studies on the effects of passively transferred serum antibodies in animal models and in infants at high risk of severe RSV disease (Prince et al., 1985a; Groothuis et al., 1993; Graham et al., 1993a; Hemming et al., 1995). Serum IgG antibodies gain access to the lungs via transudation, but this process appears to be less efficient in the nasal passages. Thus, in animal models, passive transfer of serum antibodies protected the lungs against RSV infection, but had little effect on URT infection. Studies in passively immunised cotton rats demonstrated that whereas serum neutralising antibody titres $\leqslant$ 1:380 conferred complete protection against virus replication in the lungs, there was only a partial reduction in nasal virus titres (Prince et al., 1985b). Similarly, while monthly infusions of RSV-neutralising polyclonal antibodies (RSV-IVIG) to infants at high risk of severe RSV disease, did not influence the incidence of RSV infection, RSV-IVIG reduced both the frequency and duration of hospitalisation by approximately 55% (Groothuis et al., 1993; Groothuis et al., 1995).

Although polyclonal sera contain antibodies to various viral proteins, only antibodies to the surface glycoproteins, F and G proteins, confer resistance to RSV infection. Monoclonal antibodies (mAbs) specific to the F or G proteins protect against pulmonary virus replication in mice, cotton rats and calves (Taylor et al., 1984; Walsh et al., 1984; Thomas et al., 1998). Anti-F mAbs that are virus-neutralising and inhibit the formation of multinucleated giant cells are highly effective not only at preventing RSV infection but also at eliminating virus from the lungs when given therapeutically (Taylor et al., 1992; Taylor, 1994). Even Fab fragments of these neutralising, fusion-inhibiting mAbs are able to protect against RSV infection, indicating that protection is not dependent upon complement activation or antibody-dependent cell-mediated cytotoxicity (Prince et al., 1990; Taylor, 1994). A humanised, neutralising, fusion-inhibiting mAb is now in use for the prophylactic treatment of infants at high risk of severe RSV infection (Impact-RSV Study Group, 1998).

Passively transferred mAbs specific for the G protein were also effective at protecting against RSV infection in mice and cotton rats (Taylor et al., 1984; Walsh et al., 1984). However, the majority of G-specific mAbs that protected against RSV in mice were not neutralising and were markedly less effective than F-specific mAbs when given therapeutically (Taylor, 1994). Apart from one neutralising G-specific mAb that recognised both subgroups of RSV, the protective anti-G mAbs were RSV subgroup specific, recognised the central conserved cysteine-rich region of the G protein (Taylor et al., 1984; Trudel et al., 1991; Taylor, 1994) and appeared to mediate their protective effects by means of complement activation or antibody-dependent cell-mediated cytotoxicity (Taylor, 1994).

Role of mucosal antibody in protection against RSV infection

Although parenteral administration of neutralising polyclonal or monoclonal antibodies was effective against pulmonary RSV infection, intranasal administration of antibodies was at least 160-fold more potent (Prince et al., 1987). These observations suggest that locally produced antibodies may be more effective than serum antibodies against pulmonary RSV infection. Furthermore, in contrast to the inefficiency of serum antibodies at restricting RSV replication in the URT, RSV infection at this site provides a high level of resistance to nasal reinfection (Graham et al., 1995; Johnson et al., 1996). Intranasal administration of a neutralising, F protein-specific, IgA mAb to mice 24 h prior to RSV challenge, reduced virus titres in the lungs and in the nose when given 1 h, but not 24 h, before challenge (Weltzin et al., 1994). However, a comparison of the ability of topical and parenteral administration of this IgA mAb with an IgG mAb, specific for the same antigenic site, to protect mice against RSV infection, demonstrated that administration of RSV-specific IgG was more effective in reducing RSV titres in the lung than IgA when given intranasally immediately prior to infection (Fisher et al., 1999). Since the neutralising titre of the IgG mAb was greater than that of the IgA mAb, these observations suggest that prevention of infection may be more dependent on the neutralisation titre of the passive antibody than on its isotype.

High levels of neutralising antibodies in nasal secretions appear to limit virus replication in the URT, independently of the level of serum antibodies (Mills et al., 1971). Similarly, nasal secretory antibody appears to have an important role in protection against experimental BRSV challenge in calves (Mohanty et al., 1976; Kimman et al., 1987). While virus-specific IgG, IgM and IgA antibodies can be detected in nasal secretions in both infants and calves (McIntosh et al., 1978; Kimman et al., 1987; Wright et al., 2002) following RSV infection, there is a poor correlation between the presence of these antibodies and virus neutralisation (McIntosh et al., 1978). Although virus-specific secretory IgA antibodies are short-lived, when compared with serum antibodies, repeated RSV infection induces higher levels of mucosal IgA and a more sustained response (Henderson et al., 1979; Welliver et al., 1980). Nevertheless, secretory IgA antibodies may be only partially protective since adult volunteers could still be infected even in the presence of moderate levels of such antibodies (Mills et al., 1971).

A clinical trial of a live-attenuated RSV vaccine in 1–2-month infants demonstrated that vaccine recipients that had developed a serum IgA response to the G protein were protected against infection with a second dose of vaccine virus, whereas all those that failed to mount such a response became infected (Wright et al., 2000). Presumably, the serum IgA antibody reflected the mucosal IgA response, which appears to be more difficult to measure. Mucosal IgA antibodies to the G protein may mediate protection by a mechanism other than, or in addition to, virus neutralisation, such as antibody-dependent cell-mediated cytotoxicity (Cranage et al., 1981) or intracellular disruption of virus replication during transcytosis of IgA across the epithelial mucosa (Mazanec et al., 1993). It has been proposed that the greater susceptibility of the URT compared with the lungs may be related to the avidity and/or specificity of mucosal antibody, such that local defences could be easily overwhelmed by strains of RSV exhibiting minor antigenic variations in the G protein.

Studies in calves in which the primary mucosal response is inhibited by maternally acquired antibody, have suggested that the ability to mount a rapid secondary mucosal IgA response may be more important in resistance to reinfection than the level of pre-existing mucosal antibodies (Kimman et al., 1987).

The role of antibody in recovery from RSV

Studies in BALB/c mice depleted of B cells suggest that RSV-specific antibody is not required to terminate RSV replication in a primary infection (Graham et al., 1991a). However, as discussed previously, parenteral or topical administration of polyclonal or monoclonal antibodies to RSV-infected mice, cotton rats or primates can significantly reduce pulmonary RSV titres. Similarly, parenteral administration of RSV-IG or humanised anti-F mAb to infants hospitalised with RSV can reduce the level of nasopharyngeal RSV excretion, but has little or no effect on clinical outcome (Hemming et al., 1987; Rodriguez et al., 1997; Malley et al., 1998; Saez-Llorens et al., 2004). The finding that although prophylactic or therapeutic treatment of RSV-infected, immunosuppressed cotton rats with high titre anti-F neutralising mAb was highly effective in reducing pulmonary viral replication, multiple sequential therapeutic doses of the mAb were necessary to control rebound viral replication in continually suppressed animals, suggests that T cells are required to eliminate virus completely (Ottolini et al., 1999). However, similar studies with a high titre anti-F neutralising mAb in nude (nu^+/nu^+) and SCID/beige mice indicated that mAb treatment can effectively eliminate RSV from the lungs (Taylor, 1994 and unpublished observations).

Although these studies demonstrate that neutralising antibodies can mediate recovery from RSV infection, the relatively slow kinetics and poor quality of the primary antibody response suggest that the contribution of antibody to virus clearance in a primary RSV infection may be minimal. Nevertheless, the development of RSV-specific IgA in nasal secretions appears to correlate with the elimination of virus from the nasopharynx (McIntosh et al., 1978).

In summary, antibody is an important mediator of protection against primary infection and reinfection, however protection is incomplete and of short duration. Local immunity appears to be important in protecting the URT, while high levels of serum antibodies play a major role in resistance to RSV infection in the LRT.

Role of T cells in recovery from and resistance to RSV infection

T-cell responses to RSV

Following HRSV infection of BALB/c mice, the early pulmonary NK cell response is followed by an influx of $CD4^+$ and $CD8^+$ T cells (Hussell et al., 1996). $CD8^+$ T cells predominate in the lungs at about day 10 post-infection and virus clearance is temporally associated with an increase in RSV-specific $CD8^+$ CTL activity in the lungs (Taylor et al., 1985; Anderson et al., 1990). Similarly, an increase in the proportion of $CD8^+$ T cells in the respiratory tract of BRSV antibody-negative calves, 10 days after BRSV infection (McInnes et al., 1999), correlated with BRSV-specific CTL activity in the lungs (Gaddum et al., 1996a). Although primary BRSV-specific CTLs could be detected in the lungs of all BRSV-infected calves, primary BRSV-CTLs could only be detected in the peripheral blood of 50–60% of calves.

Following restimulation with RSV, *in vitro*, RSV-specific CTLs could be detected in the peripheral blood of approximately 35% of infants less than 5 months of age within 1 week after the infection and in more than 65% infants, 6–24 months of age (Chiba et al., 1989). The lower proportion of younger infants responding with a virus-specific CTL response could be related either to immunological immaturity, a Th2 environment in the lungs during primary infection and/or to a suppressive effect of maternal antibody. Mice vaccinated with rVV expressing the M2 protein together with IL-4 developed lower levels of M2-specific primary CTL activity and diminished RSV-specific memory CTLs than those infected with rVVM2 (Aung et al., 1999). Similarly, studies using recombinant (r)RSV expressing IL-4 demonstrated that the induction of a strong Th2 environment during primary pulmonary immunisation with live RSV resulted in early inflammation and a largely non-functional primary CTL response (Bukreyev et al., 2005). However, in contrast to mice vaccinated with rVVM2/IL-4, the secondary CTL response in mice infected with rRSV/IL-4 was at least as great as that in mice infected with wild-type

RSV. Systemic overproduction of IL-4 by transgenic mice was also associated suppression of the pulmonary CTL response and in these animals there was delayed clearance of RSV infection (Fischer et al., 1997). The suppressive effects of passive antibody on CTL priming following RSV infection have also been demonstrated in mice (Bangham, 1986). Alternatively, the failure to detect CTL activity in peripheral blood of all RSV-infected individuals may be related to redistribution from the circulation towards the lungs (De Weerd et al., 1998). The high proportion of RSV-specific memory CTLs detected in the peripheral blood of infants aged 6–24 months, contrasts with the finding that RSV-specific memory CTLs could only be detected in approximately 25% of healthy adults (Isaacs et al., 1990). However, following experimental RSV challenge, 70% of previously healthy adults developed a CTL response to RSV. In a study of RSV-infected infants and their mothers over 3 epidemic seasons, RSV-specific memory CTLs could be detected in 80% of mothers and in a similar proportion of infants during or after their first RSV season (Mbawuike et al., 2001).

The pulmonary $CD4^+$ T-cell response to primary RSV infection in BALB/c mice or to BRSV infection in BRSV antibody-negative calves is less marked than that of $CD8^+$ T cells (Hussell et al., 1996; McInnes et al., 1999). Nevertheless, an increase in activated $CD4^+$ T cells, predominantly producing Th1 cytokines such as IFNγ, can be detected in the lungs of mice from day 4 to 10 post-infection (Hussell et al., 1996). The $CD4^+$ T cell bias in infants with RSV infection is unclear, with some studies demonstrating a Th2 cytokine bias (Roman et al., 1997; Bendelja et al., 2000; Legg et al., 2003), others a predominant Th1 cytokine response (Bont et al., 1999; Brandenburg et al., 2000b) and others a mixed response (Tripp et al., 2002; de Waal et al., 2003). The reasons for these discrepancies may be related to differences in the tissues sampled and differences in the assays used.

Role of T cells in recovery from RSV infection

Although antibody is important in resistance to reinfection, T-cell-mediated immune responses are probably of greater importance in virus clearance. RSV infection of immunocompromised patients, of any age, is prolonged, often severe and can be fatal (Fishaut et al., 1980; Milner et al., 1985; Hall et al., 1986). Immunocompromised individuals can shed virus for several months, compared with the typical period of 3 weeks in young infants (Fishaut et al., 1980; Hall et al., 1986). Prolonged virus shedding has also been demonstrated in athymic (nu/nu) BALB/c mice, immunodeficient irradiated BALB/c mice (Cannon et al., 1987) and in mice depleted of both $CD4^+$ and $CD8^+$ T cells (Graham et al., 1991b). Although depletion of $CD4^+$ or $CD8^+$ T cells resulted in slightly increased RSV titres in the lung at day 7 post-infection, virus was cleared from both the nose and lungs by day 11. However, depletion of both $CD4^+$ and $CD8^+$ T cells resulted in prolonged virus excretion from both the nose and lungs for at least 28 days. Despite prolonged virus excretion in mice depleted of both T-cell subsets, signs of clinical illness and pulmonary histological changes were minimal (Graham et al., 1991b). These findings indicate that the T-cell response is the primary cause of RSV disease in the mouse and contrasts with the severe and often fatal RSV infection seen in immunosuppressed humans. Studies in calves depleted of T-cell subsets showed that whereas depletion of $CD4^+$ or γ/δ^+ T cells had little effect on RSV infection, depletion of $CD8^+$ T cells resulted in delayed clearance from both the nasopharynx and lungs (Taylor et al., 1995). Furthermore, the prolonged virus excretion was associated with increased pneumonic lesions (Taylor et al., 1995; Thomas et al., 1996). Thus, the T-cell response appears to play a more important role in the pathogenesis of RSV-induced disease in the mouse than in the natural host.

Role of T cells in protection against RSV infection

The role of RSV-specific memory $CD8^+$ T cells in resistance to reinfection is not clear. Priming of BALB/c mice by simultaneous intranasal and intraperitoneal inoculation with rVVM2 demonstrated that pulmonary resistance to RSV challenge was significantly greater 9 days after immunisation than at 28 days and was mediated predominantly by $CD8^+$ T cells (Connors et al., 1991, 1992b). In these mice, the peak of pulmonary CTL activity correlated with the peak of resistance to RSV replication, and there was little resistance or accelerated clearance of virus at 45 days after immunisation (Kulkarni et al., 1993a). These findings indicate that resistance to RSV induced by immunisation with rVVM2, 9 days previously, was mediated predominantly by primary pulmonary CTLs and suggest that RSV-specific memory $CD8^+$ T cells are not very effective against pulmonary RSV replication, at least in mice.

There is evidence from the BALB/c mouse model of RSV infection that $CD8^+$ T cells are partially functionally inactivated in the RSV-infected respiratory tract (Chang et al., 2001; Chang and Braciale, 2002). Thus, only 50% of viral antigen-specific $CD8^+$ T cells, as determined by MHC class I tetramer staining, isolated from the lung at the peak of the response, secreted IFNγ. In contrast, RSV-specific effector $CD8^+$ T cells in draining lymph nodes or spleen had no deficit in effector function. Furthermore, there was a rapid decrease in the frequency of RSV-specific memory $CD8^+$ T cells in the lungs during the resolution of infection. These observations may help to explain the limited duration of immunity to RSV infection. The mechanisms by which $CD8^+$ T-cell effector function is impaired are not known. However, functional inactivation has also been described for other paramyxoviruses, such as SV5 (Gray et al., 2005) and pneumonia virus of mice (PVM) (Claassen et al., 2005), but is not seen with influenza virus (Chang and Braciale, 2002), suggesting that functional dysregulation is mediated by a property of the virus rather than an effect of the lung environment. One possibility that could explain the loss of IFNγ production by virus antigen-specific $CD8^+$ T cells in the lung is a switch to a Tc2 phenotype, with production of Th2 cytokines. However, Th2 cytokine producing $CD8^+$ T cells were not detected in the lungs of mice infected with SV5 (Gray et al., 2005). The altered effector activity of RSV-specific pulmonary $CD8^+$ T cells appears to be associated with a defect in T-cell antigen receptor signalling and both effector activity and memory $CD8^+$ T cell development could be improved by IL-2 expression in the lungs during RSV infection (Chang et al., 2004).

Studies of RSV-specific $CD8^+$ T cells in adults have demonstrated that the frequency of these cells is higher in the lungs than in the peripheral blood (de Bree et al., 2005). These resident pulmonary RSV-specific $CD8^+$ T cells are characterised by a relatively late differentiation, non-cytotoxic, long-lived memory phenotype, reflected by low levels of expression of CD28, CD27 and ganzyme B and high levels of IL-7Rα expression. Influenza virus-specific human lung $CD8^+$ T cells are able to expand readily upon reexposure to virus antigen *in vitro* (de Bree et al., 2005) and studies in mice indicate that defence against a secondary pulmonary 'flu infection is achieved mainly by reactivation of local 'flu-specific $CD8^+$ T cells, and to a lesser extent by recruitment of circulating virus-specific cells (Hogan et al., 2001). These observations suggest that the resident RSV-specific $CD8^+$ T cells may be able to provide immediate immunological protection against pulmonary virus infection. However, studies in BALB/c mice indicate that although RSV-specific memory $CD8^+$ T cells persist in the lungs for at least 50 days after an RSV infection, amplification of RSV-specific memory $CD8^+$ T cells following reinfection occurs preferentially in the draining lymph node (Ostler et al., 2001). Following activation in the draining lymph nodes, the T cells immediately migrate from the node to the site of RSV infection in the respiratory tract.

Although an RSV-specific CTL response did not appear to protect healthy adults against an experimental RSV infection or influence the duration of virus shedding, individuals that mounted a CTL response tended to have lower symptom scores that non-responders (Isaacs et al., 1990). Similarly, infants that developed an RSV-specific CTL response in the first year of life were less likely to have RSV LRT disease in the second year (Mbawuike et al., 2001). In addition, the numbers of RSV-specific IFNγ producing cells in peripheral blood from elderly healthy volunteers are significantly less than those in younger adults (Looney et al., 2002). These observations suggest that the increased morbidity observed with RSV infection in the elderly may be associated with a defect in the T-cell response to RSV. Taken together, these observations indicate a role for RSV-specific memory T cells in limiting reinfection with RSV in man. The effectiveness of RSV-specific memory T cells in protecting against reinfection with RSV may be dependent upon the speed of the secondary T-cell response in relation to the course of RSV infection.

Role of the immune response in the pathogenesis of RSV infection

RSV replicates primarily in the superficial layers of the respiratory epithelium and induces bronchiolitis and pneumonia (Aherne et al., 1970; Neilson and Yunis, 1990). The pathology of RSV in infants is similar to that of BRSV in young calves and is characterised by proliferation, necrosis and desquamation of ciliated epithelial cells accompanied by a peribronchioloar accumulation of lymphocytes and a bronchial exudate composed of mucus, desquamated epithelia cells, neutrophils, lymphocytes and macrophages (Bryson et al., 1983; Thomas et al., 1984; Viuff et al., 1996). Chapter 5 of this volume reviews the current knowledge of RSV pathogenesis in children.

RSV also replicates in type II epithelial cells and induces thickening of the alveolar wall with infiltration by macrophages and neutrophils. Direct virus-mediated cytopathology was thought to be an important component of the pathogenesis of RSV infection. However, there is little or no cytopathology following infection of differentiated, ciliated human airway epithelial cells with HRSV, *in vitro* (Zhang et al., 2002) or following infection of differentiated bovine airway epithelial cells with BRSV, *in vitro* (unpublished observations), suggesting that the host response to virus infection plays a major role in RSV pathogenesis.

Severe RSV infection in the first 6 months of life is often associated with an increased risk of wheezing, up to the age of 11 to 13 years (Sims et al., 1978; Pullan and Hey, 1982; Stein et al., 1999; Silvestri et al., 2004). Although the mechanisms responsible for this effect are not known, administration of RSV-IG to children at high risk of RSV disease improved asthmas scores and reduced atopy (Wenzel et al., 2002), suggesting that RSV-bronchiolitis leads to long-term changes to the lung that cause recurrent wheezing episodes. The mechanisms that mediate these effects are not clear and will not be discussed further in this chapter.

As mentioned previously, since severe disease occurs in immunosuppressed individuals, the adaptive immune response may not be a major component of RSV disease in man. Severe pulmonary pathology is also observed in RSV-infected, immunosuppressed cotton rats (Wong et al., 1985) and is enhanced in BRSV-infected calves depleted of $CD8^+$ T cells (Taylor et al., 1995; Thomas et al., 1996). The inflammatory response initiated by RSV infection of epithelial cells may be the main mediator of RSV pathology, and the granulocytes recruited to RSV-infected airways may be responsible for the destruction of virus-infected cells. In contrast, illness and pulmonary pathology in the mouse model of RSV infection is mediated predominantly by the adaptive T-cell response (Graham et al., 1991b). Although there are limitations to the mouse model of RSV infection, the mouse has nevertheless, been of value in investigating the types of immune responses that may contribute to the pathogenesis of RSV infection.

Role of T cells in the pathogenesis of RSV infection in the mouse

A major role for T cells in the pathogenesis of RSV infection in BALB/c mice has been demonstrated by analysis of the T-cell response in mice vaccinated with rVV expressing individual RSV proteins and from studies on T-cell depletion and T-cell transfer. RSV-infected BALB/c mice depleted of either $CD4^+$ or $CD8^+$ T cells have decreased weight loss and illness scores compared with control mice and mice depleted of both T-cell subsets have no weight loss or detectable illness, despite persistent virus replication (Graham et al., 1991b).

The adoptive transfer of $CD4^+$ Th2 cell lines from mice primed with RSV or the G protein to RSV-infected mice reduced pulmonary virus titres, but led to severe disease, characterized by pulmonary neutrophil recruitment, intense pulmonary eosinophilia and lung haemorrhage, which was often fatal (Alwan et al., 1992, 1994). Similarly, RSV-specific $CD8^+$ T-cell lines or clones reduced virus titres but produced augmented, and sometimes fatal, acute respiratory disease (Cannon et al., 1988; Alwan et al., 1994), whereas T-cell lines, composed of both $CD4^+$ Th1 and $CD8^+$ T cells, reduced virus titres and produced less severe augmented pathology than that induced by RSV-specific CTL or Th2 cell lines (Alwan et al., 1994). These observations suggest that in the mouse model of RSV infection, T-cell mediated illness is the price paid for virus clearance and augmented pulmonary pathology is mediated by an over-exuberant T-cell response.

The molecular mechanisms involved in $CD8^+$ T-cell-mediated virus control and immunopathology are unclear. However, virus control and immunopathology proceeded unimpaired in RSV-infected mice inoculated with M2-specific $CD8^+$ T cells lacking either perforin, the CD95 ligand (TNF receptor) or TNF (Ostler et al., 2002). In contrast, virus control was largely abolished and pathology was significantly reduced by depletion of IFNγ or inoculation of $CD8^+$ T cells from IFNγ-deficient mice. These studies demonstrate that IFNγ is the key mediator of virus clearance and of virus-induced immunopathology in the mouse.

Studies in BALB/c mice scarified with rVV expressing either the F, G or M2 protein demonstrated that the different patterns of T-cell priming induced in these mice resulted in different patterns of pulmonary pathology following RSV challenge (Openshaw et al., 1988; Openshaw et al., 1992; Alwan and Openshaw, 1993). Thus, following challenge with RSV, mice vaccinated with rVVM2, which primes $CD8^+$ T cells, or with rVVF, which primes $CD8^+$ T cells and a Th1-biased $CD4^+$ T-cell response, developed a pulmonary inflammatory response that was composed of lymphocytes and neutrophils. In contrast, the pulmonary inflammatory response in mice primed with rVVG, which neither induces nor is recognised by $CD8^+$ T cells but induces a more Th2-biased $CD4^+$ T-cell response, was characterised by lymphocytes and eosinophils. The influence of rVV expressing different RSV proteins and the route of vaccination on T-cell priming and immunopathology in BALB/c mice, following RSV infection is illustrated in Fig. 1.

Although virus clearance and immunopathology induced by RSV-specific $CD8^+$ T cells are mediated by IFNγ, virus-specific $CD8^+$ T cell secretion of IFNγ plays an important role in regulating the differentiation and activation of Th2 $CD4^+$ T cells. Thus, the severity of pulmonary eosinophilia in RSV-infected mice receiving G-specific Th2 cells could be reduced by co-transfer of M2-specific $CD8^+$ T cells (Alwan et al., 1994). Induction of a CTL response by vaccination with rVVG together with rVVM2 or rVV expressing the G protein in which the $CD8^+$ T-cell epitope from the M2 protein was inserted, suppressed the recruitment of eosinophils to the lung following RSV challenge (Srikiatkhachorn and Braciale, 1997). Furthermore, depletion of $CD8^+$ T cells or IFNγ in mice vaccinated with rVVF, in strains of mice normally resistant to eosinophil induction by rVVG, or in mice undergoing a primary RSV infection, resulted in pulmonary eosinophilia (Hussell et al., 1997; Srikiatkhachorn and Braciale, 1997). These observations

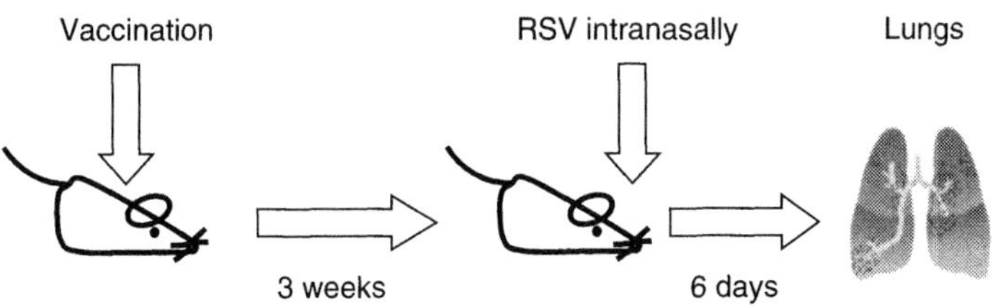

Vaccine	Route	Pulmonary inflammation		Ab	T-cell priming	Cytokines	
		PMN	Eosinophil			IFNγ	IL-5
rVV-M2	Scar.	+++	-	-	CD8	++++	-
rVV-F	Scar.	+++	-	+	CD8 + CD4	++++	-
rVV-G	Scar.	++	++	+	CD4	++	++
rVV-Gm	Scar.	+++	+	+	CD4	+++	+
rVV-Gs	Scar.	++	+++	-/+	CD4	+	+++
rVV-Fs	Scar.	++	+/-	+	CD8 + CD4	+++	++++
rVV-G	i.p.	+++	-	+	CD4	++++	+/-

Fig. 1 Influence of recombinant vaccinia viruses expressing different RSV proteins and the route of vaccination on T-cell priming and immunopathology in BALB/c mice, following RSV infection. Vaccination of mice either by scarification (scar.) or the intraperitoneal (i.p.) route with recombinant vaccinia virus (rVV) expressing the M2, F, G, membrane-anchored form of G (Gm), secreted form of G (Gs) or a secreted form of the F (Fs) protein primes either $CD8^+$, $CD4^+$ or $CD8^+$ and $CD4^+$ T cells, an antibody (Ab) response and either a more Th1- or Th2-biased cytokine response. A more biased Th2-cytokine response and/or lack of $CD8^+$ T-cell priming resulted in a pulmonary inflammatory response characterised by eosinophils following RSV challenge.

suggest that virus-specific $CD8^+$ T-cell secretion of IFNγ downregulates Th2-cytokine secretion and pulmonary eosinophilia and suggest that the balance of the T-cell response determines the outcome of RSV infection. Priming of a poor RSV-specific $CD8^+$ T-cell response in infants could contribute to a Th2-biased response and severe disease.

The different pattern of $CD4^+$ T-cell priming in BALB/c mice by rVV expressing the F or G protein may be related, at least in part, to the form of the antigen. The G protein is synthesised as two forms, a membrane-anchored form and a secreted form (Hendricks et al., 1988; Roberts et al., 1994). Priming of BALB/c mice with rVV expressing only the secreted form of the G protein (Gs) induced a more biased Th2 response and enhanced numbers of pulmonary eosinophils following RSV challenge than rVV expressing either wild-type G or membrane-anchored G (Gm) (Bembridge et al., 1998; Johnson et al., 1998). Furthermore, vaccination of mice with rVV expressing an F protein that had been engineered to be secreted (rVVFs) was associated with a shift to a more biased Th2 response. However, the extent of eosinophil recruitment in rVVFs-vaccinated mice was not as great as that in mice vaccinated with rVVG, probably because RSV-specific CTLs able to downregulate Th2-driven pathology, were still induced by rVVFs, but are not induced by rVVG (Bembridge et al., 1999) (Fig. 1).

Another possible mechanism for the differential T-cell priming by the F and G proteins is that certain MHC-peptide–ligand complexes preferentially induce a Th1 or Th2 response (Murray, 1998). Using rVV expressing frame-shift mutants of the G protein, a region corresponding to G protein residues 193–203 was shown to be responsible for induction of pulmonary eosinophilia in BALB/c mice (Sparer et al., 1998). Other studies demonstrated that immunisation of BALB/c mice with a peptide corresponding to G protein residues 184 to 198, which overlaps with the region identified by Sparer and colleagues, induced pulmonary eosinophilia following RSV challenge (Tebbey et al., 1998). Taken together these findings suggested the presence of a Th2 epitope in the G protein. However, both Th1 and Th2 $CD4^+$ T cells recognise the immunodominant region of the G protein, which encompasses the region 183 to 197 (Varga et al., 2000). Furthermore, induction of Th1 and Th2 responses by the G protein is epitope and MHC independent (Srikiatkhachorn et al., 1999; Hancock et al., 2003b). $CD4^+$ T cells recognising this immunodminant epitope are oligclonal and predominantly express Vβ14 TCR (Varga et al., 2000) and depletion of these cells *in vivo* significantly reduces pulmonary eosinophilia following RSV challenge of rVVG-vaccinated mice (Varga et al., 2000).

The demonstration of an oligoclonal T-cell response capable of eliciting both Th1 and Th2 effector cells and mediating pulmonary eosinophilia suggests that the environment in which the T cells are primed determines the balance of the effector T-cell response to the G protein. This suggestion is supported by the observations that priming for pulmonary eosinophilia is influenced by the route of vaccination. Thus, whereas administration of rVVG by the intradermal route primes for an eosinophil response, administration by either the intraperitoneal (i.p.) or intranasal (i.n.) route does not (Bembridge et al., 1998; Mackay, 2001). Following RSV challenge of intradermally vaccinated mice, the pulmonary cytokine response was characterised by high levels of IL-5 and IFNγ. In contrast, levels of IL-5 produced by pulmonary lymphocytes from mice vaccinated by either the i.p. or i.n. routes were significantly reduced while IFNγ levels remained elevated (Mackay, 2001) (Fig. 1).

The ability of the G protein to prime a Th2 response and sensitise for pulmonary eosinophilia following RSV challenge is not unique among RSV proteins. Thus, immunisation of mice with purified F or G protein formulated with alum adjuvant primes a Th2 response and pulmonary eosinophilia following RSV challenge (Hancock et al., 1995, 1996). However, whereas this Th2-biased response can be modulated to a more balanced T-cell response by formulation of the F protein with QS-21 as adjuvant, recruitment of eosinophils to the lungs is enhanced following RSV challenge of mice vaccinated with G and QS-21 (Hancock et al., 1996). These observations support the suggestion that there are intrinsic differences in the

F and G proteins that are responsible for differential T-cell priming. Analysis of the ability of a variety of adjuvants to modulate the polarised Th2 response induced by purified G protein demonstrated that adjuvants that are recognised by TLRs significantly diminished Th2 responses and reduced pulmonary eosinophilia in BALB/c mice (Hancock et al., 2003a). Thus, it is possible that induction of a Th2-biased response by the G protein may be related to the ability of the conserved cysteine-rich region to inhibit innate responses of monocytes to virus or LPS (Polack et al., 2005). These observations together with those demonstrating that the route of vaccination influences T-cell priming by the G protein suggest an important role for innate immune responses in influencing the pattern of subsequent T-cell priming and pulmonary pathology.

In summary, the priming of a Th2-biased response and pulmonary eosinophilia by the G protein in mice is dependent upon the form of the protein, with a soluble protein favouring a Th2 response; a failure of the G protein to prime $CD8^+$ T cells, which are able to downregulate Th2 responses and pulmonary eosinophilia; the route of immunisation, which suggests that the local innate response influences T-cell priming; and the genetic background of the mouse.

Augmented disease in recipients of an FI-RSV vaccine

In the 1960s, trials of a formalin-inactivated RSV (FI-RSV) vaccine were carried out in the United States in infants and children. Following natural exposure of infants less than 18 months of age to natural RSV infection, an increased frequency and severity of RSV infection, and a greater incidence of hospitalisation compared with infants vaccinated with FI-PIV-3 was observed (Chin et al., 1969; Fulginiti et al., 1969; Kapikian et al., 1969; Kim et al., 1969). RSV disease in the vaccinated infants was characterised by airway hyper responsiveness and the lung pathology in the two vaccinated infants that died was described as a peribronchiolar mononuclear cell infiltration with some excess of eosinophils (Kim et al., 1969). FI-RSV-vaccinated infants hospitalised with severe RSV infections also had increased numbers of eosinophils in the blood (Chin et al., 1969). However, a review of the lung sections in 2001 revealed that neutrophils and mononuclear cells were predominant and that eosinophils accounted for less than 2% of the pulmonary inflammatory response (Prince et al., 2001).

The immune mechanisms responsible for vaccine-augmented disease have been studied extensively in animal models of RSV infection. Vaccination with FI-RSV induces augmented pulmonary pathology following RSV challenge of BALB/c mice, cotton rats, calves and primates. The pulmonary pathology in FI-RSV-vaccinated BALB/c mice challenged with RSV is composed of monocytes, lymphocytes and large numbers (>30% of bronchoalveolar cells) of eosinophils (Graham et al., 1993b). Pulmonary eosinophilia is also a feature of vaccine-augmented disease in *rhesus macaques* (de Swart et al., 2002) and in FI-BRSV-vaccinated calves following experimental BRSV challenge (Antonis et al., 2003). Pulmonary eosinophilia was also associated with a natural outbreak of severe BRSV infection in calves vaccinated with a BRSV vaccine inactivated with β-propiolactone (Schreiber et al., 2000). During this natural BRSV outbreak, 30% of the vaccinated calves died compared with percentage of unvaccinated animals. In contrast, eosinophils were not a feature of enhanced pulmonary pathology in cotton rats (Prince et al., 2001), African green monkeys (Kakuk et al., 1993), bonnet monkeys (Ponnuraj et al., 2001) or in another study of vaccine-enhanced BRSV disease in calves (Gershwin et al., 1998). Caution must be exercised in the interpretation of some of these studies, since prior sensitisation to foetal calf serum (FCS) or other tissue culture components, present in the vaccine preparation and in the virus challenge, can lead to pulmonary eosinophilia in BALB/c mice (Boelen et al., 2000) or augmented pulmonary pathology (Ponnuraj, 2001; Ostler and Ehl, 2002).

Vaccine-augmented disease was also seen following measles virus (MV) infection of children vaccinated with a FI-MV vaccine (Fulginiti et al., 1967) and as mentioned above was seen in calves vaccinated with a *β*-propiolactone-inctivated BRSV vaccine (Schreiber et al., 2000). However, exacerbation of respiratory disease was not seen in infants or children vaccinated with FI-PIV3 (Fulginiti et al., 1969; Kim et al., 1969), suggesting that formalin-inactivation *per se* does not contribute to the development of vaccine-augmented disease for all viruses.

Role of virus-specific antibody in the pathogenesis of FI-RSV vaccine-augmented RSV disease

Children vaccinated with FI-RSV developed high titres of antibodies to the F, but not the G, protein of RSV. However, the level of neutralising antibodies was lower than that induced in children of a comparable age following a natural RSV infection (Murphy et al., 1986b), suggesting that the antibodies induced by vaccination with FI-RSV were poorly neutralising. Similarly, the neutralising antibody response in FI-RSV-vaccinated cotton rats was 1/30 of that in animals infected with RSV (Prince et al., 1986). It has been suggested that chemical inactivation may have disrupted critical epitopes on the F and/or G proteins, leading to the induction of high levels of non-neutralising antibodies, which failed to protect against RSV infection. Following RSV infection, these antibodies reacted with viral antigens in the lung leading to deposition of immune complexes and complement activation resulting in airway hyper-responsiveness and pneumonia. A role for immune complexes and complement activation in airway hyper-responsiveness has been demonstrated in mice and evidence of complement activation was detected in post-mortem lung sections from FI-RSV-vaccinated children with enhanced RSV disease (Polack et al., 2002) and in the lungs of cotton rats with vaccine-augmented pulmonary pathology (see Delgado and Polack, 2004). Activation of complement by immune complexes in the lungs could elicit bronchoconstriction, mucus secretion, attract polymorphonuclear leukocytes, promote T-cell activation and affect the level of pro-inflammatory cytokines.

FI-MV also elicited non-protective antibodies, which were of low avidity, and immune complexes were detected in affected tissues (lungs and skin) from vaccinated children with atypical measles (Polack et al., 1999, 2003). In contrast, the observations that enhanced pulmonary pathology was not seen following RSV challenge of cotton rats passively immunised with sera from FI-RSV vaccinated animals (Connors et al., 1992a), or in mice or calves passively immunised with non-protective mAbs (Taylor et al., 1984; Thomas et al., 1998), suggest that antibodies do not play a role in vaccine-augmented disease. However, airway hyper-responsiveness, which was not analysed in the studies of passively immunised animals, is not associated with the extent of the pulmonary inflammatory response. Thus, complement or antibody-deficient mice had a similar pulmonary inflammatory response as wild-type mice, but had significantly different airway responses (Polack et al., 2002).

The exaggerated response to RSV infection in FI-RSV recipients could also have arisen as a result of antibody-mediated enhancement of virus replication. The relative ease with which RSV was recovered from vaccinated infants who developed RSV disease compared with infants vaccinated with FI-PIV3, suggests that these children may have been shedding more virus (Chin et al., 1969). Higher titres of RSV were detected in the lungs of bonnet monkeys immunised with FI-RSV than in those undergoing a primary infection (Ponnuraj et al., 2001) and antibody-dependent enhancement of RSV replication in a macrophage cell line was observed with sera from these monkeys, but not in sera from animals undergoing a primary RSV infection (Ponnuraj et al., 2003). These observations suggest that non-neutralising antibodies enhance the uptake and replication of virus in monocytes, which are known to be permissive for RSV replication. Human polyclonal sera and mouse monoclonal antibodies have also been shown to enhance replication of RSV by human monocytes or macrophage cell lines, *in vitro* (Gimenez et al., 1989; Krilov et al., 1989; Osiowy et al., 1994; Gimenez et al., 1996).

Role of T cells in the pathogenesis of FI-RSV vaccine-augmented disease

A detailed analysis of the immune response induced in BALB/c mice vaccinated with FI-RSV suggests that the enhanced disease is related to a Th2-biased response, typified by recruitment of eosinophils to the lungs. Thus, mice immunised with FI-RSV had an increased number of granulocytes, eosinophils and $CD4^+$ T cells in the lungs following RSV challenge, but a decreased number of $CD8^+$ T cells, compared with control animals (Waris et al., 1996). This lung pathology was completely abrogated by depletion of $CD4^+$ T cells (Connors et al., 1992c) or by treatment with mAbs to IL-4 and IL-10 (Connors et al., 1994), suggesting a role for $CD4^+$ Th2 cells in the pathogenesis of FI-RSV-augmented disease. Whereas live RSV infection primes mice for a Th1 response, $CD4^+$ T cells primed by FI-RSV showed a predominantly Th2 cytokine profile (Graham et al., 1993b; Waris et al., 1996).

Studies from a number of laboratories have demonstrated a similar pattern of Th2 cytokine production and pulmonary eosinophilia in mice vaccinated with rVVG and challenged with RSV, or in recipients of G-specific $CD4^+$ T cells (see above). This has led to the suggestion that the G protein component of FI-RSV is responsible for the enhanced pulmonary inflammatory response. However, the cytokine requirements for pulmonary eosinophilia induced by vaccination with rVVG differ from that induced by FI-RSV. Thus, IL-4 expression predominates in vaccine-enhanced disease in mice immunised with FI-RSV and pulmonary pathology and disease is reduced by inhibition of either IL-4 or IL-13 (Tang and Graham, 1994; Johnson and Graham, 1999; Johnson et al., 2003). In contrast, pulmonary eosinophilia and disease in mice vaccinated with rVVG is only reduced when both IL-4 and IL-13 are blocked (Johnson et al., 2003). In addition, whereas some aspects of priming for a Th2 response and pulmonary eosinophilia by rVVG appear to be genetically restricted (Hussell et al., 1998; Srikiatkhachorn et al., 1999), FI-RSV vaccine-enhanced disease does not appear to be dependent upon a specific genetic background. Thus, vaccine-enhanced disease was observed in 80% of recipients of the FI-RSV vaccine (Kapikian et al., 1969; Kim et al., 1969) and can be induced in a variety of animal models. Furthermore, studies in mice vaccinated with preparations of FI-RSV containing deletions in either the entire G protein or the immunodominant region (187–197) of the G protein demonstrated that the G protein is not necessary for vaccine-enhanced disease (Polack et al., 2002; Johnson and Graham, 2004). These findings contrast with other studies which used FI preparations of RSV that either lacked both the G and SH proteins, lacked just the G protein or expressed a mutant form of the G protein containing a point mutation that disrupts the CXC3 motif of the G protein, to vaccinate mice. These latter studies suggested an important role for the G protein in Th2 priming and vaccine-augmented pulmonary pathology (Tripp et al., 1999; Haynes et al., 2003). The discrepancies between these studies may be explained, in part, by the use of challenge viruses that differ in their ability to replicate, *in vivo*, and by differences in the time after challenge when the pulmonary inflammatory response was analysed (see Johnson and Graham, 2004). Subsequent studies have demonstrated that the T-cell repertoire mediating vaccine-enhanced disease induced by rVVG and FI-RSV is different. Thus, whereas the $CD4^+$ T cells from BALB/c mice immunised with rVVG respond to a single G peptide (aa 183–195) and predominantly express Vβ14 TCR, $CD4^+$ T cells from FI-RSV-immunised mice did not respond to this G peptide and expressed a divers array of Vβ chains (Johnson et al., 2004). Furthermore, deletion of $V\beta14^+$ T cells prior to RSV challenge reduced pulmonary eosinophilia and Th2 cytokine production in rVVG-immunised mice but not in FI-RSV-immunised mice (Varga et al., 2001; Johnson et al., 2004), further supporting the suggestion that immune responses induced by the G protein are not the basis for FI-RSV vaccine-enhanced disease.

It is likely that a number of different factors contributed to the lack of protection and augmented respiratory disease in recipients of the FI-RSV vaccine. Since the vaccine was administered parenterally, it probably failed to induce an appreciable level of mucosal immunity. In addition, it appears that the serum antibody response was poorly neutralising. Therefore, in the absence of either a mucosal or systemic neutralising antibody response, the vaccinees were susceptible to RSV infection. There would have been little or no priming of RSV-specific $CD8^+$ T cells by inactivated virus. Nevertheless, vaccination appears to have primed $CD4^+$ T cells as there was a greater RSV-specific T-cell proliferative response in vaccinees after RSV infection than that observed after a natural infection (Kim et al., 1976). Since FI-RSV was administered in alum, which is known to bias the immune response towards Th2, it is likely that extensive virus replication occurred in individuals with primed Th2 cells. The activation of Th2 cells by replicating virus would have resulted in an inflammatory response possibly composed of increased numbers of eosinophils. However, analysis of lung sections from FI-RSV vaccines suggests that eosinophils were not a major contributor to pulmonary pathology (Prince et al., 2001). The reaction of replicating virus with the poorly neutralising antibodies, may not only have enhanced virus replication, but may also have resulted in deposition of immune complexes, activation of complement and induction of airway hyper-responsiveness, which together with a Th2-mediated inflammatory response resulted in severe disease.

Conclusions

Many components of the innate immune system are activated following RSV infection and these not only contribute to the pulmonary inflammatory response but also instruct the development of antigen-specific acquired immunity by influencing DC maturation, the expansion and activation of NK cells, the differentiation, survival and function of T cells and the immunoglobulin isotype of the antibody response. The relatively poor immune response of infants to RSV, which is a significant obstacle to successful vaccination, may be due to a variety of factors such as the inhibitory effects of maternal antibodies, a defect in the ability of young infants to somatically hypermutate their antibody genes and generate high affinity neutralising antibodies and/or to immature T cell responses. Other contributory factors to the poor duration of immunity to RSV may be related to the limited tissue tropism of RSV infection, the reduced capacity of RSV-infected DCs to activate naïve T cells and to antigenic variability in the G protein. Neutralising serum antibodies are an important mediator of protection against LRT disease, whereas mucosal IgA responses, particularly to the G protein, may be important in mediating protection against RSV infection in the URT. Studies in calves infected with BRSV demonstrated that $CD8^+$ T cells play a crucial role in the elimination of virus from both the upper and lower airways and studies from mice suggest that $CD4^+$ T cells may also contribute to virus clearance. However, small animal models of RSV infection have demonstrated that T cells can also contribute to the severity of vaccine-augmented disease and that the balance of the T-cell response is important in determining the outcome of RSV infection. Nevertheless it remains unclear if severe LRT disease during primary RSV infection in infants is mediated by damage induced by the virus itself, as a consequence of an inadequate immune response, or to T-cell mediated pathology. Certainly, the severe disease seen in immunocompromised individuals and the possible association between a poor T-cell response in the elderly and more severe RSV disease in this age group support the former suggestion. Further exploration of the factors that influence the induction and effector function of RSV-specific T cells within the respiratory tract and that influence the induction, duration and specificity of the mucosal IgA response will be critical for the development of safe and effective vaccines against this important pathogen.

References

Aherne W, Bird T, Court SD, Gardner PS, McQuillin J. Pathological changes in virus infections of the lower respiratory tract in children. J Clin Pathol 1970; 231: 7.

Alexopoulou L, Holt AC, Medzhitov R, Flavell RA. Recognition of double-stranded RNA and activation of NF-kappaB by Toll-like receptor 3. Nature 2001; 4136857: 732.

Alwan WH, Kozlowski WJ, Openshaw PJM. Distinct types of lung disease caused by functional subsets of antiviral T cells. J Exp Med 1994; 179: 81.

Alwan WH, Openshaw PJM. Distinct patterns of T- and B-cell immunity to respiratory syncytial virus induced by individual viral proteins. Vaccine 1993; 11: 431.

Alwan WH, Record FM, Openshaw PJ. Phenotypic and functional characterization of T cell lines specific for individual respiratory syncytial virus proteins. J. Immunol 1993; 15012: 5211.

Alwan WH, Record FM, Openshaw PJM. $CD4^+$ T-cells clear virus but augment disease in mice infected with respiratory syncytial virus. Comparison with the effects of $CD8^+$ T-cells. Clin Exp Immunol 1992; 88: 527.

Anderson JJ, Norden J, Saunders D, Toms GL, Scott R. Analysis of the local and systemic immune responses induced in BALB/c mice by experimental respiratory syncytial virus infection. J Gen Virol 1990; 71: 1561.

Anderson JJ, Serin M, Harrop J, Amin S, Toms GL, Scott R. Natural killer cell response to respiratory syncytial virus in the Balb/c mouse model. Adv Exp Med Biol 1989; 257: 211.

Antonis AF, Schrijver RS, Daus F, Steverink PJ, Stockhofe N, Hensen EJ, Langedijk JP, van der Most RG. Vaccine-induced immunopathology during bovine respiratory syncytial virus infection: exploring the parameters of pathogenesis. J Virol 2003; 7722: 12067.

Arbiza J, Taylor G, Lopez JA, Furze J, Wyld S, Whyte P, Stott EJ, Wertz G, Sullender W, Trudel M, et al. Characterization of two antigenic sites recognized by neutralizing monoclonal antibodies directed against the fusion glycoprotein of human respiratory syncytial virus. J Gen Virol 1992; 739: 2225.

Atreya PL, Kulkarni S. Respiratory syncytial virus strain A2 is resistant to the antiviral effects of type I interferons and human MxA. Virol 1999; 261: 227.

Aung S, Tang YW, Graham BS. Interleukin-4 diminishes CD8(+) respiratory syncytial virus-specific cytotoxic T-lymphocyte activity *in vivo*. J Virol 1999; 7311: 8944.

Bancroft GJ. The role of natural killer cells in innate resistance to infection. Curr Opin Immunol 1993; 54: 503.

Bangham CR, Openshaw PJ, Ball LA, King AM, Wertz GW, Askonas BA. Human and murine cytotoxic T cells specific to respiratory syncytial virus recognize the viral nucleoprotein (N), but not the major glycoprotein (G), expressed by vaccinia virus recombinants. J Immunol 1986; 13712: 3973.

Bangham CRM. Passively acquired antibodies to respiratory syncytial virus impair the secondary cytotoxic T cell response in the neonatal mouse. Immunology 1986; 59: 37.

Barr F, Pedigo H, Johnson TR, Shepherd VL. Surfactant protein-A enhances uptake of respiratory syncytial virus by monocytes and U937 macrophages. Am J Respir Cell Mol Biol 2000; 23: 586.

Bartz H, Buning-Pfaue F, Turkel O, Schauer U. Respiratory syncytial virus induces prostaglandin E2, IL-10 and IL-11 generation in antigen presenting cells. Clin Exp Immunol 2002; 1293: 438.

Bartz H, Turkel O, Hoffjan S, Rothoeft T, Gonschorek A, Schauer U. Respiratory syncytial virus decreases the capacity of myeloid dendritic cells to induce interferon-gamma in naive T cells. Immunology 2003; 1091: 49.

Beeler JA, Van Wyke Coelingh K. Neutralisation epitopes of the F glycoprotein of respiratory syncytial virus: effect of mutation upon fusion function. J Virol 1989; 63: 2941.

Belz GT, Smith CM, Kleinert L, Reading P, Brooks A, Shortman K, Carbone FR, Heath WR. Distinct migrating and nonmigrating dendritic cell populations are involved in MHC class I-restricted antigen presentation after lung infection with virus. Proc Natl Acad Sci USA 2004; 10123: 8670.

Bembridge GP, Garcia-Beato R, Lopez JA, Melero JA, Taylor G. Subcellular site of expression and route of vaccination influence pulmonary eosinophilia following respiratory syncytial virus challenge in BALB/c mice sensitized to the attachment G protein. J Immunol 1998; 161: 2473.

Bembridge GP, Lopez JA, Bustos R, Meleros JA, Cook R, Mason H, Taylor G. Priming with a secreted form of the fusion protein of respiratory syncytial virus (RSV) promotes interleukin-4 (IL-4) and IL-5 production but not pulmonary eosinophilia following RSV challenge. J Virol 1999; 7312: 10086.

Bendelac A, Rivera MN, Park SH, Roark JH. Mouse CD1-specific NK1 T cells: development, specificity, and function. Annu Rev Immunol 1997; 15: 535.

Bendelja K, Gagro A, Bace A, Lokar-Kolbas R, Krsulovic-Hresic V, Drazenovic V, Mlinaric-Galinovic G, Rabatic S. Predominant type-2 response in infants with respiratory syncytial virus (RSV) infection demonstrated by cytokine flow cytometry. Clin Exp Immunol 2000; 1212: 332.

Biron CA, Cousens LP, Ruzek MC, Su HC, Salazar-Mather TP. Early cytokine responses to viral infections and their roles in shaping endogenous cellular immunity. Adv Exp Med Biol 1998; 452: 143.

Biron CA, Nguyen KB, Pien GC, Cousens LP, Salazar-Mather TP. Natural killer cells in antiviral defense: function and regulation by innate cytokines. Ann Rev Immunol 1999; 17: 189.

Bitko V, Velazquez A, Yang L, Yang YC, Barik S. Transcriptional induction of multiple cytokines by human respiratory syncytial virus requires activation of NF-kappa B and is inhibited by sodium salicylate and aspirin. Virology 1997; 2322: 369.

Boelen A, Andeweg A, Kwakkel J, Lokhorst W, Bestebroer T, Dormans J, Kimman T. Both immunisation with a formalin-inactivated respiratory syncytial virus (RSV) vaccine and a mock antigen vaccine induce severe lung pathology and a Th2 cytokine profile in RSV-challenged mice. Vaccine 2000; 19: 982.

Bont L, Heijnen CJ, Kavelaars A, van Aalderen WM, Brus F, Draaisma JT, Geelen SM, van Vught HJ, Kimpen JL. Peripheral blood cytokine responses and disease severity in respiratory syncytial virus bronchiolitis. Eur Respir J 1999; 141: 144.

Bossert B, Marozin S, Conzelmann KK. Nonstructural proteins NS1 and NS2 of bovine respiratory syncytial virus block activation of interferon regulatory factor 3. J Virol 2003; 7716: 8661.

Brandenburg AH, de Waal L, Timmerman HH, Hoogerhout P, de Swart RL, Osterhaus AD. HLA class I-restricted cytotoxic T-cell epitopes of the respiratory syncytial virus fusion protein. J Virol 2000a; 7421: 10240.

Brandenburg AH, Kleinjan A, van Het Land B, Moll HA, Timmerman HH, de Swart RL, Neijens HJ, Fokkens W, Osterhaus AD. Type 1-like immune response is found in children with respiratory syncytial virus infection regardless of clinical severity. J Med Virol 2000b; 622: 267.

Brigl M, Bry L, Kent SC, Gumperz JE, Brenner MB. Mechanism of CD1d-restricted natural killer T cell activation during microbial infection. Nat Immunol 2003; 412: 1230.

Brinkmann V, Geiger T, Alkan S, Heusser CH. Interferon α increases the frequency of interferon γ-producing human CD4+ T cells. J Exp Med 1993; 178: 1655.

Bryson DG, McNulty MS, Logan EF, Cush PF. Respiratory syncytial virus pneumonia in young calves: clinical and pathologic findings. Am J Vet Res 1983; 44: 1648.

Bukreyev A, Belyakov IM, Prince GA, Yim KC, Harris KK, Berzofsky JA, Collins PL. Expression of interleukin-4 by recombinant respiratory syncytial virus is associated with accelerated inflammation and a nonfunctional cytotoxic T-lymphocyte response following primary infection but not following challenge with wild-type virus. J Virol 2005; 7915: 9515.

Calder LJ, Gonzalez-Reyes L, Garcia-Barreno B, Bharton SA, Skehel JJ, Wiley, DC, Melero JA. . Electron microscopy of the human respiratory syncytial virus fusion protein and complexes that it forms with monoclonal antibodies. Virology 2000; 2711: 122.

Cannon MJ, Openshaw PJM, Askonas BA. Cytotoxic T-cells clear virus but augment lung pathology in mice infected with respiratory syncytial virus. J Exp Med 1988; 168: 1163.

Cannon MJ, Stott EJ, Taylor G, Askonas BA. Clearance of persistent respiratory syncytial virus infections in immunodeficient mice following transfer of primed T cells. Immunology 1987; 621: 133.

Cella M, Jarrossay D, Facchetti F, Alebardi O, Nakajima H, Lanzavecchia A, Colonna M. Plasmacytoid monocytes migrate to inflamed lymph nodes and produce large amounts of type I interferon. Nat Med 1999; 58: 919.

Chang J, Braciale TJ. Respiratory syncytial virus infection suppresses lung $CD8^+$ T-cell effector activity and peripheral $CD8^+$ T-cell memory in the respiratory tract. Nat Med 2002; 8: 54.

Chang J, Choi SY, Jin HT, Sung YC, Braciale TJ. Improved effector activity and memory CD8 T cell development by IL-2 expression during experimental respiratory syncytial virus infection. J Immunol 2004; 1721: 503.

Chang J, Srikiatkhachorn A, Braciale TJ. Visualization and characterization of respiratory syncytial virus F-specific CD8+ T cells during experimental virus infection. J Immunol 2001; 167: 4254.

Cherrie AH, Anderson K, Wertz GW, Openshaw PJ. Human cytotoxic T cells stimulated by antigen on dendritic cells recognize the N, SH, F, M, 22K, and 1b proteins of respiratory syncytial virus. J Virol 1992; 664: 2102.

Chiba Y, Higashidate Y, Suga K, Honjo K, Tsutsumi H, Ogra PL. Development of cell-mediated immunity to respiratory syncytial virus in human infants following naturally acquired infection. J Med Virol 1989; 28: 133.

Chin J, Magoffin RL, Shearer LA, Schieble JH, Lennette EH. Field evaluation of a respiratory syncytial virus vaccine and a trivalent parainfluenza virus vaccine in a pediatric population. Am J Epidemiol 1969; 894: 449.

Claassen EA, van der Kant PA, Rychnavska ZS, van Bleek GM, Easton AJ, van der Most RG. Activation and inactivation of antiviral CD8 T cell responses during murine pneumovirus infection. J Immunol 2005; 17510: 6597.

Connors M, Collins PL, Firestone C-Y, Murphy BR. Respiratory syncytial virus (RSV) F, G, M2 (22K) and N proteins each induce resistance to RSV challenge, but resistance induced by the M2 and N proteins is short-lived. J Virol 1991; 65: 1634.

Connors M, Collins PL, Firestone CY, Sotnikov AV, Waitze A, Davis AR, Hung PP, Chanock RM, Murphy BR. Cotton rats previously immunized with a chimeric RSV FG glycoprotein develop enhanced pulmonary pathology when infected with RSV, a phenomenon not encountered following immunization with vaccinia-RSV recombinants or RSV. Vaccine 1992a; 10: 475.

Connors M, Giese NA, Kulkarni AB, Firestone CY, Morse HC, Murphy BR. Enhanced pulmonary histopathology induced by respiratory syncytial virus (RSV) challenge of formalin-inactivated RSV-immunized BALB/c mice is abrogated by depletion of interleukin-4 (IL-4) and IL-10. J Virol 1994; 688: 5321.

Connors M, Kulkarni AB, Collins PL, Firestone C-Y, Holmes KL, Morse III HC, Murphy BR. Resistance to respiratory syncytial virus (RSV) challenge induced by infection with a vaccinia virus recombinant expressing the RSV M2 protein is mediated by CD8+ T cells, while that induced by Vac-F or Vac-G recombinants is mediated by antibodies. J Virol 1992b; 66: 1277.

Connors M, Kulkarni AB, Firestone C-Y, Holmes KL, Morse III HC, Sotnkov AV, Murphy BR. Pulmonary histopathology induced by respiratory syncytial virus (RSV) challenge of formalin-inactivated RSV-immunused BALB/c mice is abrogated by depletion of CD4+ T-cells. J Virol 1992c; 66: 7444.

Cranage MP, Gardner PS, McIntosh K. *In vitro* cell-dependent lysis of respiratory syncytial virus-infected cells mediated by antibody from local respiratory secretions. Clin Exp Immunol 1981; 431: 28.

Crowe JE, Firestone C-Y, Crim R, Beeler JA, Coelingh KL, Barbas CF, Burton DR, Chanock RM, Murphy BR. Monoclonal antibody-resistant mutants selected with a respiratory syncytial virus-neutralizing human antibody Fab fragment (Fab 19) define a unique epitope on the fusion (F) glycoprotein. Virology 1998; 252: 373.

Crowe JE, Firestone C-Y, Murphy BR. Passively acquired antibodies suppress humoral but not cell-mediated immunity in mice immunized with live attenuated respiratory syncytial virus vaccines. J Immunol 2001; 167: 3910.

de Bree GJ, van Leeuwen EM, Out TA, Jansen HM, Jonkers RE, van Lier RA. Selective accumulation of differentiated CD8+ T cells specific for respiratory viruses in the human lung. J Exp Med 2005; 20210: 1433.

de Graaff PM, de Jong EC, van Capel TM, van Dijk ME, Roholl PJ, Boes J, Luytjes W, Kimpen JL, van Bleek GM. Respiratory syncytial virus infection of monocyte-derived dendritic cells decreases their capacity to activate CD4 T cells. J Immunol 2005; 1759: 5904.

de Graaff PM, Heidema J, Poelen MC, van Dijk ME, Lukens MV, van Gestel SP, Reinders J, Rozemuller E, Tilanus M, Hoogerhout P, van Els CA, van der Most RG, Kimpen JL, van Bleek GM. HLA-DP4 presents an immunodominant peptide from the RSV G protein to CD4 T cells. Virology 2004; 3262: 220.

de Jong EC, Smits HH, Kapsenberg ML. Dendritic cell-mediated T cell polarization. Springer Semin Immunopathol 2005; 263: 289.

de Swart RL, Kuiken T, Timmerman HH, van Amerongen G, Van Den Hoogen BG, Vos HW, Neijens HJ, Andeweg AC, Osterhaus AD. Immunization of macaques with formalin-inactivated respiratory syncytial virus (RSV) induces interleukin-13-associated hypersensitivity to subsequent RSV infection. J Virol 2002; 76: 11561.

de Waal L, Koopman LP, van Benten IJ, Brandenburg AH, Mulder PG, de Swart RL, Fokkens WJ, Neijens HJ, Osterhaus AD. Moderate local and systemic respiratory syncytial virus-specific T-cell responses upon mild or subclinical RSV infection. J Med Virol 2003; 702: 309.

de Waal L, Yuksel S, Brandenburg AH, Langedijk JP, Sintnicolaas K, Verjans GM, Osterhaus AD, de Swart RL. Identification of a common HLA-DP4-restricted T-cell epitope in the conserved region of the respiratory syncytial virus G protein. J Virol 2004; 784: 1775.

De Weerd W, Twilhaar WN, Kimpen JL. T cell subset analysis in peripheral blood of children with RSV bronchiolitis. Scand J Infect Dis 1998; 301: 77.

Delgado MF, Polack FP. Involvement of antibody, complement and cellular immunity in the pathogenesis of enhanced respiratory syncytial virus disease. Expert Rev Vaccines 2004; 36: 693.

Ehl S, Bischoff R, Ostler T, Vallbracht S, Schulte-Monting J, Poltorak A, Freudenberg M. The role of Toll-like receptor 4 versus interleukin-12 in immunity to respiratory syncytial virus. Eur J Immunol 2004; 344: 1146.

Falsey AR, Cunningham CK, Barker WH, Kouides RW, Yuen JB, Menegus M, Weiner LB, Bonville CA, Betts RF. Respiratory syncytial virus and influenza A infections in the hospitalized elderly. J Infect Dis 1995; 1722: 389.

Falsey AR, Walsh EE. Relationship of serum antibody to risk of respiratory syncytial virus infection in elderly adults. J Infect Dis 1998; 1772: 463.

Falsey AR, Walsh EE, Looney RJ, Kolassa JE, Formica MA, Criddle MC, Hall WJ. Comparison of respiratory syncytial virus humoral immunity and response to infection in young and elderly adults. J Med Virol 1999; 592: 221.

Fischer JE, Johnson JE, Kuli-Zade RK, Johnson TR, Aung S, Parker RA, Graham BS. Overexpression of interleukin-4 delays virus clearance in mice infected with respiratory syncytial virus. J Virol 1997; 7111: 8672.

Fishaut M, Tubergen D, McIntosh K. Cellular responses to respiratory syncytial viruses with particular reference to children with disorders of cell-mediated immunity. J Pediatr 1980; 96: 179.

Fisher RG, Crowe Jr, JE, Johnson TR, Tang Y-W. Graham BS. Passive IgA mononclonal antibody is no more effective than IgG at protecting mice from mucosal challenge with respiratory syncytial virus. J Infect Dis 1999; 180: 1324.

Fogg M. Identification of Bovine Respiratory Syncytial Virus Proteins and Epitopes recognised by Bovine CD4+ T Cells. PhD thesis, University of Reading, Berkshire, UK; 1999.

Fogg MH, Parsons KR, Thomas LH, Taylor G. Identification of $CD4^+$ T cell epitopes on the fusion (F) and attachment (G) proteins of bovine respiratory syncytial virus (BRSV). Vaccine 2001; 19: 3226.

Fulginiti VA, Eller JJ, Downie AW, Kempe CH. Altered reactivity to measles virus. Atypical measles in children previously immunized with inactivated measles virus vaccines.. JAMA 1967; 20212: 1075.

Fulginiti VA, Eller JJ, Sieber OF, Joyner JW, Minamihani M, Meikeiejohn G. Respiratory virus immunisation. I. A field trial of two inactivated respiratory vaccines: an aqueous trivalent parainfluenza virus vaccine and an alum-precipitated respiratory syncytial virus vaccine. Am J Epidemiol 1969; 89: 435.

Furze J, Wertz G, Lerch R, Taylor G. Antigenic heterogenicity of the attachment protein of bovine respiratory syncytial virus. J Gen Virol 1994; 75: 363.

Furze JM, Roberts SR, Wertz GW, Taylor G. Antigenically distinct G glycoproteins of BRSV strains share a high degree of genetic homogeneity. Virology 1997; 2311: 48.

Gaddum RM, Cook RS, Furze JM, Ellis SA, Taylor G. Recognition of bovine respiratory syncytial virus proteins by bovine CD8+ T lymphocytes. Immunology 2003; 1082: 220.

Gaddum RM, Cook RS, Thomas LH, Taylor G. Primary cytotoxic T cell responses to bovine respiratory syncytial virus in calves. Immunology 1996a; 88: 421.

Gaddum RM, Cook RS, Wyld SG, Lopez JA, Bustos R, Melero JA, Taylor G. Mutant forms of the F protein of human respiratory syncytial (RS) virus induce a cytotoxic T lymphocyte response but not a neutralizing antibody response and only transient resistance to RS virus infection. J Gen Virol 1996b; 77: 1239.

Gershwin LJ, Schelegle ES, Gunther RA, Anderson ML, Woolums AR, Larochelle DR, Boyle GA, Friebertshauser KE, Singer RS. A bovine model of vaccine enhanced respiratory syncytial virus pathophysiology. Vaccine 1998; 1611–1612: 1225.

Ghildyal R, Hartley C, Varrasso A, Meanger J, Voelker DR, Anders EM, Mills J. Surfactant protein A binds to the fusion glycoprotein of respiratory syncytial virus and neutralizes virion infectivity. J Infect Dis 1999; 180: 2009.

Gimenez HB, Chisholm S, Dornan J, Cash P. Neutralizing and enhancing activities of human respiratory syncytial virus-specific antibodies. Clin Diagn Lab Immunol 1996; 33: 280.

Gimenez HB, Keir HM, Cash P. *In vitro* enhancement of respiratory syncytial virus infection of U937 cells by human sera. J Gen Virol 1989; 70: 89.

Glezen WP, Denny FW. Epidemiology of acute lower respiraotry disease in children. N Eng J Med 1973; 288: 498.

Glezen WP, Paredes A, Allison JE, Taber LH, Frank AL. Risk of respiratory syncytial virus infection for infants from low-income families in relationship to age, sex, ethnic group, and maternal antibody level. J Pediatr 1981; 985: 708.

Goulder PJR, Lechner F, Klenerman P, McIntosh K, Walker BD. Characterization of a novel respiratory syncytial virus-specific human cytotoxic T-lymphocyte epitope. J Virol 2000; 74: 7694.

Graham BS, Bunton LA, Rowland J, Wright PF, Karzon DT. Respiratory syncytial virus infection in anti-μ-treated mice. J Virol 1991a; 65: 4936.

Graham BS, Bunton LA, Wright PF, Karzon DT. Role of T-lymphocyte subsets in the pathogenesis of primary infection and rechallenge with respiratory syncytial virus in mice. J Clin Invest 1991b; 88: 1026.

Graham BS, Davis TH, Tang YW, Gruber WC. Immunoprophylaxis and immunotherapy of respiratory syncytial virus-infected mice with respiratory syncytial virus-specific immune serum. Pediatr Res 1993a; 342: 167.

Graham BS, Henderson GS, Tang YW, Lu X, Neuzil KM, Colley DG. Priming immunization determines T helper cytokine mRNA expression patterns in lungs of mice challenged with respiratory syncytial virus. J Immunol 1993b; 1514: 2032.

Graham BS, Tang YW, Gruber WC. Topical immunoprophylaxis of respiratory syncytial virus (RSV)-challenged mice with RSV-specific immune globulin. J Infect Dis 1995; 1716: 1468.

Gray PM, Arimilli S, Palmer EM, Parks GD, Alexander-Miller MA. Altered function in CD8+ T cells following paramyxovirus infection of the respiratory tract. J Virol 2005; 796: 3339.

Groothuis JR, Simoes EA, Hemming VG. Respiratory syncytial virus (RSV) infection in preterm infants and the protective effects of RSV immune globulin (RSVIG). Respiratory syncytial virus immune globulin study group. Pediatr 1995; 954: 463.

Groothuis JR, Simoes EAF, Levin MJ, Hal, CB, Long CE, Rodriguez WJ, Arrobio J, Meissner HC, Fulton DR, Welliver RC, Tristram DA, Siber GR, Prince GA, van Raden M, Hemming VG, Group TRSV.I.G.S. Prophylactic administration of respiratory syncytial virus immune globulin to high-risk infants and young children. N Engl J Med 1993; 329: 1524.

Haeberle HA, Casola A, Gatalica Z, Petronella S, Dieterich HJ, Ernst PB, Brasier AR, Garofalo RP. IkappaB kinase is a critical regulator of chemokine expression and lung inflammation in respiratory syncytial virus infection. J Virol 2004; 785: 2232.

Haeberle HA, Takizawa R, Casola A, Brasier AR, Dieterich HJ, Van Rooijen N, Gatalica Z, Garofalo RP. Respiratory syncytial virus-induced activation of nuclear factor-kappaB in the lung involves alveolar macrophages and toll-like receptor 4-dependent pathways. J Infect Dis 2002; 1869: 1199.

Hall CB, Kopelman AE, Douglas Jr. RG, Geiman JM, Meagher MP. Neonatal respiratory syncytial virus infection. N Engl J Med 1979; 3008: 393.

Hall CB, Powell KR, MacDonald NE, Gala CL, Menegus ME, Suffin SC, Cohen HJ. Respiratory syncytial viral infection in children with compromised immune function. N Engl J Med 1986; 3152: 77.

Hancock GE, Heers KM, Pryharski KS, Smith JD, Tiberio L. Adjuvants recognized by toll-like receptors inhibit the induction of polarized type 2 T cell responses by natural attachment (G) protein of respiratory syncytial virus. Vaccine 2003a; 2127–2130: 4348.

Hancock GE, Speelman DJ, Frenchick PJ, Mineo-Kuhn MM, Baggs RB, Hahn DJ. Formulation of the purified fusion protein of respiratory syncytial virus with the saponin QS-21 induces protective immune responses in mice that are similar to those generated by experimental infection. Vaccine 1995; 13: 391.

Hancock GE, Speelman DJ, Heers K, Bortell E, Smith J, Cosco C. Generation of atypical pulmonary inflammatory responses in BALB/c mice after immunization with the native attachment (G) glycoprotein of respiratory syncytial virus. J Virol 1996; 7011: 7783.

Hancock GE, Tebbey PW, Scheuer CA, Pryharski KS, Heers KM, LaPierre NA. Immune responses to the nonglycosylated ectodomain of respiratory syncytial virus attachment glycoprotein mediate pulmonary eosinophilia in inbred strains of mice with different MHC haplotypes. J Med Virol 2003b; 702: 301.

Harrison AM, Bonville CA, Rosenberg HF, Domachowske JB. Respiratory syncytical virus-induced chemokine expression in the lower airways: eosinophil recruitment and degranulation. Am J Respir Crit Care Med 1999; 1596: 1918.

Harrop JA, Anderson JJ, Hayes P, Serin N, Scott R. Characteristics of the pulmonary natural killer (NK) cell response to respiratory syncytial virus infection in BALB/c mice. Immunol Infect Dis 1994; 4: 179.

Haynes LM, Moore D, Kurt-Jones E, Finberg RW, Anderson LJ, Tripp RA. Involvement of Toll-like receptor 4 in innate immunity to respiratory syncytial virus. J Virol 2001; 75: 10730.

Haynes LM, Jones LP, Barskey A, Anderson LJ, Tripp RA. Enhanced disease and pulmonary eosinophilia associated with formalin-inactivated respiratory syncytial virus vaccination are linked to G glycoprotein CX3C-CX3CR1 interaction and expression of substance P. J Virol 2003; 7718: 9831.

Heidema J, de Bree GJ, De Graaff PM, van Maren WW, Hoogerhout P, Out TA, Kimpen JL, van Bleek GM. Human CD8(+) T cell responses against five newly identified respiratory syncytial virus-derived epitopes. J Gen Virol 2004; 85: 2365.

Hemming VG, Prince GA, Groothuis JR, Siber GR. Hyperimmune globulins in prevention and treatment of respiratory syncytial virus infections. Clin Microbiol Rev 1995; 81: 22.

Hemming VG, Rodriguez W, Kim HW, Brandt CD, Parrott RH, Burch B, Prince GA, Baron PA, Fink RJ, Reaman G. Intravenous immunoglobulin treatment of respiratory syncytial virus infections in infants and young children. Antimicrob Agents Chemother 1987; 3112: 1882.

Henderson FW, Collier AM, Clyde WA, Denny FW. Respiratory syncytial virus infections, reinfections and immunity: a prospective, longitudinal study in young children. N Engl J Med 1979; 3000: 530.

Hendricks DA, McIntosh K, Patterson JL. Further characterization of the soluble form of the G glycoprotein of respiratory syncytial virus. J Virol 1988; 627: 2228.

Hickling TP, Bright H, Wing K, Gower D, Martin SL, Sim RB, Malhotra R. A recombinant trimeric surfactant protein D carbohydrate recognition domain inhibits respiratory syncytial virus infection *in vitro* and *in vivo*. Eur J Immunol 1999; 29: 3478.

Hogan RJ, Usherwood EJ, Zhong W, Roberts AA, Dutton RW, Harmsen AG, Woodland DL. Activated antigen-specific CD8+ T cells persist in the lungs following recovery from respiratory virus infections. J Immunol 2001; 1663: 1813.

Holberg CJ, Wright AL, Martinez FD, Ray CG, Taussig LM, Lebowitz MD. Risk factors for respiratory syncytial virus-associated lower respiratory illnesses in the first year of life. Am J Epidemiol 1991; 13311: 1135.

Hornung V, Schlender J, Guenthner-Biller M, Rothenfusser S, Endres S, Conzelmann KK, Hartmann G. Replication-dependent potent IFN-alpha induction in human plasmacytoid dendritic cells by a single-stranded RNA virus. J Immunol 2004; 17310: 5935.

Howard CJ, Sopp P, Brownlie J, Kwong LS, Parsons KR, Taylor G. Identification of two distinct populations of dendritic cells in afferent lymph that vary in their ability to stimulate T cells. J. Immunol. 1997; 159: 5372.

Hussell T, Baldwin CJ, O'Garra A, Openshaw PJ. CD8+ T cells control Th2-driven pathology during pulmonary respiratory syncytial virus infection. Eur J Immunol 1997; 2712: 3341.

Hussell T, Georgiou A, Sparer TE, Matthews S, Pala P, Openshaw PJ. Host genetic determinants of vaccine-induced eosinophilia during respiratory syncytial virus infection. J Immunol 1998; 16111: 6215.

Hussell T, Openshaw PJ. Intracellular IFN-gamma expression in natural killer cells precedes lung CD8+ T cell recruitment during respiratory syncytial virus infection. J Gen Virol 1998; 7911: 2593.

Hussell T, Spender LC, Georgiou A, O'Garra A, Openshaw PJM. Th1 and Th2 cytokine induction in pulmonary T cells during infection with respiratory syncytial virus. J Gen Virol 1996; 77: 2447.

Isaacs D, MacDonald NE, Bangham CRM, McMichael AJ, Higgins PG, Tyrrell D. The specific cytotoxic T-cell response of adult volunteers to infection with respiratory syncytial virus. Immunol Infect Dis 1990; 1: 5.

Impact-RSV Study Group. Palivizumab, a humanized respiratory syncytial virus monoclonal antibody, reduces hospitalization from respiratory syncytial virus infection in high-risk infants. Pediatrics 102, 531.

Jackson M, Scott R. Different patterns of cytokine induction in cultures of respiratory syncytial (RS) virus-specific human TH cell lines following stimulation with RS virus and RS virus proteins. J Med Virol 1996; 493: 161.

Jahnsen FL, Gran E, Haye R, Brandtzaeg P. Human nasal mucosa contains antigen-presenting cells of strikingly different functional phenotypes. Am J Respir Cell Mol Biol 2004; 301: 31.

Jiang S, Borthwick NJ, Morrison P, Gao GF, Steward MW. Virus-specific CTL responses induced by an H-2K(d)-restricted, motif-negative 15-mer peptide from the fusion protein of respiratory syncytial virus. J Gen Virol 2002; 83: 429.

Johnson KM, Chanock RM, Rifkind D, Kravetz HM, Knight V. Respiratory syncytial virus IV. Correlation of virus shedding, serologic response, and illness in adult volunteers. JAMA 1961; 176: 663.

Johnson Jr. PR, Olmsted RA, Prince GA, Murphy BR, Alling DW, Walsh EE, Collins PL. Antigenic relatedness between glycoproteins of human respiratory syncytial virus subgroups A and B: evaluation of the contributions of F and G glycoproteins to immunity. J Virol 1987; 6110: 3163.

Johnson SA, Ottolini MG, Darnell ME, Porter DD, Prince GA. Unilateral nasal infection of cotton rats with respiratory syncytial virus allows assessment of local and systemic immunity. J Gen Virol 1996; 77: 101.

Johnson TR, Graham BS. Secreted respiratory syncytial virus G glycoprotein induces interleukin-5 (IL-5), IL-13, and eosinophilia by an IL-4-independent mechanism. J Virol 1999; 7310: 8485.

Johnson TR, Graham BS. Contribution of respiratory syncytial virus G antigenicity to vaccine-enhanced illness and the implications for severe disease during primary respiratory syncytial virus infection. Pediatr Infect Dis J 2004; 231(Suppl): S46.

Johnson TR, Hong S, Van Kaer L, Koezuka Y, Graham BS. NK T cells contribute to expansion of CD8(+) T cells and amplification of antiviral immune responses to respiratory syncytial virus. J Virol 2002; 769: 4294.

Johnson TR, Johnson JE, Roberts SR, Wertz GW, Parker RA, Graham BS. Priming with secreted glycoprotein G of respiratory syncytial virus (RSV) augments interleukin-5 production and tissue eosinophilia after RSV challenge. J Virol 1998; 724: 2871.

Johnson TR, Mertz SE, Gitiban N, Hammond S, Legallo R, Durbin RK, Durbin JE. Role for innate IFNs in determining respiratory syncytial virus immunopathology. J Immunol 2005; 17411: 7234.

Johnson TR, Parker RA, Johnson JE, Graham BS. IL-13 is sufficient for respiratory syncytial virus G glycoprotein-induced eosinophilia after respiratory syncytial virus challenge. J Immunol 2003; 1704: 2037.

Johnson TR, Varga SM, Braciale TJ, Graham BS. Vbeta14(+) T cells mediate the vaccine-enhanced disease induced by immunization with respiratory syncytial virus (RSV) G glycoprotein but not with formalin-inactivated RSV. J Virol 2004; 7816: 8753.

Johnstone C, de Leon P, Medina F, Melero JA, Garcia-Barreno B, Del Val M. Shifting immunodominance pattern of two cytotoxic T-lymphocyte epitopes in the F glycoprotein of the Long strain of respiratory syncytial virus. J Gen Virol 2004; 85: 3229.

Kakuk TJ, Soike K, Brideau RJ, Zaya RM, Cole SL, Zhang JY, Roberts ED, Wells PA, Wathen MW. A human respiratory syncytial virus (RSV) primate model of enhanced pulmonary pathology induced with a formalin-inactivated RSV vaccine but not a recombinant FG subunit vaccine. J Infect Dis 1993; 1673: 553.

Kapikian AZ, Mitchell RH, Chanock RM, Shvedoff RA, Stewart CE. An epidemiologic study of altered clinical reactivity to respiratory syncytial (RS) virus infection in children previously vaccinated with an inactivated RS virus vaccine. Am J Epidemiol 1969; 894: 405.

Kerr MH, Paton JY. Surfactant protein levels in severe respiratory syncytial virus infection. Am J Respir Crit Care Med 1999; 1594: 1115.

Kim HW, Canchola JG, Brandt CD, Pyles G, Chanock RM, Jensen K, Parrott RH. Respiratory syncytial virus disease in infants despite prior administration of antigenic inactivated vaccine. Am J Epidemiol 1969; 89: 422.

Kim HW, Leikin SL, Arrobio J, Brandt CD, Chanock RM, Parrott RH. Cell-mediated immunity to respiratory syncytial virus induced by inactivated vaccine or by infection. Pediatr Res 1976; 101: 75.

Kimman TG, Westenbrink F, Schreuder BE, Straver PJ. Local and systemic antibody response to bovine respiratory syncytial virus infection and reinfection in calves with and without maternal antibodies. J Clin Microbiol 1987; 256: 1097.

Kimman TG, Westenbrink F, Straver PJ. Priming for local and systemic antibody memory responses to bovine respiratory syncytial virus: effect of amount of virus, virus replication, route of administration and maternal antibodies. Vet Immunol Immunopathol 1989; 222: 145.

Kos FJ, Engleman EG. Immune regulation: a critical link between NK cells and CTLs. Immunol Today 1996; 174: 174.

Kravetz HM, Knight V, Chanock RM, Morris JA, Johnson KM, Rifkind D, Utz JP. Respiratory syncytial virus. III. Production of illness and clinical observations in adult volunteers. JAMA 1961; 176: 657.

Krilov LR, Anderson LJ, Marcoux L, Bonagura VR, Wedgwood JF. Antibody-mediated enhancement of respiratory syncytial virus infection in two monocyte/macrophage cell lines. J Infect Dis 1989; 160: 777.

Kulkarni AB, Collins PL, Bacik I, Yewdell JW, Bennink JR, Crowe Jr. JE, Murphy BR. Cytotoxic T cells specific for a single peptide on the M2 protein of respiratory syncytial virus are the sole mediators of resistance induced by immunization with M2 encoded by a recombinant vaccinia virus. J Virol 1995; 692: 1261.

Kulkarni AB, Connors M, Firestone CY, Morse 3rd HC, Murphy BR. The cytolytic activity of pulmonary CD8+ lymphocytes, induced by infection with a vaccinia virus recombinant expressing the M2 protein of respiratory syncytial virus (RSV), correlates with resistance to RSV infection in mice. J Virol 1993a; 672: 1044.

Kulkarni AB, Morse HCd, Bennink JR, Yewdell JW, Murphy BR. Immunization of mice with vaccinia virus-M2 recombinant induces epitope-specific and cross-reactive Kd-restricted CD8+ cytotoxic T cells. J Virol 1993b; 677: 4086.

Kurt-Jones EA, Popova L, Kwinn L, Haynes LM, Jones LP, Tripp RA, Walsh EE, Freeman MW, Golenbock DT, Anderson LJ, Finberg RW. Pattern recognition receptors TLR4 and CD14 mediate response to respiratory syncytial virus. Nat Immunol 2000; 1: 398.

Lahti M, Lofgren J, Marttila R, Renko M, Klaavuniemi T, Haataja R, Ramet M, Hallman M. Surfactant protein D gene polymorphism associated with severe respiratory syncytial virus infection. Pediatr Res 2002; 51: 696.

Lamprecht CL, Krause HE, Mufson MA. Role of maternal antibody in pneumonia and bronchiolitis due to respiratory syncytial virus. J Infect Dis 1976; 1343: 211.

Langedijk JP, de Groot BL, Berendsen HJ, van Oirschot JT. Structural homology of the central conserved region of the attachment protein G of respiratory syncytial virus with the fourth subdomain of 55-kDa tumor necrosis factor receptor. Virology 1998; 2432: 293.

Langedijk JP, Meloen RH, Taylor G, Furze JM, van Oirschot JT. Antigenic structure of the central conserved region of protein G of bovine respiratory syncytial virus. J Virol 1997; 715: 4055.

Le Bon A, Tough DF. Link between innate and adaptative immunity via type I interferon. Curr Opin Immunol 2002; 14: 432.

Legg JP, Hussain IR, Warner JA, Johnston SL, Warner JO. Type 1 and type 2 cytokine imbalance in acute respiratory syncytial virus bronchiolitis. Am J Respir Crit Care Med 2003; 1686: 633.

Levely ME, Bannow CA, Smith CW, Nicholas JA. Immunodominant T-cell epitopes on the F protein of respiratory syncytial virus recognised by human lymphocytes. J Virol 1991; 65: 3789.

LeVine AM, Gwozdz J, Stark J, Bruno M, Whitsett J, Korfhagen T. Surfactant protein-A enhances respiratory syncytial virus clearance *in vivo*. J Clin Invest 1999; 103: 1015.

Lofgren J, Ramet M, Renko M, Marttila R, Hallman M. Association between surfactant protein A gene locus and severe respiratory syncytial virus infection in infants. J Infect Dis 2002; 185: 283.

Looney RJ, Falsey AR, Walsh E, Campbell D. Effect of aging on cytokine production in response to respiratory syncytial virus infection. J Infect Dis 2002; 1855: 682.

Lopez JA, Andreu D, Carreno C, Whyte P, Taylor G, Melero JA. Conformational constraints of conserved neutralizing epitopes from a major antigenic area of human respiratory syncytial virus fusion glycoprotein. J Gen Virol 1993; 74: 2567.

Lopez JA, Bustos R, Orvell C, Berois M, Arbiza J, Garcia-Barreno BA, Melero JA. Antigenic structure of human respiratory syncytial virus fusion glycoprotein. J Virol 1998; 728: 6922.

Mackay LJ. Induction and Regulation of Pulmonary Eosinophilia in Mice Primed with the G Protein of RSV. PhD thesis, University of Bristol, Bristol, UK; 2001.

Malley R, DeVincenzo J, Ramilo O, Dennehy PH, Meissner HC, Gruber WC, Sanchez PJ, Jafri H, Balsley J, Carlin D, Buckingham S, Vernacchio L, Ambrosino DM. Reduction of respiratory syncytial virus (RSV) in tracheal aspirates in intubated infants by use of humanized monoclonal antibody to RSV F protein. J Infect Dis 1998; 1786: 1555.

Martinez I, Dopazo J, Melero JA. Antigenic structure of the human respiratory syncytial virus G glycoprotein and relevance of hypermutation events for the generation of antigenic variants. J Gen Virol 1997; 78: 2419.

Martinez I, Melero JA. Enhanced neutralization of human respiratory syncytial virus by mixtures of monoclonal antibodies to the attachment (G) glycoprotein. J Gen Virol 1998; 79: 2215.

Mazanec MB, Nedrud JG, Kaetzel CS, Lamm ME. A three-tiered view of the role of IgA in mucosal defences. Immunol Today 1993; 14: 430.

Mbawuike IN, Wells J, Byrd R, Cron SG, Glezen WP, Piedra PA. HLA-restricted CD8+ cytotoxic T lymphocyte, interferon-gamma, and interleukin-4 responses to respiratory syncytial virus infection in infants and children. J Infect Dis 2001; 1835: 687.

McGuirk P, Mills KH. Pathogen-specific regulatory T cells provoke a shift in the Th1/Th2 paradigm in immunity to infectious diseases. Trends Immunol 2002; 239: 450.

McInnes E, Sopp P, Howard CJ, Taylor G. Phenotypic analysis of local cellular responses in calves infected with bovine respiratory syncytial virus. Immunology 1999; 963: 396.

McIntosh K, Masters HB, Orr I, Chao RK, Barkin RM. The immunologic response to infection with respiratory syncytial virus in infants. J Infect Dis 1978; 1381: 24.

Melero J, Garcia-Barreno B, Martinez I, Pringle CR, Cane PA. Antigenic structure, evolution and immunobiology of human respiratory syncytial virus attachment (G) protein. J Gen Virol 1997; 78: 2411.

Meurman O, Waris M, Hedman K. Immunoglobulin G antibody avidity in patients with respiratory syncytial virus infection. J Clin Microbiol 1992; 306: 1479.

Miller AL, Bowlin TL, Lukacs NW. Respiratory syncytial virus-induced chemokine production: linking viral replication to chemokine production *in vitro* and *in vivo*. J Infect Dis 2004; 1898: 1419.

Mills JT, Van Kirk JE, Wright PF, Chanock RM. Experimental respiratory syncytial virus infection of adults. Possible mechanisms of resistance to infection and illness. J Immunol 1971; 1071: 123.

Milner ME, de la Monte SM, Hutchins GM. Fatal respiratory syncytial virus infection in severe combined immunodeficiency syndrome. Am J Dis Child 1985; 13911: 1111.

Mohanty SB, Lillie MG, Ingling AL. Effect of serum and nasal neutralizing antibodies on bovine respiratory syncytial virus infection in calves. J Infect Dis 1976; 1344: 409.

Monick MM, Yarovinsky TO, Powers LS, Butler NS, Carter AB, Gudmundsson G, Hunninghake GW. Respiratory syncytial virus up-regulates TLR4 and sensitizes airway epithelial cells to endotoxin. J Biol Chem 2003; 27852: 53035.

Murphy BR, Alling DW, Snyder MH, Walsh EE, Prince GA, Chanock RM, Hemming VG, Rodriguez WJ, Kim HW, Graham BS, Wright PF. Effect of age and preexisting antibody on serum antibody response of infants and children to the F and G glycoproteins during respiratory syncytial virus infection. J Clin Microbiol 1986a; 245: 894.

Murphy BR, Collins PL, Lawrence L, Zubak J, Chanock RM, Prince GA. Immunosuppression of the antibody response to respiratory syncytial virus (RSV) by pre-existing serum antibodies: partial prevention by topical infection of the respiratory tract with vaccinia virus-RSV recombinants. J Gen Virol 1989; 70: 2185.

Murphy BR, Olmsted RA, Collins PL, Chanock RM, Prince GA. Passive transfer of respiratory syncytial virus (RSV) antiserum suppresses the immune response to the RSV fusion (F) and large (G) glycoproteins expressed by recombinant vaccinia viruses. J Virol 1988; 6210: 3907.

Murphy BR, Prince GA, Walsh EE, Kim HW, Parrott RH, Hemming VG, Rodriguez WJ, Chanock RM. Disassociation between serum neutralisng and glycoprotein antibody responses of infants and children who received inactivated respiratory syncytial virus vaccine. J Clin Microbiol 1986b; 24: 197.

Murray JS. How the MHC selects Th1/Th2 immunity. Immunol Today 1998; 194: 157.

Neilson KA, Yunis EJ. Demonstration of respiratory syncytial virus in an autopsy series. Pediatr Pathol 1990; 104: 491.

Noah T, Becker S. Chemokines in nasal secretions of normal adults experimentally infected with respiratory syncytial virus. Clin. Immunol. 2000; 97: 43.

Ogilvie MM, Vathenen AS, Radford M, Codd J, Key S. Maternal antibody and respiratory syncytial virus infection in infancy. J Med Virol 1981; 7: 263.

Openshaw PJ, Anderson K, Wertz GW, Askonas BA. The 22,000-kilodalton protein of respiratory syncytial virus is a major target for Kd-restricted cytotoxic T lymphocytes from mice primed by infection. J Virol 1990; 644: 1683.

Openshaw PJ, Clarke SL, Record FM. Pulmonary eosinophilic response to respiratory syncytial virus infection in mice sensitized to the major surface glycoprotein G. Int Immunol 1992; 44: 493.

Openshaw PJ, Pemberton RM, Ball LA, Wertz GW, Askonas BA. Helper T cell recognition of respiratory syncytial virus in mice. J Gen Virol 1988; 69: 305.

Osiowy C, Horne D, Anderson R. Antibody-dependent enhancement of respiratory syncytial virus infection by sera from young infants. Clin Diagn Lab Immunol 1994; 16: 670.

Ostler T, Davidson W, Ehl S. Virus clearance and immunopathology by CD8(+) T cells during infection with respiratory syncytial virus are mediated by IFN-gamma. Eur J Immunol 2002; 328: 2117.

Ostler T, Ehl S. A cautionary note on experimental artefacts induced by fetal calf serum in a viral model of pulmonary eosinophilia. J Immunol Methods 2002; 2682: 211.

Ostler T, Hussell T, Surh CD, Openshaw P, Ehl S. Long-term persistence and reactivation of T cell memory in the lung of mice infected with respiratory syncytial virus. Eur J Immunol 2001; 319: 2574.

Ottolini MG, Porter DD, Hemming VG, Zimmerman MN, Schwab NM, Prince GA. Effectiveness of RSVIG prophylaxis and therapy of respiratory syncytial virus in an immunosuppressed animal model. Bone Marrow Transplant 1999; 241: 41.

Parrott RH, Kim HW, Arrobio JO, Hodes DS, Murphy BR, Brandt CD, Camargo E, Chanock RM. Epidemiology of respiratory syncytial virus infection in Washington, D.C. II. Infection and disease with respect to age, immunologic status, race and sex. Am J Epidemiol 1973; 984: 289.

Pemberton RM, Cannon MJ, Openshaw PJ, Ball LA, Wertz GW, Askonas BA. Cytotoxic T cell specificity for respiratory syncytial virus proteins: fusion protein is an important target antigen. J Gen Virol 1987; 68: 2177.

Polack FP, Auwaerter PG, Lee SH, Nousari HC, Valsamakis A, Leiferman KM, Diwan A, Adams RJ, Griffin DE. Production of atypical measles in rhesus macaques: evidence for disease mediated by immune complex formation and eosinophils in the presence of fusion-inhibiting antibody. Nat Med 1999; 56: 629.

Polack FP, Hoffman SJ, Crujeiras G, Griffin DE. A role for nonprotective complement-fixing antibodies with low avidity for measles virus in atypical measles. Nat Med 2003; 99: 1209.

Polack FP, Irusta PM, Hoffman SJ, Schiatti MP, Melendi GA, Delgado MF, Laham FR, Thumar B, Hendry RM, Melero JA, Karron RA, Collins PL, Kleeberger SR. The cysteine-rich region of respiratory syncytial virus attachment protein inhibits innate immunity elicited by the virus and endotoxin. Proc Natl Acad Sci U S A 2005; 10225: 8996.

Polack FP, Teng MN, Collins PL, Prince GA, Exner M, Regele H, Lirman DD, Rabold R, Hoffman SJ, Karp CL, Kleeberger SR, Wills-Karp M, Karron RA. A role for immune complexes in enhanced respiratory syncytial virus disease. J Exp Med 2002; 196: 859.

Ponnuraj EM, Hayward AR, Raj A, Wilson H, Simoes EA. Increased replication of respiratory syncytial virus (RSV) in pulmonary infiltrates is associated with enhanced histopathological disease in bonnet monkeys (*Macaca radiata*) pre-immunized with a formalin-inactivated RSV vaccine. J Gen Virol 2001; 82: 2663.

Ponnuraj EM, Springer J, Hayward AR, Wilson H, Simoes EA. Antibody-dependent enhancement, a possible mechanism in augmented pulmonary disease of respiratory syncytial virus in the Bonnet monkey model. J Infect Dis 2003; 1878: 1257.

Preston FM, Beier PL, Pope JH. Identification of the respiratory syncytial virus-induced immunosuppressive factor produced by human peripheral blood mononuclear cells in vitro as interferon-γ. J Infect Dis 1995; 172: 919.

Prince GA, Curtis SJ, Yim KC, Porter DD. Vaccine-enhanced respiratory syncytial virus disease in cotton rats following immunization with Lot 100 or a newly prepared reference vaccine. J Gen Virol 2001; 82: 2881.

Prince GA, Hemming VG, Horswood RL, Baron PA, Chanock RM. Effectiveness of topically administered neutralizing antibodies in experimental immunotherapy of respiratory syncytial virus infection in cotton rats. J Virol 1987; 616: 1851.

Prince GA, Hemming VG, Horswood RL, Baron PA, Murphy BR, Chanock RM. Mechanism of antibody-mediated viral clearance in immunotherapy of respiratory syncytial virus infection of cotton rats. J Virol 1990; 646: 3091.

Prince GA, Hemming VG, Horswood RL, Chanock RM. Immunoprophylaxis and immunotherapy of respiratory syncytial virus infection in the cotton rat. Virus Res 1985a; 33: 193.

Prince GA, Horswood RL, Camargo E, Koenig D, Chanock RM. Mechanisms of immunity to respiratory syncytial virus in cotton rats. Infect Immunol 1983; 42: 81.

Prince GA, Horswood RL, Chanock RM. Quantitative aspects of passive immunity to respiratory syncytial virus infection in infant cotton rats. J Virol 1985b; 553: 517.

Prince GA, Jenson AB, Hemming VG, Murphy B, Walsh EE, Horswood RL, Chanock RM. Enhancement of respiratory syncytial virus pulmonary pathology in cotton rats by prior intramuscular inoculation of formalin-inactivated virus. J Virol 1986; 57: 721.

Proietti E, Bracci L, Puzelli S, Di Pucchio T, Sestili P, De Vincenzi E, Venditti M, Capone I, Seif I, Maeyer E, Tough DF, Donatelli I, Bellardelli F. Type I IFN as a natural adjuvant for a protective immune response: lessons from the influenza vaccine model. J Immunol 2002; 169: 375.

Pullan CR, Hey EN. Wheezing, asthma, and pulmonary dysfunction 10 years after infection with respiratory syncytial virus in infancy. Br Med J (Clin Res Ed) 1982; 2846330: 1665.

Richardson LS, Yolken RH, Belshe RB, Camargo E, Kim HW, Chanock RM. Enzyme-linked immunosorbent assay for measurement of serological response to respiratory syncytial virus infection. Infect Immunol 1978; 20: 660.

Roberts SR, Compans RW, Wertz GW. Respiratory syncytial virus matures at the apical surfaces of polarized epithelial cells. J Virol 1995; 694: 2667.

Roberts SR, Lichtenstein D, Ball LA, Wertz GW. The membrane-associated and secreted forms of the respiratory syncytial virus attachment glycoprotein G are synthesized from alternative initiation codons. J Virol 1994; 687: 4538.

Rodriguez WJ, Gruber WC, Welliver RC, Groothuis JR, Simoes EA, Meissner HC, Hemming VG, Hall CB, Lepow ML, Rosas AJ, Robertsen C, Kramer AA. Respiratory syncytial virus (RSV) immune globulin intravenous therapy for RSV lower respiratory tract infection in infants and young children at high risk for severe RSV infections: respiratory syncytial virus immune globulin study group. Pediatrics 1997; 993: 454.

Romagnani S. Induction of TH1 and TH2 responses: a key role for the 'natural' immune response? Immunol Today 1992; 13: 379.

Roman M, Calhoun WJ, Hinton KL, Avendano LF, Simon V, Escobar AM, Gaggero A, Diaz PV. Respiratory syncytial virus infection in infants is associated with predominant Th-2-like response. Am J Respir Crit Care Med 1997; 1561: 190.

Rudd BD, Burstein E, Duckett CS, Li X, Lukacs NW. Differential role for TLR3 in respiratory syncytial virus-induced chemokine expression. J Virol 2005; 796: 3350.

Rudd BD, Smit JJ, Flavell RA, Alexopoulou L, Schaller MA, Gruber A, Berlin AA, Lukacs NW. Deletion of TLR3 alters the pulmonary immune environment and mucus production during respiratory syncytial virus infection. J Immunol 2006; 1763: 1937.

Rutigliano JA, Rock MT, Johnson AK, Crowe Jr. JE, Graham BS. Identification of an H-2D(b)-restricted CD8+ cytotoxic T lymphocyte epitope in the matrix protein of respiratory syncytial virus. Virology 2005; 3372: 335.

Saez-Llorens X, Moreno MT, Ramilo O, Sanchez PJ, Top Jr. FH, Connor EM. Safety and pharmacokinetics of palivizumab therapy in children hospitalized with respiratory syncytial virus infection. Pediatr Infect Dis J 2004; 238: 707.

Sakurai H, Williamson RA, Crowe JE, Beeler JA, Poignard P, Bastidas RB, Chanock RM, Burton DR. Human antibody responses to mature and immature forms of viral envelope in respiratory syncytial virus infection: significance for subunit vaccines. J Virol 1999; 734: 2956.

Salkind AR, McCarthy DO, Nichols JE, Domurat FM, Walsh EE, Roberts Jr. NJ. Interleukin-1-inhibitor activity induced by respiratory syncytial virus: abrogation of virus-specific and alternate human lymphocyte proliferative responses. J Infect Dis 1991; 1631: 71.

Schlender J, Bossert B, Buchholz U, Conzelmann K-K. Bovine respiratory syncytial virus nonstructural proteins NS1 and NS2 cooperatively antagonize alpha/beta interferon-induced antiviral response. J Virol 2000a; 74: 8234.

Schlender J, Hornung V, Finke S, Gunthner-Biller M, Marozin S, Brzozka K, Moghim S, Endres S, Hartmann G, Conzelmann KK. Inhibition of toll-like receptor 7- and 9-mediated alpha/beta interferon production in human plasmacytoid dendritic cells by respiratory syncytial virus and measles virus. J Virol 2005; 799: 5507.

Schlender J, Walliser G, Conzelmann K-K. Contact inhibition of PBL proliferation by respiratory syncytial virus (RSV) fusion (F) protein. 11th International Conference on Negative Strand Viruses, 2000b; 200.

Schreiber P, Matheise JP, Dessy F, Heimann M, Letesson JJ, Coppe P, Collard A. High mortality rate associated with bovine respiratory syncytial virus (BRSV) infection in Belgian white blue calves previously vaccinated with an inactivated vaccine. J Vet Med B, Infect Dis Vet Public Health 2000; 47: 535.

Sha Q, Truong-Tran AQ, Plitt JR, Beck LA, Schleimer RP. Activation of airway epithelial cells by toll-like receptor agonists. Am J Respir Cell Mol Biol 2004; 313: 358.

Silvestri M, Sabatini F, Defilippi AC, Rossi GA. The wheezy infant—immunological and molecular considerations. Paediatr Respir Rev 2004; 5(Suppl A): S81.

Sims DG, Downham MA, Gardner PS, Webb JK, Weightman D. Study of 8-year-old children with a history of respiratory syncytial virus bronchiolitis in infancy. Br Med J 1978; 16104: 11.

Spann KM, Tran KC, Chi B, Rabin RL, Collins PL. Suppression of the induction of alpha, beta, and lambda interferons by the NS1 and NS2 proteins of human respiratory syncytial virus in human epithelial cells and macrophages [corrected]. J Virol 2004; 788: 4363.

Sparer TE, Matthews S, Hussell T, Rae AJ, Garcia Barreno B, Melero JA, Openshaw PJ. Eliminating a region of respiratory syncytial virus attachment protein allows induction of protective immunity without vaccine-enhanced lung eosinophilia. J Exp Med 1998; 18711: 1921.

Srikiatkhachorn A, Braciale TJ. Virus-specific CD8+ T lymphocytes downregulate T helper cell type 2 cytokine secretion and pulmonary eosinophilia during experimental murine respiratory syncytial virus infection. J Exp Med 1997; 1863: 421.

Srikiatkhachorn A, Chang W, Braciale TJ. Induction of Th-1 and Th-2 responses by respiratory syncytial virus attachment glycoprotein is epitope and major histocompatibility complex independent. J Virol 1999; 73: 6590.

Stein RT, Sherrill D, Morgan WJ, Holberg CJ, Halonen M, Taussig LM, Wright AL, Martinez FD. Respiratory syncytial virus in early life and risk of wheeze and allergy by age 13 years. Lancet 1999; 3549178: 541.

Stott EJ, Taylor G. Respiratory syncytial virus. Brief Rev Arch Virol 1985; 841-842: 1.

Stott EJ, Thomas LH, Taylor G, Collins AP, Jebbett J, Crouch S. A comparison of three vaccines against respiratory syncytial virus in calves. J Hyg Camb 1984; 93: 251.

Takeda K, Kaisho T, Akira S. Toll-like receptors. Ann Rev Immunol 2003; 21: 335.

Tal G, Mandelberg A, Dalal I, Cesar K, Somekh E, Tal A, Oron A, Itskovich S, Ballin A, Houri S, Beigelman A, Lider O, Rechavi G, Amariglio N. Association between common Toll-like receptor 4 mutations and severe respiratory syncytial virus disease. J Infect Dis 2004; 18911: 2057.

Tang YW, Graham BS. Anti-IL-4 treatment at immunization modulates cytokine expression, reduces illness, and increases cytotoxic T lymphocyte activity in mice challenged with respiratory syncytial virus. J Clin Invest 1994; 945: 1953.

Taylor G. The role of antibody in controlling and/ or clearing virus infections. In: Strategies Vaccine Design (Ada GL, editor). Austin, TX: R.G. Landes Company; 1994; p. 17.

Taylor G, Stott EJ, Bew M, Fernie BF, Cote PJ, Collins AP, Hughes M, Jebbett J. Monoclonal antibodies protect against respiratory syncytial virus infection in mice. Immunology 1984; 521: 137.

Taylor G, Stott EJ, Furze J, Ford J, Sopp P. Protective epitopes on the fusion protein of respiratory syncytial virus recognized by murine and bovine monoclonal antibodies. J Gen Virol 1992; 739: 2217.

Taylor G, Stott EJ, Hayle AJ. Cytotoxic lymphocytes in the lungs of mice infected with respiratory syncytial virus. J Gen Virol 1985; 66: 2533.

Taylor G, Thomas LH, Furze JM, Cook RS, Wyld SG, Lerch R, Hardy R, Wertz GW. Recombinant vaccinia viruses expressing the F, G or N, but not the M2, protein of bovine respiratory syncytial virus (BRSV) induce resistance to BRSV challenge in the calf and protect against the development of pneumonic lesions. J Gen Virol 1997; 7812: 3195.

Taylor G, Thomas LH, Wyld SG, Furze J, Sopp P, Howard CJ. Role of T-lymphocyte subsets in recovery from respiratory syncytial virus infection in calves. J Virol 1995; 69: 6658.

Tebbey PW, Hagen M, Hancock GE. Atypical pulmonary eosinophilia is mediated by a specific amino acid sequence of the attachment (G) protein of respiratory syncytial virus. J Exp Med 1998; 18810: 1967.

Thomas LH, Cook RS, Howard CJ, Gaddum RM, Taylor G. Influence of selective T-lymphocyte depletion on the lung pathology of gnotobiotic calves and the distribution of different T-lymphocyte subsets following challenge with bovine respiratory syncytial virus. Res Vet Sci 1996; 611: 38.

Thomas LH, Cook RS, Wyld SG, Furze JM, Taylor G. Passive protection of gnotobiotic calves using monoclonal antibodies directed at different epitopes on the fusion protein of bovine respiratory syncytial virus. J Infect Dis 1998; 1774: 874.

Thomas LH, Stott EJ, Collins AP, Jebbett J. Experimental pneumonia in gnotobiotic calves produced by respiratory syncytial virus. Br J Exp Pathol 1984; 65: 19.

Tripp R, Moore D, Jones L, Sullender W, Winter J, Anderson LJ. Respiratory syncytial virus G and/or SH protein alters Th1 cytokines, natural killer cells, and neutrophils responding to pulmonary infection in BALB/c mice. J Virol 1999; 739: 7099.

Tripp RA, Anderson LJ. Respiratory syncytial virus G and/or SH glycoproteins modify CC and CXC chemokine mRNA expression in the BALB/c mouse. J Virol 2000; 74: 6227.

Tripp RA, Moore D, Barskey At, Jones L, Moscatiello C, Keyserling H, Anderson LJ. Peripheral blood mononuclear cells from infants hospitalized because of respiratory syncytial virus infection express T helper-1 and T helper-2 cytokines and CC chemokine messenger RNA. J Infect Dis 2002; 18510: 1388.

Trudel M, Nadon F, Seguin C, Binz H. Protection of BALB/c mice from respiratory syncytial virus infection by immunization with a synthetic peptide derived from the G glycoprotein. Virology 1991; 1852: 749.

Tsutsumi H, Matsuda K, Sone S, Takeuchi R, Chiba S. Respiratory syncytial virus-induced cytokine production by neonatal macrophages. Clin Exp Immunol 1996; 106: 442.

Valarcher J-F, Furze J, Wyld S, Cook R, Conzelmann K-K, Taylor G. Role of type I interferons in the attenuation and immunogenicity of recombinant bovine respiratory syncytial viruses (BRSV) lacking NS proteins. J Virol 2003; 77: 8426.

van Bleek GM, Poelen MC, van der Most R, Brugghe HF, Timmermans HAM, Boog CJ, Hoogerhout P, Otten HG, van Els CACM. Identification of immunodominant epitopes derived from the respiratory syncytial virus fusion protein that are recognized by human CD4 T cells. J Virol 2003; 77: 980.

Varga SM, Wang X, Welsh RM, Braciale TJ. Immunopathology in RSV infection is mediated by a discrete oligoclonal subset of antigen-specific CD4(+) T cells. Immunity 2001; 154: 637.

Varga SM, Wissinger EL, Braciale TJ. The attachment (G) glycorprotein of respiratory syncytial virus contains a single immunodominant epitope that elicits both Th1 and Th2 CD4+ T cell responses. J Immunol 2000; 165: 6487.

Venter M, Rock M, Puren AJ, Tiemessen CT, Crowe Jr. JE. Respiratory syncytial virus nucleoprotein-specific cytotoxic T-cell epitopes in a South African population of diverse HLA types are conserved in circulating field strains. J Virol 2003; 7713: 7319.

Viuff B, Uttenthal A, Tegtmeier C, Alexandersen S. Sites of replication of bovine respiratory syncytial virus in naturally infected calves as determined by *in situ* hybridisation. Vet Pathol 1996; 33: 383.

Walsh EE, Peterson DR, Falsey AR. Risk factors for severe respiratory syncytial virus infection in elderly persons. J Infect Dis 2004; 1892: 233.

Walsh EE, Schlesinger JJ, Brandriss MW. Protection from respiratory syncytial virus infection in cotton rats by passive transfer of monoclonal antibodies. Infect Immunol 1984; 43: 756.

Waris ME, Tsou C, Erdman DD, Zaki SR, Anderson LJ. Respiratory synctial virus infection in BALB/c mice previously immunized with formalin-inactivated virus induces enhanced pulmonary inflammatory response with a predominant Th2-like cytokine pattern. J Virol 1996; 705: 2852.

Watt PJ, Zardis M, Lambden PR. Age related IgG subclass response to respiratory syncytial virus fusion protein in infected infants. Clin Exp Immunol 1986; 643: 503.

Weitkamp JH, Lafleur BJ, Greenberg HB, Crowe Jr. JE. Natural evolution of a human virus-specific antibody gene repertoire by somatic hypermutation requires both hotspot-directed and randomly directed processes. Hum Immunol 2005; 666: 666.

Welliver RC, Kaul TN, Putnam TI, Sun M, Riddlesberger K, Ogra PL. The antibody response to primary and secondary infection with respiratory syncytial virus: kinetics of class-specific responses. J Pediatr 1980; 965: 808.

Weltzin R, Hsu SA, Mittler ES, Georgakopoulos K, Monath TP. Intranasal monoclonal immunoglobulin A against respiratory syncytial virus protects against upper and lower respiratory tract infections in mice. Antimicrob Agents Chemother 1994; 3812: 2785.

Wenzel SE, Gibbs RL, Lehr MV, Simoes EA. Respiratory outcomes in high-risk children 7 to 10 years after prophylaxis with respiratory syncytial virus immune globulin. Am J Med 2002; 1128: 627.

Werling D, Collins RA, Taylor G, Howard CJ. Cytokine responses of bovine dendritic cells and T cells following exposure to live or inactivated bovine respiratory syncytial virus. J Leuk Biol 2002; 72: 297.

Wong DT, Rosenbrand M, Hovey K, Ogra PL. Respiratory syncytial virus infection in immunosuppressed animals: implications in human infection. J Med Virol 1985; 17: 359.

Wright PF, Gruber WC, Peters M, Reed G, Zhu Y, Robinson F, Coleman-Dockery S, Graham BS. Illness severity, viral shedding, and antibody responses in infants hospitalized with bronchiolitis caused by respiratory syncytial virus. J Infect Dis 2002; 1858: 1011.

Wright PF, Karron RA, Belshe RB, Thompson J, Crowe Jr. JE, Boyce TG, Halburnt LL, Reed GW, Whitehead SS, Anderson EL, Wittek AE, Casey R, Eichelberger M, Thumar B, Randolph VB, Udem SA, Chanock RM, Murphy BR. Evaluation of a live, cold-passaged, temperature-sensitive, respiratory syncytial virus vaccine candidate in infancy. J Infect Dis 2000; 1825: 1331.

Zhang L, Peeples ME, Boucher RC, Collins PL, Pickles RJ. Respiratory syncytial virus infection of human airway epithelial cells is polarized, specific to ciliated cells, and without obvious cytopathology. J Virol 2002; 76: 5654.

Respiratory Syncytial Virus
Patricia Cane (Editor)

DOI 10.1016/S0168-7069(06)14003-3

Molecular Epidemiology and Evolution of RSV

Patricia Cane
Virus Reference Department, Health Protection Agency, UK

Introduction

Respiratory syncytial virus (RSV) provides an excellent model for the study of the link between epidemic processes and pathogen evolution. The virus is an important human pathogen, causing considerable morbidity in infants and vulnerable adults. Almost all infants are infected before they are 2 years old, with their severity of illness ranging from a mild upper respiratory tract illness to severe lower respiratory tract disease (Hall et al., 1976; Report to the Medical Research Council Subcommittee on Respiratory Syncytial Virus Vaccines, 1978; Glezen et al., 1981; Cox et al., 1998). RSV causes predictable well-defined epidemics with many hospitalisations during which clinical samples are taken for diagnostic purposes. In addition, unlike influenza virus, there is no modulating effect of vaccination. Thus, it has been possible to undertake extensive studies on the variability of RSV strains in many epidemics and from around the world. This has allowed a detailed analysis of the molecular epidemiology and evolution of the virus and these are the topics covered in this chapter.

RSV groups and genotypes

RSV can be divided into two groups, A and B, which can be distinguished antigenically with polyclonal animal sera (Coates et al., 1966) and monoclonal antibodies (Anderson et al., 1985; Mufson et al., 1985; Gimenez et al., 1986), and which are also distinct at the nucleotide sequence level (Johnson et al., 1987; Johnson and Collins, 1988, 1989). The most variable protein between the groups is the attachment (G) protein which shows 47% amino acid differences between the prototype strains of the different groups (Johnson et al., 1987). There are conflicting reports concerning the relative severity of disease caused by the two groups of the viruses

(Walsh et al., 1997; Brandenburg et al., 2000; Martinello et al., 2002; Papadopoulos et al., 2004).

Variability of isolates within the groups A and B of RSV was initially demonstrated with respect to differences in reactions with monoclonal antibodies (Orvell et al., 1987; Storch and Park, 1987; Akerlind et al., 1988; Anderson et al., 1991; Nagai et al., 1993), and then by using ribonuclease (RNase) A mismatch cleavage methods (Storch et al., 1989, 1991; Cristina et al., 1991). Nucleotide sequencing of the G gene showed that the amino acid variability was up to 20% within the groups (Cane et al., 1991; Sullender et al., 1991).

Reverse transcription of viral RNA followed by amplification using the polymerase chain reaction (RT-PCR) of part of the G gene and then restriction digestion analysis (RFLP) is a rapid technique that can be used to screen large numbers of clinical samples from epidemics in order to obtain an estimate of the variability within an epidemic (Cane et al., 1991, 1992; Sullender et al., 1993). Phylogenetic analysis of G gene nucleotide sequences has allowed the definition of a number of genotypes or lineages of RSV belonging to both groups A and B (Cane et al., 1992, 1994; Peret et al., 1998). The nomenclature of the genotypes is not consistent between laboratories, and it is clear that new genotypes are continuing to emerge while others are no longer detectable (see section on Evolution of RSV).

Structure of epidemics

It has been known for many years that RSV causes annual epidemics during the winter in temperate climates. In the UK the annual epidemic usually peaks around December. Similar annual epidemics occur in many temperate countries, though there are exceptions such as Finland where every two years there is a minor peak of RSV activity in April followed by a major peak in December (Waris, 1991). In the USA, RSV activity often peaks slightly later, around February, but the cause of these variations is unknown (Felton et al., 2004). In the tropics, RSV outbreaks are often associated with the rainy season in those countries with seasonal rainfall and have also been associated with religious festivals (Hazlett et al., 1988; Nwankwo et al., 1988; Cherian et al., 1990; Sung et al., 1992; Weber et al., 1998). In South Africa, RSV epidemics also occur in the autumn and winter in HIV-negative children. However, it was found that in HIV-positive infants RSV isolation was not limited by season, but instead could occur throughout the year (Madhi et al., 2000). It may be that this is due to prolonged excretion of virus by these immune-compromised individuals.

The cause of the strict seasonality of RSV epidemics is not known but it seems likely that social conditions such as the return to school after the long summer break in developed countries or indoor crowding during the rainy seasons in the tropics are contributing factors.

There has been extensive analysis of strain variability within epidemics. These studies have almost invariably focused on isolates obtained from hospitalised infants. Initial studies using monoclonal antibodies showed that both groups of RSV co-circulate in epidemics, although their relative incidence may vary. In general, throughout the world, group A isolates are more often detected than group B isolates (Hendry et al., 1986, 1989; Tsutsumi et al., 1988; Hall et al., 1990; Freymuth et al., 1991; Salomon et al., 1991; Mlinaric-Galinovic et al., 1994; Carballal et al., 2000; Rajala et al., 2003; Fodha et al., 2004). In Birmingham, UK, a cyclic triennial pattern in groups A and B has been observed (Cane, 2001), while in Finland the group dominance appears to alternate every two years (Waris, 1991). Mathematical modelling of these data has suggested that the group dominance patterns can be explained by reductions in susceptibility to, and infectiousness of, secondary homologous and heterologous infections (White et al., 2005).

The constitution of epidemics over 11 years from 1989 in Birmingham, UK, was examined using RT-PCR and RFLP, combined with G gene sequencing (Cane and Pringle, 1992; Cane et al., 1994; Cane, 2001). The results are shown in Fig. 1. Group A isolates were most commonly detected in eight of the epidemics, but with group B predominating every third year, namely in 1992–1993, 1995–1996, and 1998–1999. Each epidemic was made up of multiple genotypes, with the proportions varying year by year. There appeared to be yearly replacement of the most common genotype with genotypes predominating in one year being usually less abundant the following season. One genotype (A:5 in Fig. 1) that was common at the beginning of the study was not detected at all after a couple of years.

A community-based study of RSV variability was carried out in Birmingham between 1995 and 1998, to compare the strains being detected in hospitalised babies with those in patients presenting to their general practitioner with influenza-like illness. It was found that very similar viruses were circulating in these two groups of patients (Zambon et al., 2001). A study conducted in South Africa compared RSV isolates from infants attending rural community clinics with isolates from hospitalised infants in Soweto near Johannesburg. This found that the same RSV strains could cause mild upper-respiratory tract infections, lower-respiratory tract infections, and severe RSV disease in infants (Venter et al., 2002). Similar results were obtained from a study of a cohort of babies in Kenya (Nokes et al., 2004; Scott et al., 2004). These results suggest that it is reasonable to conclude that although analyses of samples from hospitalised babies provide information about only a highly selected subset of infections, such data can be extrapolated to the epidemics as a whole.

Analyses of the genotypic make-up of RSV epidemics world-wide have yielded mainly similar overall results. For example, Choi and Lee (2000) looked at epidemics in Seoul, Korea and found that multiple strains were present in each epidemic and that the dominant strain was repeatedly replaced. Seki et al. (2001) and Kuroiwa et al. (2005) found similar results from studies of 15–20 years of RSV epidemics in Japan. Interestingly, in the Japanese studies, the genotype A5 (also designated GA1 in some studies), which had been common in Birmingham, UK, in the 1980s and then disappeared as mentioned above, was likewise detected in the1980s in Japan but was subsequently undetectable. In addition, the Korean group failed to detect group A genotype A5 in their study which commenced in 1990.

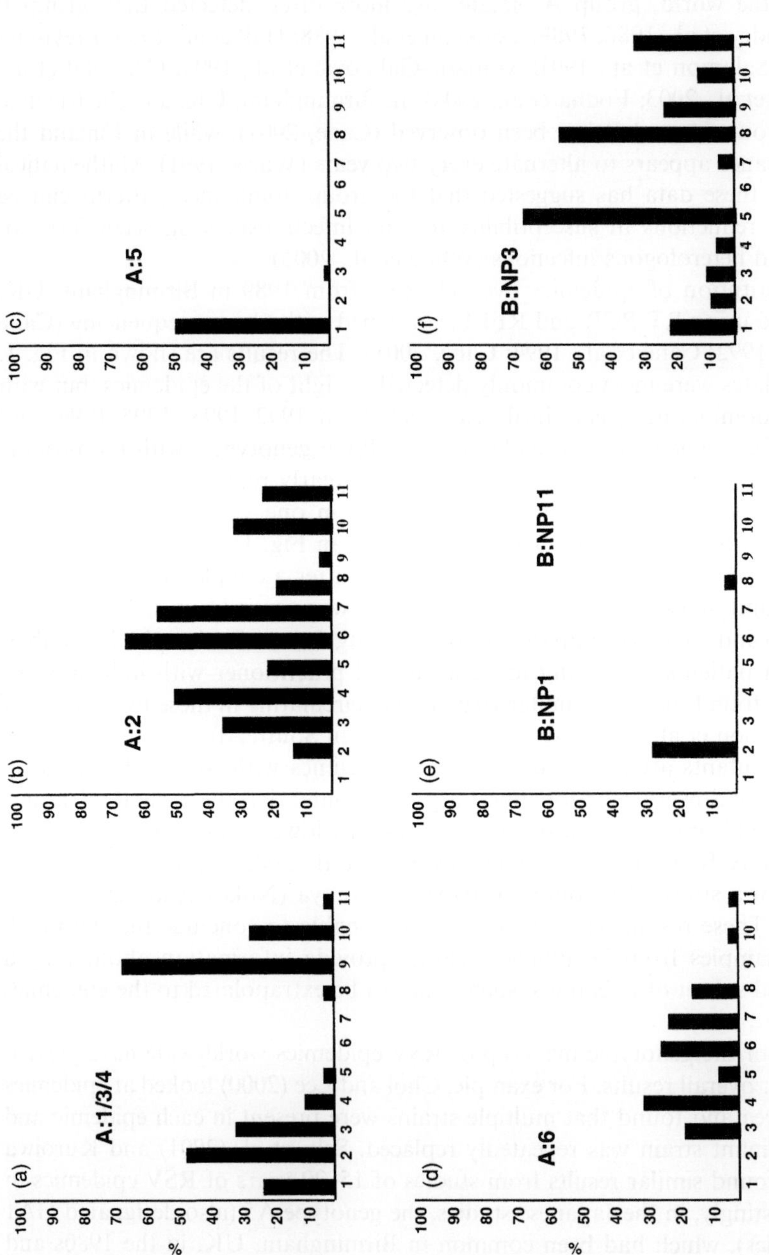

Fig. 1 The relative incidence of different genotypes of RSV in epidemics in Birmingham, UK, from 1988 to 1999 inclusive. The vertical axes show the percent of the genotypes in each epidemic while the horizontal axes represent the epidemics. Panels (a)–(f) present the data for a single genotype except panel (e) in which two group B genotypes are shown (Cane et al., 1994; Cane, 2001; and unpublished data).

Peret et al. (1998) looked at five RSV epidemics in Rochester USA from 1990. They also found multiple genotypes in each epidemic, with no particular genotype predominating for more than one season. Similar results were also obtained over three years of the same period in Birmingham, Alabama (Coggins et al., 1998). In these studies in the USA, the group A genotype A5 was abundant in Rochester in the 1994–1995 epidemic, and was detected in Birmingham, Alabama in 1993 and 1995.

In contrast, a study of RSV variability from Stockholm found that one group A genotype was predominant in four epidemics between 2000 and 2004, but the numbers of samples examined for each epidemic were small and only group A viruses were analysed (Rafiefard et al., 2004). Again this study found genotype A5 only in the early years of the study. Thus, it would appear that a genotype A5 (or GA1 in the designation of Peret et al., 1998) was common before the mid-1990s but has been rarely detected since. This observation is of particular interest as the candidate vaccine strains based on the prototype laboratory strain A2 belong to this genotype.

RSV epidemics in the tropics tend to be less predictable in terms of date of occurrence but the patterns of multiple strains of virus in the epidemics continue to be observed including in the Gambia, Kenya, Mozambique, and South Africa (Cane et al., 1999; Roca et al., 2001; Venter et al., 2001; Scott et al., 2004).

A number of studies have examined the extent to which epidemics within the same country are caused by similar strains. Christensen et al. (1999) compared epidemics in Copenhagen with those in other districts of Denmark: they found that almost identical results were obtained from different hospitals in Copenhagen, but that differences were observed between the regions. The variability of RSV during one epidemic season was also examined in geographically diverse locations in North America (Rochester, Houston, Birmingham, St Louis, and Winnipeg). As expected, each community showed a number of distinct genotypes but the predominant strains and overall patterns of circulating genotypes were different for three of the five communities. Thus, there was no detection of one predominant genotype for North America for that season (Peret et al., 2000).

Variability of RSV during outbreaks among small groups of individuals has been examined using monoclonal antibodies and RNase A mismatching. RSV was isolated from residents living in two separate halls of an institution and it was found that different strains of virus were circulating in each of the halls (Finger et al., 1987). RSV can be responsible for outbreaks of severe disease in bone marrow transplant units. In these outbreaks, several different strains have been observed and it was concluded that there was some nosocomial transmission within the outbreaks combined with independent introductions into the units (Harrington et al., 1992; McCarthy et al., 1999).

The mechanism underlying the commonly observed replacement of the predominant genotype year-on-year is unknown. It could be that there is accumulation of herd immunity, which then restricts the circulation of a previously dominant strain but it is not known whether emergence of a new predominant variant is a necessary prerequisite for an epidemic to occur. The most common strain observed in a particular epidemic has frequently been observed at low levels in the previous season. It is possible that a high level of maternal immunity present in the population after an epidemic of a particular strain of virus may result in diminution of severity of disease caused by that strain in infants born after the epidemic. Since most isolates analysed come from hospitalised babies this would result in an apparent decline in that strain, although, as mentioned above, there is little evidence of molecular differences between strains causing mild and severe disease within particular epidemics.

Geographic distribution of RSV strains

As described above, there is a considerable body of evidence showing that RSV epidemics are made up of multiple strains and that usually the predominant strain is replaced each year. The generation of nucleotide sequence data from viruses such as RSV became much easier and cheaper in the late 1980s with the development of RT-PCR combined with population sequencing of PCR products. This has provided a very large amount of nucleotide sequence data, which allow comparison of isolates from around the world at different times. The vast majority of sequencing has been performed on the G gene with smaller contributions from the F and SH genes (Cane and Pringle, 1991; Agenbach et al., 2005).

Although individual epidemics usually consist of multiple strains such that babies within the same clinics at the same time may be infected with distinct strains of RSV, it is clear that infections with very similar viruses may be occurring worldwide during the same season. For example, it was initially reported that very similar viruses had been isolated around the same time in Europe, USA, The Gambia, Malaysia, Uruguay and Australia (Cane et al., 1992; Cane and Pringle, 1995). This lack of geographical restriction of RSV strains has been repeatedly confirmed. Similar viruses have now been described in USA, Uruguay, Argentina, Brasil, Japan, many countries in Northern Europe, Mozambique, Korea, China, India, Kenya, The Gambia and Southern Africa (Garcia et al., 1994; Peret et al., 1998; Cane et al., 1999; Martinez et al., 1999; Choi and Lee, 2000; Roca et al., 2001; Seki et al., 2001; Venter et al., 2001; Baumeister et al., 2003; Frabasile et al., 2003; Madhi et al., 2003; Rajala et al., 2003; Kuroiwa et al., 2005; Scott et al., 2004; Blanc et al., 2005; Galiano et al., 2005). On occasions apparently new versions of the virus have been found which appeared to be geographically restricted, for example some strains described from The Gambia (Cane et al., 1999), Mozambique (Roca et al., 2001) and South Africa (Venter et al., 2001) but then similar strains are subsequently reported in other countries such as Japan and Brasil following more extensive analysis (Kuroiwa et al., 2005; Moura et al., 2004).

Thus, overall there appears to be very little geographic clustering of RSV strains and where this has been reported it may often be due to inadequate sampling or delayed reporting of strain variability, particularly from less developed parts of the world. As the virus is constantly accumulating genetic and antigenic change (see below), this implies that when a new strain arises it is able to spread very rapidly around the world.

The G protein

The RSV attachment (G) protein is a type II glycoprotein which is produced in two forms (Wertz et al., 1985, 1989): first, a transmembrane form with an N terminal cytoplasmic tail and second, a soluble form which is truncated at the N terminus. The full-length G molecule is synthesised as a 32 kDa precursor, which is then modified including the addition of O- and N-linked oligosaccharides to give a molecule with a final mobility on SDS-PAGE equivalent to 80–90 kDa. The soluble form is generated by initiation at an alternative in-frame AUG triplet located in the hydrophobic domain followed by proteolytic removal of the signal/anchor domain (Hendricks et al., 1988; Roberts et al., 1994) and then secreted extracellularly.

The ectodomain of the G protein has two highly variable mucin-like domains, which are separated by a short conserved central region which includes a 13 amino acid segment (amino acids 164–176) which is identical between virtually all wild-type isolates. This segment overlaps with a short conserved cysteine-rich region with cysteine residues at codons 173, 176, 182 and 186 (Johnson et al., 1987; Cane et al., 1991; Sullender et al., 1991). Recent evidence suggests that this cysteine-rich region can inhibit innate immunity by modulation of cytokine production and thus this may be a key function of the secreted form of the G protein (Polack et al., 2005). The G protein has also been shown to have structural similarities with the CX3C chemokine fractaline and to induce leucocyte chemotaxis *in vitro* (Tripp et al., 2001). The molecular biology of the G protein is described in more detail in the first chapter of this volume.

The diversity of the G protein lies in the mucin-like regions, both in the amino acid variation and in the length of the protein. The mucin-like nature of the protein is derived from the high proline, serine and threonine content with the latter residues allowing high levels of O-linked glycosylation (Wertz et al., 1985). The transmembrane form of this protein varies between 254 and 319 amino acids in length, according to the position of the stop codon as illustrated in Fig. 2 for group B viruses (Cane and Pringle, 1995; Martinez et al., 1999; Zlateva et al., 2004, 2005).

Evolution of RSV

When we started looking at the variability of the G gene in clinical isolates from the late 1980s and early 1990s, it was immediately apparent that currently circulating strains had G gene nucleotide sequences that were markedly different from those of the prototype strains isolated in the 1950s and 1960s (Cane et al., 1991; Sullender et al., 1991). A collection of group A samples from across this time range was therefore sequenced (Cane and Pringle, 1995) and it was possible to show that

1. In the variable domains of the G gene non-synonymous changes were more frequent than synonymous changes.
2. There was an accumulation of nucleotide and amino acid changes with time. The rate of accumulation of amino acid changes over the whole molecule was estimated at about 0.25% per year.

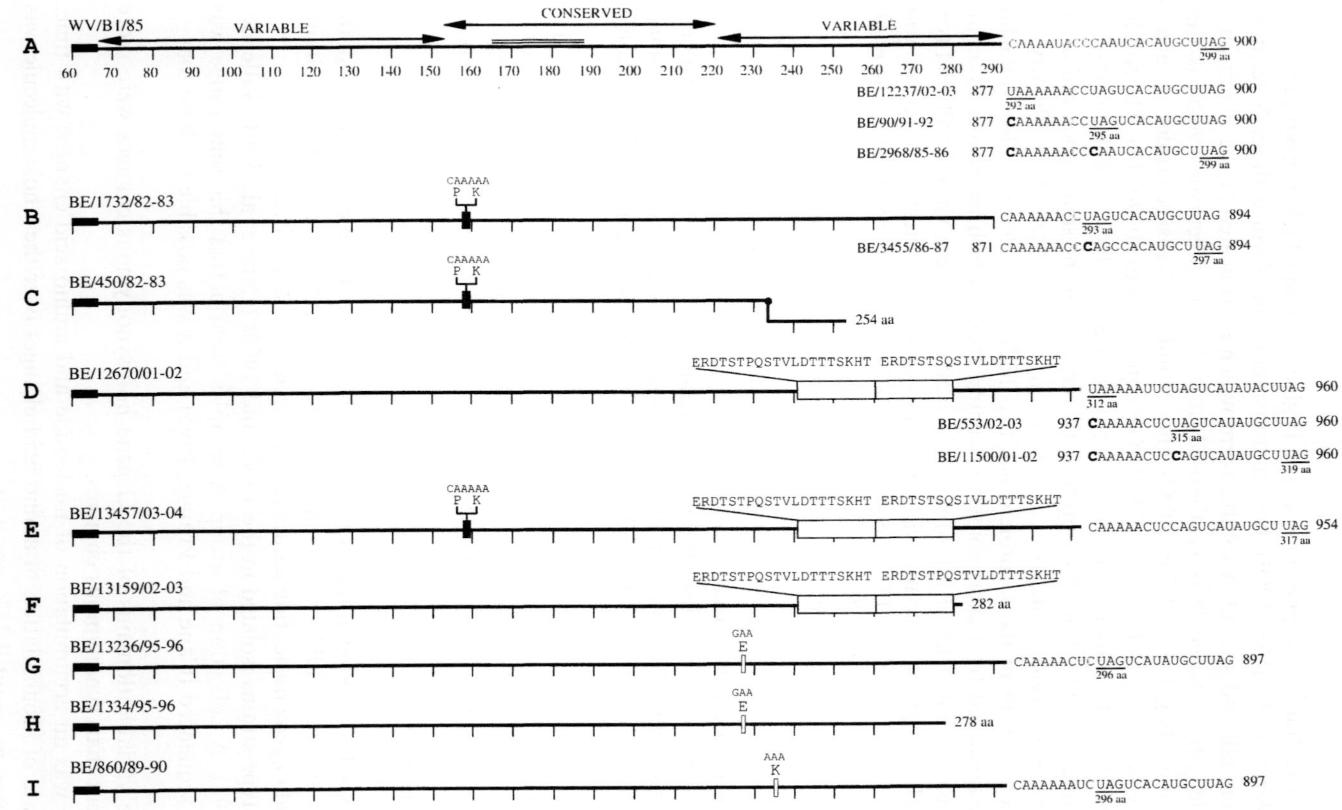

A
WV/B1/85
VARIABLE
CONSERVED
VARIABLE
60 70 80 90 100 110 120 130 140 150 160 170 180 190 200 210 220 230 240 250 260 270 280 290
CAAAAUACCCAAUCACAUGCUUAG 900
299 aa
BE/12237/02-03 877 UAAAAAACCUAGUCACAUGCUUAG 900
292 aa
BE/90/91-92 877 CAAAAAACCUAGUCACAUGCUUAG 900
295 aa
BE/2968/85-86 877 CAAAAAACCCAAUCACAUGCUUAG 900
299 aa
B
BE/1732/82-83
CAAAAA
P K
CAAAAAACCUAGUCACAUGCUUAG 894
293 aa
BE/3455/86-87 871 CAAAAAACCCAGCCACAUGCUUAG 894
297 aa
C
BE/450/82-83
CAAAAA
P K
254 aa
D
BE/12670/01-02
ERDTSTPQSTVLDTTTSKHT ERDTSTSQSIVLDTTTSKHT
UAAAAAUUCUAGUCAUAUACUUAG 960
312 aa
BE/553/02-03 937 CAAAAACUCUAGUCAUAUGCUUAG 960
315 aa
BE/11500/01-02 937 CAAAAACUCCAGUCAUAUGCUUAG 960
319 aa
E
BE/13457/03-04
CAAAAA
P K
ERDTSTPQSTVLDTTTSKHT ERDTSTSQSIVLDTTTSKHT
CAAAAACUCCAGUCAUAUGCUUAG 954
317 aa
F
BE/13159/02-03
ERDTSTPQSTVLDTTTSKHT ERDTSTPQSTVLDTTTSKHT
282 aa
G
BE/13236/95-96
GAA
E
CAAAAACUCUAGUCAUAUGCUUAG 897
296 aa
H
BE/1334/95-96
GAA
E
278 aa
I
BE/860/89-90
AAA
K
CAAAAAAUCUAGUCACAUGCUUAG 897
296 aa

3. The changes resulted in the emergence of new lineages with a "cactus"-like shape to the phylogenetic tree.
4. The accumulation of amino acid change was associated with changes in the reaction of the strains with a panel of monoclonal antibodies.
5. The hypothetical ancestor of the group A viruses was estimated to have been present in the 1940s.

This pattern of human RSV evolution resembles that of influenza B viruses (Rota et al., 1992; McCullers et al., 2004). Subsequently, these observations have been extended and G gene sequences subject to stringent analysis for positive selection. Woelk and Holmes (2001) identified six positively selected sites in the G protein in both A and B group, although only one site was shared by both groups but no positively selected site was identified by these workers in bovine RSV (BRSV). Zlateva et al. (2004, 2005) also examined the evolution of groups A and B RSV. They calculated a rate of accumulation of 1.83×10^{-3} nucleotide substitutions/site/year over 629 nucleotides omitting the conserved amino terminal region for the A strains, and also suggested that the most recent common ancestor (MRCA) of RSV A strains was from the early 1940s. In group B strains the rate of accumulation of nucleotide changes was found to be 1.95×10^{-3} nucleotide substitutions/site/year (as illustrated in Fig. 3), and that the MRCA of B group viruses was between 1938 and 1955. In addition, these authors suggested that the divergence of the group A and B strains occurred about 350 years ago.

However, analysis of the G genes of 23 isolates of RSV from Havana, Cuba, in 1994–1995 showed that these belonged to a strain that had only five nucleotide changes relative to the long strain isolated in 1956 in USA. So for those years it appeared that the situation on Cuba was markedly different to that observed elsewhere with relative homogeneity in the epidemics and those epidemics being made up of an ancient strain (Valdes et al., 1998), and that identical strains were detected in two epidemic seasons. It may be that the differences in seasonality of RSV infections in Cuba along with restrictions on travel may favour relative viral

Fig. 2 Schematic diagrams presenting the predicted G protein length variability among HRSV-B Belgian isolates. The linear presentations are given according to the reference strain WV/B1/85 with the two variable regions and the central conserved region (residues 153–221) indicated above the top diagram. The absolutely conserved amino acid region (amino acid positions 164–187) among the HRSV-B isolates is indicated with a double line (A). The underlined sequences present alternative termination codons described previously (Sullender et al., 1991), and the predicted full protein lengths of Belgian representative sequences are given. The six-nucleotide deletion is indicated with a filled box (B, C, and E), the 60 nucleotide duplication is indicated (see below) with a large open and divided box (D–F), and the three-nucleotide insertions are indicated with a small open box (G to I). The position of the frame shifting a frameshift mutant is indicated (•) in panel C. The two premature terminated sequences with their respective protein lengths are presented in panels F and H. Adapted from and reproduced with permission from Zlateva et al. (2005).

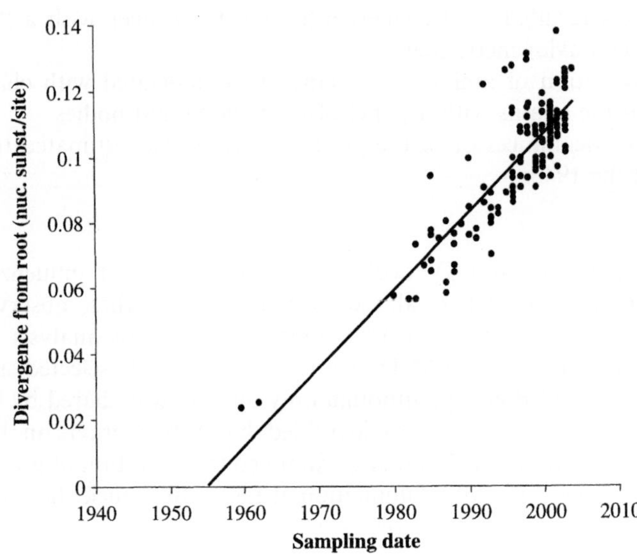

Fig. 3 Linear root-to-tip regression plot presenting the correlation between the branch lengths and the sampling dates of the HRSV-B isolates included in Zlateva et al. (2005). Reproduced with permission from Zlateva et al. (2005).

stability. It will be interesting to see if this situation persists with the increased tourism from Western Europe particularly in the winter months.

BRSV evolution has also been examined and provided intriguing results since vaccination is used in parts of Europe and thus may modify the epidemiology of the virus. Valarcher et al. (2000) showed that continuous evolution of the sequences of the N, G and F proteins of BRSV had been occurring in isolates since 1967 in countries where vaccination of cattle was widely implemented. In contrast to the analysis of Woelk and Holmes (2001), they presented evidence of positive selective pressure on the mucin-like region of the G protein and on particular sites of the N and F proteins. In addition, they observed mutations in the conserved central hydrophobic part of the ectodomain of the G protein and which resulted in the loss of the four highly conserved cysteine residues in some recent French BRSV isolates. Such loss of the conserved cysteine residues has been reported in antibody escape mutants of human RSV but never in natural human isolates (Rueda et al., 1994). Thus, it may be that use of an inactivated RSV vaccine in cattle has provided a selective pressure that has resulted in the apparent generation of escape mutants.

Emergence of new lineages

Since there appears to be a relatively steady accumulation of amino acid changes with time as illustrated in Fig. 3, it becomes increasingly difficult to designate the lineage or genotype of a particular new isolate. For example, delineation of genotypes using isolates from the 1970s would lead to very different designations than those derived using current isolates (Cane and Pringle, 1995). Thus, it would probably be more useful and flexible to move away from a rigid classification of isolates, although such schemes are very useful for comparing strains isolated during particular time periods.

In addition, the steady replacement of strains with slightly different versions makes it difficult to be sure whether a new strain has emerged and spread or whether there has simply been evolution locally of a particular lineage. However, in recent years Mother Nature has provided an excellent example of a readily identifiable new strain. This strain is a B group virus with a 60 nucleotide insertion in the G gene encoding a 20 amino acid reduplication in the variable region of the ectodomain of the G protein (Trento et al., 2003). It is highly unlikely that such a major gene "event" would have arisen more than once and this reduplication provides a readily detectable natural tag that can be used to track the dissemination and transmission of a novel strain of RSV. Isolates with this insertion were first detected in Buenos Aires in South America in June–August 1999 (Trento et al., 2003) and then in Belgium in December 1999–2000 (Zlateva et al., 2005) and in Birmingham, UK, in 2000–2001 (Cane, unpublished results). They were detected in Sapporo in Japan first in 2000 (Nagai et al., 2004; Sato et al., 2005), in North America in 2001 and in Kenya in 2003 (Scott et al., 2004). The degree of surveillance of strain variation of course varies with place and time, but such strains were not detected at all before 1999 including in epidemics intensively examined around the world in the preceding years. Fig. 4 shows distribution of this new strain worldwide with time since 1999 and illustrates how a newly emergent strain of RSV can attain world-wide distribution extremely rapidly (Trento et al., 2006). Although this novel strain was first detected in South America, we cannot of course be sure of the actual geographic origin of this new virus.

While the newly emergent B group virus with the 20 amino acid insertion on the G protein was detected in Belgium first in 1999–2000 it did not become the predominant strain there until 2001–2002, i.e., two years later. Thus, emergence of such a new variant does not automatically result in that variant becoming the predominant strain immediately.

The G genes of strains with the 60 nucleotide insertion have continued to accumulate change. Zlateva et al. (2005) have examined this further evolution in detail by comparison of isolates from Belgium from 1999 to 2003. They have observed that there has been further variation in the duplicated region along with changes in the position of the stop codon, and also a deletion of 6 nucleotides in one strain. Thus, the predicted amino acid lengths of the G proteins of these samples include 282, 312, 315, 317 and 319 amino acids. This is illustrated in Fig. 2. Trento et al. (2006) have likewise examined samples with this reduplication from Buenos Aires. They also showed further changes in the reduplicated segment at a rate apparently higher than in other regions of the G protein gene.

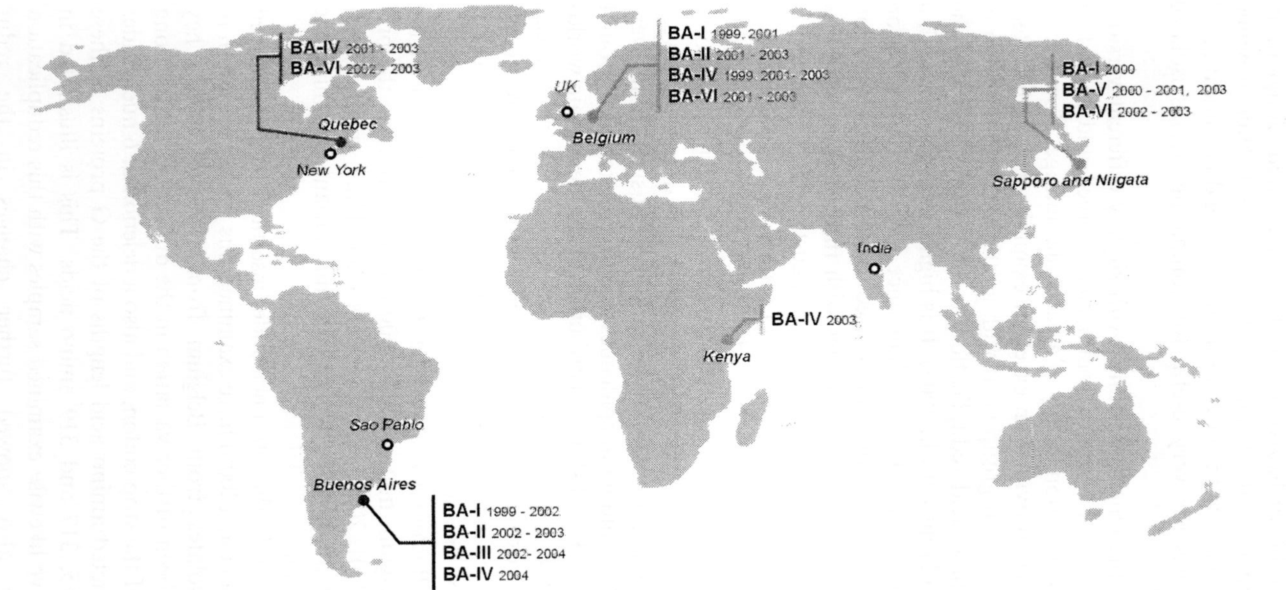

Fig. 4 The locations from which HRSV G sequences with the duplicated segment have been reported are indicated in the map indicating Buenos Aires (BA) branches and isolation years of samples. Samples from India, Rochester, New York, and Sao Paulo, and UK (indicated by empty dots in the map) containing sequences with the 60 nucleotide duplication have been reported in meetings, but details of those samples are still unavailable. Reproduced from Trento et al. (2006) with permission.

Disappearance of lineages

Phylogenetic analysis of the G gene sequences of strains from around the world isolated since 1956 showed that one group A lineage was clearly an outlier from other strains without any determinable linkage to other isolates other than clearly being group A. This cluster made up of 5 isolates from Sweden and the UK, isolated in the early 1970s (Cane and Pringle, 1995). So it appears that viruses belonging to this cluster were circulating widely at least in Northern Europe. However, in all the extensive analyses of current isolates, such viruses have never been detected since 1972, so it seems reasonable to deduce that this lineage is now extinct. Likewise as mentioned above it may be that the lineage represented by the prototype A strains A2 and Long which was common up until the late 1980s and early 1990s has not been detected in recent years in the developed world so it seems that that lineage is not a major contributor to disease at the present time. It will be interesting to determine whether this lineage reemerges at some time in the future or whether it becomes extinct.

Mechanism of selection of new strains

As discussed above, the evidence is now very strong that there can be progressive accumulation of genetic and antigenic change in the G protein of RSV isolates. One consequence of this is that the monoclonal antibody panels that can be used for characterisation of isolates have become steadily less useful since the antibodies that react with the variable epitopes tend increasingly to fail to react with any of the currently circulating strains.

Early studies on neutralisation of RSV with polyclonal animal sera showed differences between strains (Coates et al., 1966) but it is much more difficult to show such discrimination using human sera. This is largely because most RSV proteins other than the G protein show a high degree of antigenic similarity between the groups, and little variability at the lineage level. Even in the case of the highly variable G protein, the conserved central area of the protein provides cross-reactivity between the groups. Such cross-reactions mean that the dissection out of a strain specific antibody response is challenging.

The antigenic structure of the group A G protein has been extensively studied using both monoclonal antibodies and human convalescent sera. Three types of epitopes have been identified in the G protein using panels of monoclonal antibodies. These are (i) conserved epitopes which are found in all strains of RSV; (ii) group-specific epitopes which are shared by all strains belonging to the same group; and (iii) strain-specific or variable epitopes that are found in only some isolates of the same group (Melero et al., 1997). In general, the conserved and group-specific epitopes have been located in the central conserved region of the G protein while most of the strain-specific epitopes map to the carboxy-terminal variable region (Garcia-Barreno et al., 1989, 1990; Palomo et al., 1991; Rueda et al., 1991, 1995). However, although most strain-specific epitopes recognised by mouse monoclonal antibodies were mapped to the variable carboxy region of the G protein, for some time it was difficult to map any elements of the human antibody response to this region. It would be reasonable to assume that such a response would be a prerequisite for selection to be occurring in this region.

Attempts to map antigenic sites using overlapping peptides showed that only the conserved central region of the protein reacted with human convalescent sera and those authors concluded that the carboxy terminal part of the protein was not antigenically important (Norrby et al., 1987). Hence, it is difficult to imagine what the selective pressure could be that was apparently selecting for antigenic change in the variable regions of RSV G protein. However, this work used peptides whose sequence were based on old laboratory strains of RSV while, as mentioned above, current isolates have very different carboxy terminal amino acid sequences to those strains.

In order to search for potential antigenic sites in the variable regions of the G protein, it was necessary to match the infecting genotype of virus with the appropriate convalescent antiserum, i.e., to obtain paired virus isolates and acute and convalescent antisera from the same patients (Cane et al., 1996). Using recombinant fusion proteins of glutathione *S*-transferase (GST) and the carboxy terminal region of G proteins representing various lineages expressed in *Escherichia coli*, it was found that the antibody response to this region of the G protein was highly genotype specific (Cane et al., 1996). This result was confirmed using the Luminex multiplex detection system with bacterially expressed protein (Jones et al., 2002) and also by using glycosylated protease-resistant fragments of purified native G protein (Palomo et al., 2000). To further complicate the issue of antigenic variation in the G protein, it has also been shown that host cell type can affect its glycosylation and antigenicity (Garcia-Beato et al., 1996; Garcia-Beato and Melero, 2000).

These strain-specific epitopes were further analysed using overlapping peptides based on the carboxy-terminal 85 amino acids of G protein to delinate linear epitopes recognised by human convalescent antibody. As mentioned above, the recognition of the epitopes was highly dependent on both the amino acid sequence of the peptides and on the infecting genotype of virus. Four different antigenic sites in this region of the G protein (amino acids 229–240, 250–258, 265–273 and 283–291) were recognised by the convalescent baby sera tested, although only one serum was found that reacted with more than one of the sites. All the sites represent potential N-linked glycosylation sites in at least some isolates, though not necessarily in the sequence recognised by the sera (Cane, 1997).

The amino acid sequences in natural isolates of the G protein regions implicated as antigenic sites are extremely variable. Peptides were then synthesised to represent all the observed natural variants of these epitopes and the reactions of these peptides with convalescent sera examined. An example of the reactions of a convalescent baby serum with these variant peptides is shown in Fig. 5. The serum reacted with peptides derived from amino acids 265–273 and 283–291. The sequence of the infecting strain of virus was that shown in peptides 3–3 for the second of these sites. The crucial change that abrogated antibody recognition in this case

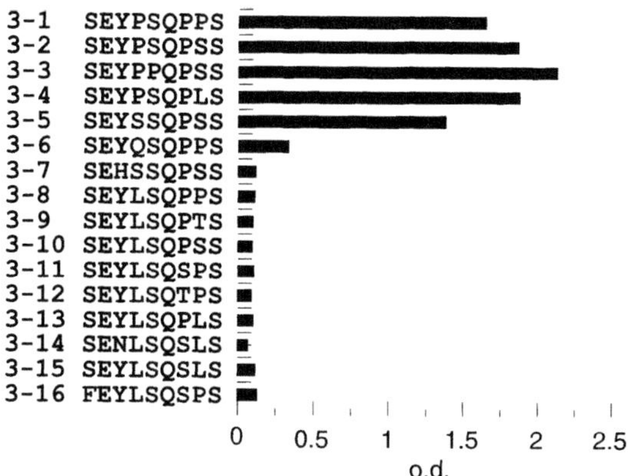

Fig. 5 Reaction in an enzyme-linked immunoassay (x-axis) of a baby RSV convalescent serum with peptides based on natural variants of residues 283-291 of the G protein of group A isolates (y-axis). Peptide 3-3 represents the sequence of the infecting virus. The crucial change that abrogated antibody recognition in this case was change of residue 4, proline, to leucine. Change of this residue to serine appeared to have no effect unless residue 3, tyrosine, was also changed to histidine (peptide 3-7) while change of the residue to glutamine reduced but did not eliminate antibody binding. Adapted from Cane (1997) (for colour version: see colour section on page 325).

was change of residue 4, proline, to leucine. Change of this residue to serine appeared to have no effect unless residue 3, tyrosine, was also changed to histidine (peptides 3–7) while change of the residue to glutamine reduced but did not eliminate antibody binding.

The antigenic sites determined using the human convalescent sera did not in the main correspond exactly with the amino acids showing mutations in murine monoclonal antibody neutralisation escape mutants and few human convalescent sera show competition in ELISA with murine monoclonals (Palomo et al., 2000). However, amino acids 283–291 do overlap with one monoclonal antibody escape mutation site. One neutralising monoclonal antibody reacts only with natural isolates that show a leucine residue at position 4 of this site while escape mutants to this monoclonal antibody change this residue to proline. Thus neutralisation escape *in vitro* was found to occur by varying the same residue that also determined the binding of a human convalescent serum as described above (Cane, 1997).

Paradox

There is a paradox with the hypothesis that antigenic drift of a virus occurs as a consequence of selection by the immune response. In the experimental version of antigenic drift, i.e., selection of an antibody escape mutant by a monoclonal antibody, this is only observed in the presence of a single monoclonal antibody. This is because the likelihood of two or more appropriate independent amino acids substitutions occurring simultaneously is vanishingly low. It is therefore difficult to envisage how a polyclonal serum induced during a natural infection with a virus such as HIV, influenza virus or RSV could select for single amino acid changes. There is some evidence that serum–antibody responses in influenza may be biased towards single epitopes (Lambkin et al., 1994; Lambkin and Dimmock, 1995; Cleveland et al., 1997) and it may be that a similar phenomenon is happening with RSV (Sullender and Edwards, 1999). Certainly, the convalescent sera examined in this study did not react equally with all the epitopes examined. Antigenic drift in RSV G protein is slow (about 0.25% amino acid change per year over the whole protein) in relation to the vast numbers of viral genomes produced during each annual epidemic which may infect most children and an estimated one in five adults. It would thus require only a rare individual with a very biased antibody response to provide the potential for selection of antigenic variants.

Reinfection with RSV

It has been known for many years that RSV can repeatedly reinfect individuals, although overall it appears that second and subsequent infections are generally less severe than the primary infection (Henderson et al., 1979; Glezen et al., 1986; Wilson et al., 2000). It has been proposed that reinfection could either be due to natural infection not providing a long lasting protective immunity or that variation in the virus enables it to evade the immune response. The observations that at the community level, the epidemics often show replacement of predominant genotype while at the same time there also appears to be positive selection on the G protein, would favour the concept of viral variation playing a role in susceptibility to reinfection. Thus, the molecular epidemiological evidence suggests that group or genotype infection prevalence influences future transmission of the homologous and heterologous variants within a population, a notion supported by recent mathematical modelling studies (White et al., 2005).

At the individual level, studies of RSV reinfection are few, particularly in the context of detailed characterisation of infecting strains. Natural reinfections with both the homologous and heterologous group of RSV have been shown. Mufson et al. (1987) reported 13 children (age range 6–49 months) with RSV infection who were subsequently reinfected at least nine months later. Six reinfections of group B occurred in 10 children initially infected with group A, and two group B reinfections occurred in three children initially infected with group B. Sullender et al. (1998) studied two children (aged 7 and 23 months at first infection) each with sequential (separated by over one year) group A virus infections, for whom the G protein amino acid sequences of the reinfecting viruses were up to 15% different. In a study of adult volunteers who were repeatedly challenged with the same strain of virus, Hall et al. (1991) found that reinfection could readily be achieved. The duration of immunity tended to increase after two closely spaced infections. Higher neutralising antibody levels before challenge correlated significantly with protection against infection. However, even in subjects with the highest antibody levels, the risk of reinfection was 25%. They suggested that humoral neutralising, F, and

G antibodies correlate with resistance to reinfection, but protection is far from complete and is of short duration.

Apparently persistent infection or repeated reinfection with RSV has been observed by Arbiza et al. (2006) in a child with immunosuppression due to HIV infection. This child had three distinct episodes of respiratory disease each two months apart, with viruses with identical G gene sequences isolated each time.

We have attempted to study natural reinfection by means of following a cohort of babies from birth and characterising the virus from each infection (Nokes et al., 2004). Apparent reinfections in the first year of life (i.e., two positive samples at least 14 days apart) were analysed from 12 infants. Four of these infants appeared to be persistently infected with the same strain of virus for up to seven weeks. Six infants were infected in both epidemics, four with RSV-A in the first epidemic followed by RSV-B in the second epidemic and two infected with RSV-A strains in both epidemics with no significant G gene sequence variability between samples. Two children showed infection and reinfection with different RSV-A strains within the same epidemic (Scott et al., 2006). Thus, there appeared to be little homologous protection detected in these babies. However, these babies were those that showed symptomatic reinfection. It may be that there were additional babies who showed solid resistance to reinfection and therefore were not included in the analysis. Further studies are ongoing to check the humoral antibody levels in a subset of the children in order to determine whether there were subclinical infections that were missed.

Conclusions

Study of the molecular epidemiology of RSV has provided considerable insight into this challenging virus, although it sometimes seems that more questions have been raised that answers provided. Clearly, the ultimate aim must be to develop a vaccine that provides protection against severe disease since the evidence indicates that it may not be possible to provide complete protection against infection. In the meantime, the use of prophylactic measures such as antibody preparations together with antiviral drugs and immune modulators will provide some defence against severe disease. These topics are reviewed and discussed in later chapters of this volume.

References

Agenbach E, Tiemessen CT, Venter M. Amino acid variation within the fusion protein of respiratory syncytial virus subtype A and B strains during annual epidemics in South Africa. Virus Genes 2005; 30: 267–278.

Akerlind B, Norrby E, Orvell C, Mufson MA. Respiratory syncytial virus: heterogeneity of subgroup B strains. J Gen Virol 1988; 69: 2145–2154.

Anderson LJ, Hendry RM, Pierik LT, Tsou C, McIntosh K. Multicentre study of strains of respiratory syncytial virus. J Infect Dis 1991; 163: 687–692.

Anderson LJ, Hierholzer JC, Tsou C, Hendry RM, Fernie BF, Stone Y, McIntosh K. Antigenic characterisation of respiratory syncytial virus strains with monoclonal antibodies. J Infect Dis 1985; 151: 626–633.

Arbiza J, Berois M, Delfraro A, Frabasile S, Mitoma FD, Milk R, Russi JC. Genetic characterization of respiratory syncytial viruses isolated from consecutive acute respiratory infections in a HIV infected child. J Clin Virol 2006; 35: 41–45.

Baumeister EG, Hunicken DS, Savy VL. RSV molecular characterization and specific antibody response in young children with acute lower respiratory infection. J Clin Virol 2003; 27: 44–51.

Blanc A, Delfraro A, Frabasile S, Arbiza J. Genotypes of respiratory syncytial virus group B identified in Uruguay. Arch Virol 2005; 150: 603–609.

Brandenburg AH, van Beek R, Moll HA, Osterhaus AD, Claas EC. G protein variation in respiratory syncytial virus group A does not correlate with clinical severity. J Clin Microbiol 2000; 38: 3849–3852.

Cane PA. Analysis of linear epitopes recognised by the primary human antibody response to a variable region of the attachment (G) protein of respiratory syncytial virus. J Med Virol 1997; 51: 297–304.

Cane PA. Molecular epidemiology of respiratory syncytial virus. Rev Med Virol 2001; 11: 103–116.

Cane PA, Matthews DA, Pringle CR. Identification of variable domains of the attachment (G) protein of subgroup A respiratory syncytial viruses. J Gen Virol 1991; 72: 2091–2096.

Cane PA, Matthews DA, Pringle CR. Analysis of relatedness of subgroup A respiratory syncytial viruses isolated worldwide. Virus Res 1992; 25: 15–22.

Cane PA, Matthews DA, Pringle CR. Analysis of respiratory syncytial virus strain variation in successive epidemics in one city. J Clin Microbiol 1994; 32: 1–4.

Cane PA, Pringle CR. Respiratory syncytial virus heterogeneity during an epidemic: analysis by limited nucleotide sequencing (SH gene) and restriction mapping (N gene). J Gen Virol 1991; 72: 349–357.

Cane PA, Pringle CR. Molecular epidemiology of respiratory syncytial virus: rapid identification of subgroup A lineages. J Virol Methods 1992; 40: 297–306.

Cane PA, Pringle CR. Evolution of subgroup A respiratory syncytial virus: evidence for progressive accumulation of amino acid changes in the attachment protein. J Virol 1995; 69: 2918–2925.

Cane PA, Thomas HM, Simpson AF, Evans JE, Hart CA, Pringle CR. Analysis of the human serological immune response to a variable region of the attachment (G) protein of respiratory syncytial virus during primary infection. J Med Virol 1996; 48: 253–261.

Cane PA, Weber M, Sanneh M, Dackour R, Pringle CR, Whittle H. Molecular epidemiology of respiratory syncytial virus in The Gambia. Epidemiol Infect 1999; 122: 155–160.

Carballal G, Videla C, Sequeira MD, Mistchenko A, Requeijo PV, Arbiza J. Respiratory syncytial virus: changes in prevalence of subgroups A and B among Argentinian children, 1990–1996. J Med Virol 2000; 61: 275–279.

Cherian T, Simoes EA, Steinhoff MC, Chitra K, John M, Raghupathy P, John TJ. Bronchiolitis in tropical south India. Am J Dis Child 1990; 144: 1026–1030.

Choi EH, Lee HJ. Genetic diversity and molecular epidemiology of the G protein of subgroups A and B of respiratory syncytial virus isolated over 9 consecutive epidemics in Korea. J Infect Dis 2000; 181: 1547–1556.

Christensen LS, Larsen LB, Johansen J, Andersen EA, Wejse C, Klug B, Hornsleth A. The fluctuating pattern of various genome types of respiratory syncytial virus in Copenhagen and some other locations in Denmark. APMIS 1999; 107: 843–850.

Cleveland SM, Taylor HP, Dimmock NJ. Selection of neutralizing antibody escape mutants with type A influenza virus HA-specific polyclonal antisera: possible significance for antigenic drift. Epidemiol Infect 1997; 118: 149–154.

Coates HV, Alling DW, Chanock RM. An antigenic analysis of respiratory syncytial virus isolates by a plaque reduction neutralisation test. Am J Epidemiol 1966; 83: 299–313.

Coggins WB, Lefkowitz EJ, Sullender WM. Genetic variability among group A and B respiratory syncytial viruses in a children's hospital. J Clin Microbiol 1998; 36: 3552–3557.

Cox MJ, Azevedo RS, Cane PA, Massad E, Medley GF. Seroepidemiological study of respiratory syncytial virus in Sao Paulo state, Brazil. J Med Virol 1998; 55: 234–239.

Cristina J, Moya A, Arbiza J, Russi J, Hortal M, Albo C, Garcia-Barreno B, Garcia O, Melero JA, Portela A. Evolution of the G and P genes of human respiratory syncytial virus (subgroup A) studied by the RNase A mismatch cleavage method. Virology 1991; 184: 210–218.

Felton KJ, Pandya-Smith I, Curns AG, Fry AM, Anderson LJ, Keeler NM. Respiratory syncytial virus activity—United States, 2003–2004. MMWR 2004; 53: 1159–1160.

Finger R, Anderson LJ, Dicker RC, Harrison B, Doan R, Downing A, Corey L. Epidemic infections caused by respiratory syncytial virus in institutionalised young adults. J Infect Dis 1987; 155: 1335–1339.

Fodha I, Vabret A, Trabelsi A, Freymuth F. Epidemiological and antigenic analysis of respiratory syncytial virus in hospitalised Tunisian children, from 2000 to 2002. J Med Virol 2004; 72: 683–687.

Frabasile S, Delfraro A, Facal L, Videla C, Galiano M, de Sierra MJ, Ruchansky D, Vitureira N, Berois M, Carballal G, Russi J, Arbiza J. Antigenic and genetic variability of human respiratory syncytial viruses (group A) isolated in Uruguay and Argentina: 1993–2001. J Med Virol 2003; 71: 305–312.

Freymuth F, Petitjean J, Pothier P, Brouard J, Norrby E. Prevalence of respiratory syncytial virus subgroups A and B in France from 1982 to 1990. J Clin Microbiol 1991; 29: 653–655.

Galiano MC, Palomo C, Videla CM, Arbiza J, Melero JA, Carballal G. Genetic and antigenic variability of human respiratory syncytial virus (groups A and B) isolated over seven consecutive seasons in Argentina (1995 to 2001). J Clin Microbiol 2005; 43: 2266–2273.

Garcia O, Martin M, Dopazo J, Arbiza J, Frabasile S, Russi J, Hortal M, Perez-Brena P, Martinez I, Garcia-Barreno B, Melero JA. Evolutionary pattern of human respiratory syncytial virus (subgroup A): cocirculating lineages and correlation of genetic and antigenic changes in the G glycoprotein. J Virol 1994; 68: 5448–5459.

Garcia-Barreno B, Palomo C, Penas C, Delgado T, Perez-Brena P, Melero JA. Marked differences in the antigenic structure of human respiratory syncytial virus F and G glycoproteins. J Virol 1989; 63: 925–932.

Garcia-Barreno B, Portela A, Delgado T, Lopez JA, Melero JA. Frame shift mutations as a novel mechanism for the generation of neutralisation resistant mutants of human respiratory syncytial virus. EMBO J 1990; 9: 4181–4187.

Garcia-Beato R, Martinez I, Franci C, Real FX, Garcia-Barreno B, Melero JA. Host cell effect upon glycosylation and antigenicity of human respiratory syncytial virus G glycoprotein. Virology 1996; 221: 301–309.

Garcia-Beato R, Melero JA. The C-terminal third of human respiratory syncytial virus attachment (G) protein is partially resistant to protease digestion and is glycosylated in a cell-type-specific manner. J Gen Virol 2000; 81: 919–927.

Gimenez HB, Hardman N, Keir HM, Cash P. Antigenic variation between human respiratory syncytial virus isolates. J Gen Virol 1986; 67: 863–870.

Glezen WP, Paredes A, Allison JE, Taber LH, Frank AL. Risk of respiratory syncytial virus infection for infants from low-income families in relationship to age, sex, ethnic group, and maternal antibody level. J Pediatr 1981; 98: 708–715.

Glezen WP, Taber LH, Frank AL, Kasel JA. Risk of primary infection and reinfection with respiratory syncytial virus. Am J Dis Child 1986; 140: 543–546.

Hall CB, Geiman JM, Biggar R, Kotok DI, Hogan PM, Douglas Jr. GR. Respiratory syncytial virus infections within families. N Engl J Med 1976; 294: 414–419.

Hall CB, Walsh EE, Long CE, Schnabel KC. Immunity to and frequency of reinfection with respiratory syncytial virus. J Infect Dis 1991; 163: 693–698.

Hall CB, Walsh EE, Schnabel KC, Long CE, McConnochie KM, Hildreth SW, Anderson LJ. Occurrence of groups A and B of respiratory syncytial virus over 15 years: associated epidemiologic and clinical characteristics in hospitalised and ambulatory children. J Infect Dis 1990; 162: 1283–1290.

Harrington RD, Hooton TM, Hackman RC, Storch GA, Osborne B, Gleaves CA, Benson A, Meyers JD. An outbreak of respiratory syncytial virus in a bone marrow transplant centre. J Infect Dis 1992; 165: 987–993.

Hazlett DT, Bell TM, Tukei PM, Ademba GR, Ochieng WO, Magana JM, Gathara GW, Wafula EM, Pamba A, Ndinya-Achola JO, Arap Siongok TK. Viral etiology and epidemiology of acute respiratory infections in children in Nairobi, Kenya. Am J Trop Med Hyg 1988; 39: 632–640.

Henderson FW, Collier AM, Clyde Jr. WA, Denny FW. Respiratory-syncytial-virus infections, reinfections and immunity. A prospective, longitudinal study in young children. N Engl J Med 1979; 300: 530–534.

Hendricks DA, McIntosh K, Patterson JL. Further characterisation of the soluble form of the G glycoprotein of respiratory syncytial virus. J Virol 1988; 62: 2228–2233.

Hendry RM, Pierik LT, McIntosh K. Prevalence of respiratory syncytial virus subgroups over six consecutive outbreaks: 1981–1987. J Infect Dis 1989; 160: 185–190.

Hendry RM, Talis AL, Godfrey E, Anderson LJ, Fernie BF, McIntosh K. Concurrent circulation of antigenically distinct strains of respiratory syncytial virus during community outbreaks. J Infect Dis 1986; 153: 291–297.

Johnson PR, Collins PL. The fusion glycoproteins of human respiratory syncytial virus of subgroups A and B: sequence conservation provides a structural basis for antigenic relatedness. J Gen Virol 1988; 69: 2623–2628.

Johnson PR, Collins PL. The 1B (NS2), 1C (NS1) and N proteins of human respiratory syncytial virus (RSV) of antigenic subgroups A and B: sequence conservation and divergence within RSV genomic RNA. J Gen Virol 1989; 70: 1539–1547.

Johnson PR, Spriggs MK, Olmsted RA, Collins PL. The G glycoprotein of human respiratory syncytial viruses of subgroups A and B: extensive sequence divergence between antigenically related proteins. Proc Natl Acad Sci USA 1987; 84: 5625–5629.

Jones LP, Zheng HQ, Karron RA, Peret TC, Tsou C, Anderson LJ. Multiplex assay for detection of strain-specific antibodies against the two variable regions of the G protein of respiratory syncytial virus. Clin Diagn Lab Immunol 2002; 9: 633–638.

Kuroiwa Y, Nagai K, Okita L, Yui I, Kase T, Nakayama T, Tsutsumi H. A phylogenetic study of human respiratory syncytial viruses group A and B strains isolated in two cities in Japan from 1980–2002. J Med Virol 2005; 762: 241–247.

Lambkin R, Dimmock NJ. All rabbits immunized with type A influenza virions have a serum haemagglutination-inhibition antibody response biased to a single epitope in antigenic site B. J Gen Virol 1995; 76: 889–897.

Lambkin R, McLain L, Jones SE, Aldridge SL, Dimmock NJ. Neutralization escape mutants of type A influenza virus are readily selected by antisera from mice immunized with whole virus: a possible mechanism for antigenic drift. J Gen Virol 1994; 75: 3493–3502.

Madhi SA, Schoub B, Simmank K, Blackburn N, Klugman KP. Increased burden of respiratory viral associated severe lower respiratory tract infections in children infected with human immunodeficiency virus type-1. J Pediatr 2000; 137: 78–84.

Madhi SA, Venter M, Alexandra R, Lewis H, Kara Y, Karshagen WF, Greef M, Lassen C. Respiratory syncytial virus associated illness in high-risk children and national characterisation of the circulating virus genotype in South Africa. J Clin Virol 2003; 27: 180–189.

Martinello RA, Chen MD, Weibel C, Kahn JS. Correlation between respiratory syncytial virus genotype and severity of illness. J Infect Dis 2002; 186: 839–842.

Martinez I, Valdes O, Delfraro A, Arbiza J, Russi J, Melero JA. Evolutionary pattern of the G glycoprotein of human respiratory syncytial viruses from antigenic group B: the use of alternative termination codons and lineage diversification. J Gen Virol 1999; 80: 125–130.

McCarthy AJ, Kingman HM, Kelly C, Taylor GS, Caul EO, Grier D, Moppett J, Foot AB, Cornish JM, Oakhill A, Steward CG, Pamphilon DH, Marks DI. The outcome of 26 patients with respiratory syncytial virus infection following allogeneic stem cell transplantation. Bone Marrow Transplant 1999; 24: 1315–1322.

McCullers JA, Saito T, Iverson AR. Multiple genotypes of influenza B virus circulated between 1979 and 2003. J Virol 2004; 78: 12817–12828.

Melero JA, Garcia-Barreno B, Martinez I, Pringle CR, Cane PA. Antigenic structure, evolution and immunobiology of human respiratory syncytial virus attachment (G) protein. J Gen Virol 1997; 78: 2411–2418.

Mlinaric-Galinovic G, Chonmaitree T, Cane PA, Pringle CR, Ogra PL. Antigenic diversity of respiratory syncytial virus subgroup B strains circulating during a community outbreak of infection. J Med Virol 1994; 42: 380–384.

Moura FE, Blanc A, Frabasile S, Delfraro A, de Sierra MJ, Tome L, Ramos EA, Siqueira MM, Arbiza J. Genetic diversity of respiratory syncytial virus isolated during an epidemic period from children of northeastern Brazil. J Med Virol 2004; 74: 156–160.

Mufson MA, Belshe RB, Orvell C, Norrby E. Subgroup characteristics of respiratory syncytial virus strains recovered from children with two consecutive infections. J Clin Microbiol 1987; 25: 1535–1539.

Mufson MA, Orvell C, Rafnar B, Norrby E. Two distinct subtypes of human respiratory syncytial virus. J Gen Virol 1985; 66: 2111–2124.

Nagai K, Kamasaki H, Kuroiwa Y, Okita L, Tsutsumi H. Nosocomial outbreak of respiratory syncytial virus subgroup B variants with the 60 nucleotides-duplicated G protein gene. J Med Virol 2004; 74: 161–165.

Nagai K, Yamazaki H, Pattamadilok S, Chiba S. Three antigenic variant groups in human respiratory syncytial virus subgroup B isolated in Japan. Arch Virol 1993; 128: 55–63.

Nokes DJ, Okiro EA, Ngama M, White LJ, Ochola R, Scott PD, Cane PA, Medley GF. Respiratory syncytial virus epidemiology in a birth cohort from Kilifi district, Kenya: infection during the first year of life. J Infect Dis 2004; 190: 1828–1832.

Norrby E, Mufson MA, Alexander H, Houghten RA, Lerner RA. Site-directed serology with synthetic peptides representing the large glycoprotein G of respiratory syncytial virus. Proc Natl Acad Sci USA 1987; 84: 6572–6576.

Nwankwo MU, Dym AM, Schuit KE, Offor E, Omene JA. Seasonal variation in respiratory syncytial virus infections in children in Benin-City, Nigeria. Trop Geogr Med 1988; 40: 309–313.

Orvell C, Norrby E, Mufson MA. Preparation and characterisation of monoclonal antibodies directed against five structural components of human respiratory syncytial virus subgroup B. J Gen Virol 1987; 68: 3125–3135.

Palomo C, Cane PA, Melero JA. Evaluation of the antibody specificities of human convalescent-phase sera against the attachment (G) protein of human respiratory syncytial virus: influence of strain variation and carbohydrate side chains. J Med Virol 2000; 60: 468–474.

Palomo C, Garcia-Barreno B, Penas C, Melero JA. The G protein of human respiratory syncytial virus: significance of carbohydrate side-chains and the C-terminal end to its antigenicity. J Gen Virol 1991; 72: 669–675.

Papadopoulos NG, Gourgiotis D, Javadyan A, Bossios A, Kallergi K, Psarras S, Tsolia MN, Kafetzis D. Does respiratory syncytial virus subtype influences the severity of acute bronchiolitis in hospitalized infants? Respir Med 2004; 98: 879–882.

Peret TC, Hall CB, Hammond GW, Piedra PA, Storch GA, Sullender WM, Tsou C, Anderson LJ. Circulation patterns of group A and B human respiratory syncytial virus genotypes in 5 communities in North America. J Infect Dis 2000; 181: 1891–1896.

Peret TC, Hall CB, Schnabel KC, Golub JA, Anderson LJ. Circulation patterns of genetically distinct group A and B strains of human respiratory syncytial virus in a community. J Gen Virol 1998; 79: 2221–2229.

Polack FP, Irusta PM, Hoffman SJ, Schiatti MP, Melendi GA, Delgado MF, Laham FR, Thumar B, Hendry RM, Melero JA, Karron RA, Collins PL, Kleeberger SR. The cysteine-rich region of respiratory syncytial virus attachment protein inhibits innate immunity elicited by the virus and endotoxin. Proc Natl Acad Sci USA 2005; 102: 8996–9001.

Rafiefard F, Johansson B, Tecle T, Orvell C. Molecular epidemiology of respiratory syncytial virus (RSV) of group A in Stockholm, Sweden, between 1965 and 2003. Virus Res 2004; 105: 137–145.

Rajala MS, Sullender WM, Prasad AK, Dar L, Broor S. Genetic variability among group A and B respiratory syncytial virus isolates from a large referral hospital in New Delhi, India. J Clin Microbiol 2003; 41: 2311–2316.

Report to the Medical Research Council Subcommittee on Respiratory Syncytial Virus Vaccines. Respiratory syncytial virus infection: admissions to hospital in industrial, urban, and rural areas. Br Med J 1978; 2(6140): 796–798.

Roberts SR, Lichtenstein D, Ball LA, Wertz GW. The membrane-associated and secreted forms of the respiratory syncytial virus attachment glycoprotein G are synthesised from alternative initiation codons. J Virol 1994; 68: 4538–4546.

Roca A, Loscertales MP, Quinto L, Perez-Brena P, Vaz N, Alonso PL, Saiz JC. Genetic variability among group A and B respiratory syncytial virus in Mozambique: identification of a new cluster of group B isolates. J Gen Virol 2001; 82: 103–111.

Rota PA, Hemphill ML, Whistler T, Regnery HL, Kendal AP. Antigenic and genetic characterization of the haemagglutinins of recent cocirculating strains of influenza B virus. J Gen Virol 1992; 73: 2737–2742.

Rueda P, Delgado T, Portela A, Melero JA, Garcia-Barreno B. Premature stop codons in the G glycoprotein of human respiratory syncytial viruses resistant to neutralisation by monoclonal antibodies. J Virol 1991; 65: 3374–3378.

Rueda P, Garcia-Barreno B, Melero JA. Loss of conserved cysteine residues in the attachment (G) glycoprotein of two human respiratory syncytial virus escape mutants that contain multiple A–G substitutions (hypermutations). Virology 1994; 198: 653–662.

Rueda P, Palomo C, Garcia-Barreno B, Melero JA. The three C-terminal residues of human respiratory syncytial virus G glycoprotein (Long strain) are essential for integrity of multiple epitopes distinguishable by antiidiotypic antibodies. Viral Immunol 1995; 8: 37–46.

Salomon HE, Avila MM, Cerqueiro MC, Orvell C, Weissenbacher M. Clinical and epidemiological aspects of respiratory syncytial virus antigenic variants in Argentinian children. J Infect Dis 1991; 163: 1167.

Sato M, Saito R, Sakai T, Sano Y, Nishikawa M, Sasaki A, Shobugawa Y, Gejyo F, Suzuki H. Molecular epidemiology of respiratory syncytial virus infections among children with acute respiratory symptoms in a community over three seasons. J Clin Microbiol 2005; 43: 36–40.

Scott PD, Ochola R, Ngama M, Okiro EA, Nokes DJ, Medley GF, Cane PA. Molecular epidemiology of respiratory syncytial virus in Kilifi district, Kenya. J Med Virol 2004; 74: 344–354.

Scott PD, Ochola R, Ngama M, Okiro EA, Nokes J, Medley GF, Cane PA. Molecular analysis of respiratory syncytial virus reinfections in infants from coastal Kenya. J Infec Dis 2006; 193: 59–67.

Seki K, Tsutsumi H, Ohsaki M, Kamasaki H, Chiba S. Genetic variability of respiratory syncytial virus subgroup A strain in 15 successive epidemics in one city. J Med Virol 2001; 64: 374–380.

Storch GA, Anderson LJ, Park CS, Tsou C, Dohner DE. Antigenic and genomic diversity within group A respiratory syncytial virus. J Infect Dis 1991; 163: 858–861.

Storch GA, Park CS. Monoclonal antibodies demonstrate heterogeneity in the G glycoprotein of prototype strains and clinical isolates of respiratory syncytial virus. J Med Virol 1987; 22: 345–356.

Storch GA, Park CS, Dohner DE. RNA fingerprinting of respiratory syncytial virus using ribonuclease protection. Application to molecular epidemiology. J Clin Invest 1989; 83: 1894–1902.

Sullender WM, Edwards KG. Mutations of respiratory syncytial virus attachment glycoprotein G associated with resistance to neutralisation by primate polyclonal antibodies. Virology 1999; 264: 230–236.

Sullender WM, Mufson MA, Anderson LJ, Wertz GW. Genetic diversity of the attachment protein of subgroup B respiratory syncytial viruses. J Virol 1991; 65: 5425–5434.

Sullender WM, Mufson MA, Prince GA, Anderson LJ, Wertz GW. Antigenic and genetic diversity among the attachment proteins of group A respiratory syncytial viruses that have caused repeat infections in children. J Infect Dis 1998; 178: 925–932.

Sullender WM, Sun L, Anderson LJ. Analysis of respiratory syncytial virus genetic variability with amplified cDNAs. J Clin Microbiol 1993; 31: 1224–1231.

Sung RY, Chan RC, Tam JS, Cheng AF, Murray HG. Epidemiology and aetiology of acute bronchiolitis in Hong Kong infants. Epidemiol Infect 1992; 108: 147–154.

Trento A, Galiano M, Videla C, Carballal G, Garcia-Barreno B, Melero JA, Palomo C. Major changes in the G protein of human respiratory syncytial virus isolates introduced by a duplication of 60 nucleotides. J Gen Virol 2003; 84: 3115–3120.

Trento A, Viegas M, Galiano M, Videla C, Carballal G, Mistchenko AS, Melero JA. Natural history of human respiratory syncytial virus inferred from phylogenetic analysis of the attachment (G) glycoprotein with a sixty nucleotide duplication. J Virol 2006; 80: 975–984.

Tripp RA, Jones LP, Haynes LM, Zheng H, Murphy PM, Anderson LJ. CX3C chemokine mimicry by respiratory syncytial virus G glycoprotein. Nat Immunol 2001; 2: 732–738.

Tsutsumi H, Onuma M, Suga K, Honjo T, Chiba Y, Chiba S, Ogra PL. Occurrence of respiratory syncytial virus subgroup A and B strains in Japan, 1980 to 1987. J Clin Microbiol 1988; 26: 1171–1174.

Valarcher J-F, Schelcher F, Bourhy H. Evolution of bovine respiratory syncytial virus. J Virol 2000; 74: 10714–10728.

Valdes O, Martinez I, Valdivia A, Cancio R, Savon C, Goyenechea A, Melero JA. Unusual antigenic and genetic characteristics of human respiratory syncytial viruses isolated in Cuba. J Virol 1998; 72: 7589–7592.

Venter M, Collinson M, Schoub BD. Molecular epidemiological analysis of community circulating respiratory syncytial virus in rural South Africa: comparison of viruses and genotypes responsible for different disease manifestations. J Med Virol 2002; 68: 452–461.

Venter M, Madhi SA, Tiemessen CT, Schoub BD. Genetic diversity and molecular epidemiology of respiratory syncytial virus over four consecutive seasons in South Africa: identification of new subgroup A and B genotypes. J Gen Virol 2001; 82: 2117–2124.

Walsh EE, McConnochie KM, Long CE, Hall CB. Severity of respiratory syncytial virus infection is related to virus strain. J Infect Dis 1997; 175: 814–820.

Waris M. Pattern of respiratory syncytial virus epidemics in Finland: two-year cycles with alternating prevalence of groups A and B. J Infect Dis 1991; 163: 464–469.

Weber MW, Dackour R, Usen S, Schneider G, Adegbola RA, Cane P, Jaffar S, Milligan P, Greenwood BM, Whittle H, Mulholland EK. The clinical spectrum of respiratory syncytial virus disease in The Gambia. Pediatr Infect Dis J 1998; 17: 224–230.

Wertz GW, Collins PL, Huang Y, Gruber C, Levine S, Ball LA. Nucleotide sequence of the G protein gene of human respiratory syncytial virus reveals an unusual type of viral membrane protein. Proc Natl Acad Sci USA 1985; 82: 4075–4079.

Wertz GW, Krieger M, Ball LA. Structure and cell surface maturation of the attachment glycoprotein of human respiratory syncytial virus in a cell line deficient in O-glycosylation. J Virol 1989; 63: 4767–4776.

White LJ, Waris M, Cane PA, Nokes DJ, Medley GF. The transmission dynamics of groups A and B human respiratory syncytial virus (hRSV) in England & Wales and Finland: seasonality and cross-protection. Epidemiol Infect 2005; 133: 279–289.

Wilson SD, Roberts K, Hammond K, Ayres JG, Cane PA. Estimation of incidence of respiratory syncytial virus infection in schoolchildren using salivary antibodies. J Med Virol 2000; 61: 81–84.

Woelk CH, Holmes EC. Variable immune-driven natural selection in the attachment (G) glycoprotein of respiratory syncytial virus (RSV). J Mol Evol 2001; 52: 182–192.

Zambon MC, Stockton JD, Clewley JP, Fleming DM. Contribution of influenza and respiratory syncytial virus to community cases of influenza-like illness: an observational study. The Lancet 2001; 358: 1410–1416.

Zlateva KT, Lemey P, Moes E, Vandamme AM, Van Ranst M. Genetic variability and molecular evolution of the human respiratory syncytial virus subgroup B attachment G protein. J Virol 2005; 79: 9157–9167.

Zlateva KT, Lemey P, Vandamme AM, Van Ranst M. Molecular evolution and circulation patterns of human respiratory syncytial virus subgroup A: positively selected sites in the attachment G glycoprotein. J Virol 2004; 78: 4675–4683.

Respiratory Syncytial Virus
Patricia Cane (Editor)

DOI 10.1016/S0168-7069(06)14004-5

Genetic Susceptibility to RSV Disease

Jeremy Hull
Oxford University Department of Paediatrics, John Radcliffe Hospital, Oxford, UK

The ability of individuals to deal successfully with infectious disease is influenced by several variables, including the nature of the pathogen, environmental factors, pre-existing illness and heritable genetic variation. A specific illustration of the latter is the lower incidence of malaria in those who have sickle cell trait.

Inherited vulnerability to infection has been shown in observations on both adopted children and twins. In inquiries on adopted children in Scandinavia it was found that children whose biological parent died under the age of 50 years of an infectious disease had an almost six-fold increased risk of dying themselves from an infectious disease (Sorensen et al., 1988). In contrast the premature death of an adoptive parent from infection had no effect on the adoptee's risk. Although the causes of death are not specified in this study, respiratory infections were prominent among the range of infectious diseases causing by death in Northern Europeans during the middle of the last century, suggesting that the heritable risk is likely to apply to respiratory infections, among others. Twin research has also been used to study the genetic effect on susceptibility to infections. Dizygotic twins arise from two fertilised eggs and 50% of their genes will be identical—the same amount as in non-twin siblings. Monozygotic twins arise from the division of a single fertilised egg and are genetically identical. If, on average, there is more variation in a trait (such as susceptibility to infection) between dizygotic twins than between monozygotic twins, then that additional variation is presumed to be due to genetic differences. This approach has been used to study several acute and chronic infectious diseases and many do show a higher concordance in monozygotic than dizygotic twins including malaria (Jepson et al., 1995), tuberculosis (Comstock, 1978), *Helicobacter pylori* (Malaty et al., 1994), rubella and measles (Gedda et al., 1984).

These studies help us understand why some individuals suffer more severe disease than others, but they say nothing about what it is that is different in the genes of these individuals that leads to susceptibility. Understanding this process is a massive undertaking and we are only just beginning to address the issues involved. The techniques being used are those of genetic epidemiology. The answers when they come are likely to lead to major changes in the way we practice medicine.

Research into variations in DNA sequences that lead to differing phenotypes has expanded dramatically since the completion of the Human Genome Project in 2003. The primary aim of the Human Genome Project was to determine the sequence of the 3 billion chemical base pairs that make up human DNA and to identify all human genes. As the project progressed it became apparent that there was more variation in the DNA sequences between different individuals that had previously been supposed. By the end of the project it was clear that *all* human genes have variations of the DNA sequences and that those are carried at *relatively high frequencies* (>1%) in the normal population. For the vast majority of variants, the consequences of the DNA change on gene function are just not known, and they have not yet been investigated. However the presence of these variants enables us for the first time to determine whether the DNA variation at a particular gene or genes is associated with observed variation in disease susceptibility. This is the first step. The second bigger step will be to determine the biological connection.

This chapter is concerned with infection in infancy with the respiratory syncytial virus (RSV). I shall review:

1. the the epidemiological evidence of genetic susceptibility to RSV;
2. evidence that the host response affects the severity of disease expression;
3. the approach required to carry out a robust genetic association study; and
4. what has been published so far on genetic associations with severe RSV disease.

All the work carried out so far on host genetics and RSV has been in relation to acute RSV bronchiolitis and its consequences, rather than on coryzal illness or pneumonia in the elderly, and the following discussion is limited to this expression of RSV disease.

Epidemiological evidence of genetic susceptibility to RSV infection in infancy

In temperate climates RSV occurs in annual winter epidemics. During these epidemics over 70% of infants are infected by the virus. All infants will be infected by the end of their second winter (Kim et al., 1973). The majority will have mild symptoms such as a runny nose with or without a dry cough. A small percentage, 1–3%, develops a severe illness, acute bronchiolitis, caused by inflammation and narrowing of the small airways of the lung. The affected babies become breathless and need hospital care for oxygen therapy and assistance with feeding. Infants who are compromised, for example due to premature birth or congenital heart disease, are more at risk of developing severe disease, but in most reports they account for a relatively small proportion (10–15%) of the children ill enough to need admission to hospital for treatment (Nielsen et al., 2003). The majority of infants with severe disease are otherwise healthy and do not have clearly identifiable environmental risk factors. These observations, of near-universal exposure to RSV with only a small proportion developing severe disease, raise the possibility of a genetic predisposition. For a relatively common disease in early childhood, twin studies are probably the most effective way of demonstrating a heritable predisposition. There are yet no published twin studies on RSV bronchiolitis, although at least one is underway. There are, however, a number of existing lines of evidence that suggest that genetically determined host responses are important.

Family studies

Several studies have shown that when a parent suffered from asthma or other respiratory illness when they were children, then their child had an increased risk of lower respiratory tract infection (LRI) in early life. In a birth cohort study of 1246 infants in the US, parents were asked at enrolment into the study whether they had suffered from asthma, bronchitis, bronchiolitis, croup or pneumonia in childhood. The infants were then followed prospectively and all respiratory illnesses were documented. Thirty percent of infants had at least one physician diagnosed LRI. Overall infants whose parents had had any respiratory illness before the age of 16 years had a 1.7 times increased risk of developing wheezy or non-wheezy LRIs (Camilli et al., 1993). The effect was strongest in those parents who had suffered from bronchiolitis or asthma in the first 3 years of their lives; 43% of the infants of these parents had at least one LRI in the first year of life (2.8 times increased risk). The potential for recall bias for the parental history of respiratory illness, which was reduced by recording this information before any LRIs occurred in the infants. Using the same questions, a different study has shown a strong positive relationship between reported childhood respiratory illness and lung function in adulthood (Burrows et al., 1977), suggesting that the questions accurately identify adults with respiratory problems. Three other prospective cohort studies that, taken together, documented respiratory symptoms in a total of over 7000 infants, have all identified parental asthma and atopy as a risk factor for wheezing and non-wheezing LRI in the infants (Leeder et al., 1976; Bosken et al., 2000; Koopman et al., 2001). The majority of LRI in the first 12 months of life is caused by viral infection and RSV accounts for 50–70% of the total. These data suggest that respiratory illness in parents increases the chance of respiratory illness in their children. An inherited genetic effect is a likely explanation for these findings.

Case–control studies of infants admitted to hospital with bronchiolitis show a similar effect of parental asthma on more severe infant LRI (McConnochie and Roghmann, 1986; Trefny et al., 2000). Goetghebuer et al. (2004) identified 92 infants treated in hospital for LRI (80% had bronchiolitis). For each case, 2 age- and sex-matched controls were selected. Questionnaires were used to record potential risk factors. In a multiple regression analysis, a maternal history of asthma was associated with a 1.9 times increased risk of infant LRI (Goetghebuer et al., 2004). Interestingly a maternal history of bronchiolitis was also associated with infant LRI using univariant analysis, although clearly this result may have been affected by recall bias. The association between maternal asthma and infant LRI was independent of the effect of subsequent wheezing illness in the child, suggesting that the effect was not due to inheritance of a predisposition to atopic disease, but rather to a genetic influence on susceptibility to respiratory viral infection in early life.

Variation among different human populations

Differences in the severity and frequency of RSV bronchiolitis have been reported in different ethnic populations. In a study of infants with their first episode of wheeze or bronchiolitis severe enough for treatment in hospital, Bradley et al. (2005), found that Black American infants had milder disease (higher mean oxygen saturations and shorter length of stay) than White American infants (Bradley et al., 2005). Black American children were no more likely to present earlier for admission after the onset of respiratory symptoms suggesting that there was not a bias towards Black American families seeking medical assistance with infants with milder disease. The effect of ethnicity persisted in a multiple regression model that included socioeconomic status, maternal smoking and maternal atopy. These findings are similar to those of DeVincenzo et al. (2005) who studied 188 infants presenting to hospital with RSV bronchiolitis. White Americans required, on average, one additional day of hospital treatment compared to Black Americans (DeVincenzo et al., 2005). Other studies have shown that American Indians, Native Alaskans and New Zealand Maoris have higher rates of hospitalisation for RSV disease in infancy, although in some studies these effects were not independent of socioeconomic factors (Holman et al., 2004). Environmental factors and pathogen strain variation may also contribute to differences in infectious disease prevalence and severity in different human populations. Nevertheless, since these populations also have marked differences in the nature of their genetic variation (shown most recently by the HapMap project www.hapmap.org), this evidence is consistent with a genetic influence on disease susceptibility.

Variation in different mouse strains

Inbred laboratory mice can be used to study the genetic factors that control phenotypic traits. If there is greater variation of the trait between different strains of mice compared to that which is seen between individual animals of the same strain, it suggests that the genetic background of the mice influences the nature of the observed phenotype. Studies of this type have identified genetic loci influencing bronchial hyper-responsiveness and pulmonary inflammation, both key features of the host response to RSV infection. RSV is not a mouse pathogen, but it can replicate in several mouse strains. Studies of the mouse model of RSV infection have provided insights into RSV pathology, immunology and vaccine biology in humans (Openshaw, 1995). When RSV disease in different mouse strains is compared, there are clear differences, dependent of the genetic background of the mice. Susceptible strains such as BALB/c and AKR/J after inoculation with RSV have viral titres 1–2 logs higher than resistant strains such as C57BL/6. Susceptible animals also show more weight loss (Stark et al., 2002), and more pulmonary inflammation, as shown on lung histology and bronchoalveolar lavage cytokine concentrations (Chavez-Bueno et al., 2005) than resistant strains. Experiments to model the genetic influence on disease severity by crossing susceptible and resistant strains suggest that the effect is multi-genetic.

Evidence that the host response rather than the virus is responsible for disease

RSV infection is associated with a profound inflammatory response

The inflammatory response to RSV has been studied using cell culture systems, animal models and in infants. These studies have all indicated that RSV elicits a rapid and pronounced innate inflammatory response. It also stimulates an adaptive response, which is essential to viral clearance.

RSV is not cytopathic

Using differentiated airway cells in culture, Zhang et al. (2002) have demonstrated that RSV can infect these cells with little cytopathic effect. The cells remain stably infected for several weeks. During this period large amounts of pro-inflammatory cytokines are produced by the cells, but in the absence of host effector cells, no cell injury is apparent. This is in stark contrast to the effect of influenza virus in the same system, which results in cell lysis within 48 h.

Viral load correlates poorly with disease severity

This has been shown in several studies, looking at viral load in both nasal secretions and tracheal secretions of ventilated infants (Hall et al., 1975; Wright et al., 2002). At the time of admission, viral load has usually reached its peak and falls at the same time as the illness becomes more severe. The anti-viral drug ribavirin is effective in reducing viral load, but does not affect disease outcome.

Effect of formalin-inactivated vaccine

The importance of the host response on disease severity was evident following the use of a formalin-inactivated vaccine in the 1960s. In these trials a formalin inactivated whole virus (FI-RSV) was used as a vaccine and given via the intramuscular route. Vaccinees produced antibodies to the virus, but these were non-neutralising. On exposure to natural infection, vaccinees developed more severe disease than controls, resulting in 80% requiring hospital admission compared to 5% of controls and 2 children died (Kim et al., 1969). This outcome indicates that an inappropriate host response to the virus can lead to enhanced disease.

The vaccine-enhanced disease has been studied extensively using mice. BALB/C mice given intranasal human RSV can develop lower respiratory tract disease. The disease is more severe in mice that have prior vaccination with formalin-inactivated RSV. Studies of the cells present in the lungs of these mice indicate that virus-specific cytotoxic T-cells are sufficient for effective virus clearance, but that CD8+ and CD4+ T-cells also contribute to disease enhancement following FI-RSV vaccination. One suggestion that arose from this work was that the immune response is unbalanced by the formalin-inactivated vaccine, leading to a Th2 weighted immune response to natural infection, which fails to clear the infection efficiently and enhances airways inflammation (Openshaw, 1995; Graham et al., 2000). Studies using the mouse models have provided possible immune mechanisms that explain vaccine-enhanced disease, and which may also be relevant in naturally occurring severe bronchiolitis. In infants, some studies have demonstrated correlation between Th2-type responses and the severity of RSV disease (Roman et al., 1997; Bont et al., 2001; Legg et al., 2003); others have not (Brandenburg et al., 2000; Welliver et al., 2002).

Taken together, these findings suggest that the damage to small airways in infants infected with RSV might not be directly due to viral presence and growth, but rather is a consequence of destructive components of a robust immune response that eventually clears the virus infection.

Requirements for effective genetic association studies

To weigh the results of studies on genetic variation it is necessary to appreciate the investigative approach. In concept genetic association studies are straightforward. A gene variant is selected and typed in cases and controls. If the frequency of the variant differs significantly between the 2 groups, it follows that the variant predisposed individuals to develop the disease. In practice there are a number of potential problems. Failure to adequately address these problems has been identified as one of the main reasons that many of the early genetic association studies were either negative or were not replicated by subsequent large studies (Hirschhorn and Altshuler, 2002; Ioannidis, 2003; Ioannidis et al., 2003; Lohmueller et al., 2003; Page et al., 2003). In this section I will discuss the important features of a successful genetic association study.

Single-nucleotide polymorphisms

The most common form of DNA variation is the single-nucleotide polymorphism (SNP). SNPs arise by mutation when one base is substituted for another (Fig. 1). There are an estimated 10 million common SNPs in the human genome, roughly one every 300 nucleotides. Between any 2 unrelated individuals there will be approximately 3 million loci where DNA bases differ.

The highly diverse nature of the genome led to questions about the origins and maintenance of the variation. Traditionally, mutations that arose were thought to be largely deleterious and would be subject to negative selection and rapidly lost from the population. To explain the observed high levels of diversity, the neutral theory of evolution was developed (Kimura, 1983), which suggested that most

Single nucleotide polymorphisms

Each person carries 2 copies of each chromosome, apart from the X and Y chromosome in males. Chromosomes are made tightly bundled DNA. The genetic information in DNA is carried by 4 bases, A, T, C and G. When a cell divides, DNA is replicated. Each of the 3 billion bases of DNA is faithfully copied and new chromosomes are made. Very rarely an error occurs, and one base is incorrectly copied. If this happens in a germ-line cell, this base change can be passed on to the next generation Base changes which have only deleterious effects will be rapidly lost from the population and never reach a measurably frequency. Base changes which are either neutral or have some beneficial effects can increase in frequency. Once they occur in at least 1% of the population they called single nucleotide polymorphisms or SNPs (pronounced "snips"). The frequency of a particular SNP depends on how long ago they arose and whether there has been any positive selection of the gene region in which they are located. Eventually most neutral SNPs will drift to 'fixation' - the point when they replace the previous base in all chromosomes in a population. SNPs occur every 100 to 300 bases along the 3-billion-base human genome. Two of every three SNPs involve the replacement of cytosine (C) with thymine (T). SNPs can occur in both coding (gene) and non-coding regions of the genome. Many SNPs have no effect on cell function, but others could predispose people to disease or influence their response to a drug.

Nearly all SNPs are bi-allelic. This means that there are 2 possible bases that can be present at the position of the SNP in the DNA sequence. The 2 different bases are called alleles. Individuals in the population will either carry 2 copies of one allele (homozygotes) or carry one copy of each (heterozygotes). The combination of the 2 alleles together is referred to as a person's genotype. The distribution of genotypes can be predicted according to the frequencies of the alleles – this is called the Hardy Weinberg distribution. The frequency of homozygotes is equal to the square of their allele frequencies and the frequency of heterozygotes is equal to the twice the product of the 2 allele frequencies – this is represented by the equation: $p^2 + 2pq + q^2 = 1$ where p and q are the common and rare allele frequencies respectively. It is expected that all SNP genotypes will conform to this distribution in both cases and controls. Significant deviation away from Hardy Weinberg frequencies can be an indication that the genotyping method is inaccurate.

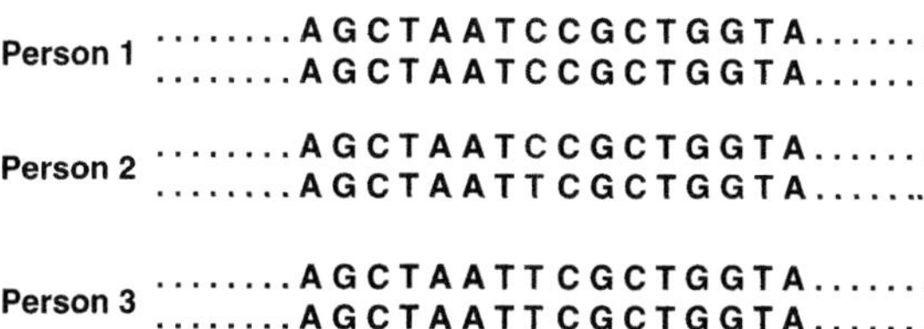

DNA sequences of 2 copies of each chromosome in each of 3 individuals are shown. Individual 1 is a CC homozygote, individual 2 is a CT heterozygote and individual 3 is TT homozygote.

Fig. 1 Single-nucleotide polymorphisms (for colour version: see colour section on page 326).

sequence variation does not directly impact phenotypic variation, and thus is not directly subjected to the forces of selection. One consequence of this theory is that most identified DNA polymorphisms will not have an associated overt or clinically relevant phenotype. Nevertheless, most human genes studied so far have structural and regulatory variants. The basis of these variants must ultimately lie in the DNA sequence. SNPs have become the method of choice for identifying the nature of the DNA variation. They have several advantages over other forms of variation:

(a) They very abundant and will occur within or in very close proximity to all genes.
(b) Technically they are easy to detect in DNA samples, making it possible to type individuals for thousands of different SNPs.
(c) They are less mutable that other forms of DNA variation making it less likely that associations will be confounded by alleles having mutated to different forms in the course of the transmission of alleles from generation to generation.
(d) SNPs are found throughout the genome, in exons, introns, promoters, enhancers, and other regulatory elements. Hence, they are more likely to yield a functional or physiologically relevant allele than other sorts of polymorphism. Thus, a SNP in the coding region may directly affect the sequence of a protein, an intronic SNP can influence splicing, and a SNP in a regulatory element can influence gene expression.
(e) Finally, because new SNP alleles arise as mutations at different loci and at different points in time, and because they occur with such great abundance over the genome, groups of neighbouring SNPs may show distinctive patterns of linkage disequilibrium (LD). LD is the phenomenon whereby the presence of one allele on a chromosome may suggest a high probability that a particular allele will be present at a neighbouring site on the same chromosome (Fig. 2).

Selection of SNPs to study

All gene regions are now known to have a large number of genetic variants. For example, in IL13, a relatively small gene, there are over 100 identified SNPs. Most SNPs are thought to be biologically inert (i.e. 'neutral'), and so using all identified SNPs in an association study would be wasteful of effort, time and money. Two approaches can be used to reduce the number of SNPs needed – using haplotypes and identifying 'functional' SNPs.

Haplotypes

Haplotypes are groups of related SNPs that occur together on the same chromosome (Fig. 2). The relationship between SNPs is described in terms of linkage disequilibrium. Identifying the haplotype structure at a particular genetic locus that provides a description of the genetic diversity at that locus, and allows a subgroup

Linkage disequilibrium and haplotypes

Each SNP will generally arise only once in human evolution – back mutations are very rare. SNPs that are on *different* chromosomes will occur together in the same individual at a frequency predicted by their respective frequencies. For example if SNP-A is present at a frequency of 0.1 and SNP-B at 0.3, they will occur together at a frequency 0.1 x 0.3 = 0.03, that is, 3% of the population. If they lie on the *same* chromosome then they may occur together more frequently than predicted by their frequencies. This phenomenon is called linkage disequilibrium. The likelihood of 2 SNPs occurring together depends on how much chromosome recombination has occurred in the local gene region. Recombination is the process where material from the 2 copies of the same chromosome is exchanged. Recombination events are more common as distance between 2 loci increases. The recombination rate also varies in different parts of the genome, so physical distance between 2 markers alone is not a reliable predictor of linkage disequilibrium.

A haplotype is a group of SNPs which occur on the same chromosome. If the SNPs were independent of each other, there would a possible 2^n different haplotypes, where n is the number of SNPs. For example, for a group of 6 SNPs there are 64 (2^6) possible arrangements. In practice the number of haplotypes observed in a local gene region is much smaller, not only because of linkage disequilibrium between SNPs but also because a number of haplotypes will have been lost from the population, or occur at very low frequency.

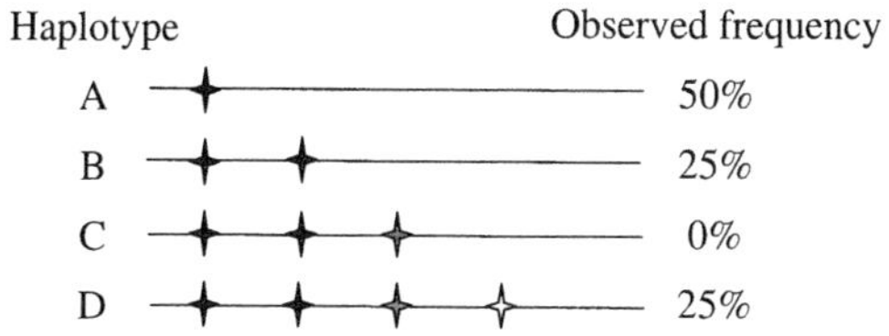

Haplotype		Observed frequency
A	—+————————	50%
B	—+——+—————	25%
C	—+——+——+——	0%
D	—+——+——+——+—	25%

In this example, 4 SNPs have arisen sequentially. The intermediate haplotype C has been lost from the population – by chance or because of a population bottleneck or because of selection – leaving only 3 observable haplotypes.

Arranging SNPs into haplotypes in gene regions permits a description of the observed diversity of that region. It also allows a subset of SNPs to be selected which fully describe that variation, with subsequent cost savings when genotyping large sample sets.

A..G..C..T..A...G
A..C..G..T..T...C
T..G..C..A..T...C
T..G..C..T..A...G

In this example, 4 common haplotypes are observed using 6 SNPs. The 4 haplotypes can be identified using only 3 of the 6 SNPs (shaded). The presence of the other SNPs can then be inferred.

Fig. 2 Linkage disequilibrium and haplotypes.

of 'tagging SNPs' to be selected which efficiently describes that diversity (see Fig. 2). Grouping SNPs into blocks or haplotypes, and then identifying tagging SNPs for the haplotypes, forms the basis of the International HapMap project (www.hapmap.org). By systematically typing common SNPs in individuals from 30 families from 4 distinct human populations, this project will develop a haplotype map of the human genome, the HapMap, which will describe the common patterns of human DNA sequence variation. There is no requirement for the selected tagging SNPs to have known functional effects. Rather they are acting as markers of genetic variation, and thereby any functional consequences of it. It has been estimated that once the HapMap is complete, between 200,000 and 1 million tagging SNPs will be needed to describe the haplotypic diversity across the genome.

Functional SNPs

The second approach is to identify which SNPs have direct effects on gene function. Since what you would like to test is the effect of variation in gene function on disease risk, knowing which SNPs affected gene function would make the process much simpler. The difficulty with this approach is that the experimental and bioinformatic tools available are not sufficiently precise to make accurate predictions of SNP function. This is particularly true for SNPs, which may affect the regulation of gene activity. There are approaches that can be applied which will enrich the SNP pool for those with functional effects. Two commonly used methods are to select SNPs which alter amino acids (non-synonymous SNPs) and SNPs in regulatory regions, such as promoters. The functional importance of regulatory elements may be increased if they show conserved homology between species. New SNPs are being identified on a daily basis and no definitive list of SNPs known to have direct effects on gene function is likely to be available for several years. Current estimates suggest there will be in excess of 30,000 non-synonymous SNPs and significantly more than that in the regulatory regions. It will only be possible to test experimentally the functional effects of a fraction of these SNPs. The effects of SNPs on gene function may depend on the tissue in which the gene is expressed, and the nature of the stimulus. The effects may also require the presence of other genetic variations (gene–gene interactions). Finally their effects on gene function may be rather subtle. Thus, it may be difficult to design effective in vitro experiments, which will 'prove', that a SNP has a direct effect on gene function.

Selection of genes to study

In an ideal situation, a genetic association study would seek to determine the effect of all genetic variation on the disease of interest. This approach has the greatest chance of identifying novel disease mechanisms. The cheapest genotyping technology now costs one cent per genotype. To account for the effects of multiple comparisons, samples sizes in excess of 1000 cases and controls are needed (see below). This means that typing a conservative 100,000 SNPs for a genome-wide study using either design would cost $2 million. So comprehensive investigation means big numbers and requires 'big bucks'. Therefore, all genetic association studies reported to date, including those on RSV disease, have used a candidate gene approach to focus on a smaller number of gene variants. The genes selected have biologically plausible roles in the disease process. Variation at the selected gene locus can then be studied with either the haplotype tagging or 'functional' SNP approach. Even using a candidate gene approach, based on what is already known about how RSV infection causes severe bronchiolitis, the list of potential candidate genes which might be critical in determining disease severity is large. These include mediators of innate host defence, cell signalling, surface molecules (including HLA molecules), cytokines, chemokines and interferons. Together this group alone comprises nearly 1000 genes.

Selection of subjects and controls

The phenotype to be studied must be well defined. Relatively modest levels of error in the phenotype will result in significantly diminished power (Ellsworth and Manolio, 1999; Terwilliger and Goring, 2000). Strict definition of phenotypes can be difficult. It is critical that various groups working on the genetic predisposition to RSV use agreed phenotypes. Sufficient clinical details should be collected about all infants enrolled in such studies to allow comparison between the same phenotype in different populations. This should include the age of the infant, the presence or absence of crackles heard on auscultation of the chest, the presence or absence of wheeze, objective markers of disease severity such as requirement for and duration of oxygen therapy, the ethnic background of the infant and parents, the presence or absence of risk factors, including prematurity, older siblings, parental smoking, use of daycare, and pre-existing heart or lung disease. Ideally the infant would also be followed up in subsequent years to determine the presence of subsequent wheezing illness. Collection of this type of clinical information will also allow subgroup analysis on larger sample sets.

Knowledge of ethnicity is particularly important. Different human populations, most commonly identified by ethnicity, often exhibit differences in frequency DNA variants, due to non-random mating such as that based on proximity or culture, population migration or selective pressure on particular populations. This substructure, or stratification, can cause problems since different proportions of ethnic groups may occur in cases compared to controls, either by chance or through systematic bias. For example, if cases are collected in a regional referral centre and controls are selected from the local population, it is quite possible for the distribution of different ethnicities to differ in the cases and controls. One method of avoiding this potential bias is to use family-based samples. By using the transmission of alleles from parents to offspring, the family-based approach completely obviates concerns about population substructure (Spielman et al., 1993; Ewens and Spielman, 1995) (Fig. 3). The disadvantage of this approach is that the design can make it harder to recruit large sample sizes (Risch and Teng, 1998) and larger

Case control study

In a case control study, cases are selected by a given phenotypic characteristic, for example blood culture proven pneumococcal septicaemia. At least an equal number of carefully matched controls are identified. Allele frequencies are then compared between the two groups. For relatively rare diseases (affecting less than 10% of the population), odds ratio gives the best estimate of true relative risk within the population.

Affected D+

Control D-

	D+	D-
Blue allele	16	10
Red allele	8	14

Odds ratio (OR) = (16/8) / (10/14) = 2.8

Note in the example that the OR is the same whether it is calculated as the odds of being affected if carrying the blue variant, or the odds of carrying the blue variant if affected. It estimates the true population risk of being affected if carrying the allele of interest. The probability (p value) is calculated by Chi square or Fishers exact test. In this example, p= 0.08

Family-based study

The family based design can be easily understood by considering the hypothetical family in (a). One of the parents is heterozygous for the marker of interest and carries a blue and a red allele. The other parent is homozygous for the red allele and therefore not informative. When we look at whether the red or blue allele is transmitted from the heterozygote parent to the ten offspring, as expected, five offspring have the red allele and five have the blue allele. If it turns out that the blue allele predisposes to the infection being studied, then more offspring carrying the blue allele will be affected (in this example three blue versus one red). If we now select families on the basis of having an affected offspring, we notice that, because we are now selecting for those offspring who are more likely to carry the blue allele, there is an apparent excess of transmission of this allele from heterozygote parents to their offspring. In the example shown in (b), instead of the 50% transmission expected if there were no effect, we observe the blue allele being transmitted on 6 out of 10 occasions (transmission of 60%). This distortion of expected transmission forms the bases of the transmission disequilibrium test (TDT) used in most family based designs. The probability of this being a non-random variation (p value) is calculated using Chi square, with 50% transmission giving the 'expected' values.

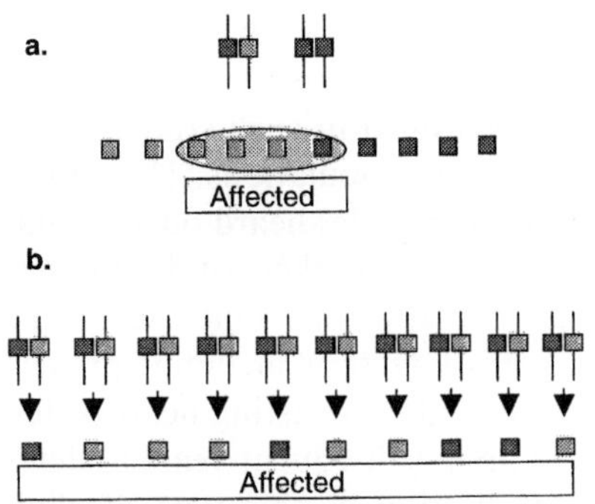

Adapted from Hull, J Genetic susceptibility to infection, in Infection and Immunity, Eds Friedland and Lightstone, publ: Martin Dunitz 2003.

Fig. 3 Case–control study (for colour version: see colour section on page 327).

numbers of samples need to be typed (2 parental controls per case). Positive associations present in both case control and family-based studies are likely to be more robust.

Sample size and method of analysis.

Analysis of genetic association studies is usually straightforward, particularly for case–control studies. The distribution of alleles or genotypes between cases and controls is compared using 2×2 or 2×3 tables, and odds ratios (ORs) are calculated with confidence intervals (Fig. 3). The OR is the odds of exposure among cases divided by the odds of exposure among controls. The OR provides a good approximation of the relative risk of the risk factor in question (that is, the ratio of risk of disease in people with the risk factor to that in people without it) using cross-sectionally selected cases and controls, provided that the disease under study is relatively rare (prevalence $< \sim 10\%$) (Kirkwood, 1988).

Complex diseases are typically characterised by high levels of genetic complexity, where multiple genes, each with a relatively small effect, may act independently or may interact with other genes to influence the diseased phenotype. Allelic influences on reasonably common, complex diseases will usually confer only modest ORs when the allele is also relatively common (above 0.05). For most genetic association studies of complex human diseases, the detected ORs have been between 1.2 and 2.0 (Ioannidis et al., 2003). To detect effects of this size with reasonable power (say 80%) will require studies of 1000 cases and 1000 controls (Risch, 2000; Botstein and Risch, 2003). The samples sizes selected must also take into account the need for correction for multiple comparisons. One practical approach to the problem of multiple comparisons is to re-test positive associations in a second cohort of similar size. Clearly the time and money required to establish DNA archives of this size are considerable. For this reason many of the preliminary studies reported so far have used smaller samples.

Genetic association studies of RSV bronchiolitis

In this section, I have summarised the published genetic association studies on RSV bronchiolitis. The section is arranged by the genes studied. A summary of the studies is shown in Table 1.

Surfactant proteins

Surfactant protein A (SPA) is a collectin and is thought to play a role in innate host defence. SPA binds to RSV via a carbohydrate recognition domain (CRD) (Ghildyal et al., 1999; Barr et al., 2000) and enhances opsonisation and receptor-mediated uptake of RSV by alveolar macrophages and monocytes (Barr et al., 2000). SPA-deficient mice have more severe RSV infection than do their wild-type littermates. Lofgren and colleagues in Finland (Lofgren et al., 2002) collected DNA

Table 1

Summary of studies on genetic associations with RSV bronchiolitis

Gene	Authors	Sample size	Study design	Analysis	Findings	Interpretation
SPA	Lofgren et al. (2002)	86	Case–control	9 SNPs sorted into alleles and haplotypes	Coding polymorphisms were associated with severe RSV ($p = 0.001$–0.023)	SPA may be important in controlling RSV infection, possibly as an opsonisation agent. Sample size rather small
SPD	Lahti et al. (2002)	84	Case–control	3 SNPs studied	One coding polymorphism was associated with severe RSV (OR 1.6, $p = 0.03$)	SPD may be important in controlling RSV infection, possibly as an opsonisation agent. Sample size rather small
MBL	Kristensen et al. (2004)	55	Case–control	3 functional SNPs which affect MBL levels	No association	Negative result. Sample size is too small to identify moderate effects
IL8	Hull et al. (2000)	580	Case–control and family study	18 SNPs	Positive association with individual SNPs and haplotypes	IL8 variants that appear to correlate with increased IL8 production are associated with severe RSV bronchiolitis
	Hull et al. (2004)			Allele, genotype and haplotype analysis	OR 1.3, $p = 0.01$	
IL9	Hoebee et al. (2004)	207	Case–control and family study	One promoter SNP	No association	Negative result. Hard to interpret since only 1 SNP of unknown functional significance was typed and the sample size is relatively small
IL10	Hoebee et al. (2004)	207	Case–control and family study	One promoter SNP	No overall effect. In subgroup analysis infants under 6 months were more likely to carry IL10-590C	Some conflict in results. Hull et al were unable to confirm the findings of Hoebee. Both effects were only seen in subgroups
	Wilson et al. (2005)	580	Case–control	4 haplotype-tagging SNPs	No overall effect. In subgroup analysis IL10-1117 was more frequent in infant who required mechanical ventilation (OR 1.7 $p = 0.004$)	

IL4	Choi et al. (2002)	105	Case–control	4 promoter and 2 intronic SNPs assorted into haplotypes	Positive association with IL4-589T (OR 1.6, $p = 0.02$)	Supports a role of IL4 in determining disease outcome. Similar result in 2 different populations increases likelihood of genuine effect
	Hoebee et al. (2003)	207	Case–control and family study	Single promoter SNP	Positive association with IL4-589T (OR 1.4, $p = 0.04$)	
IL4 receptor	Hoebee et al. (2003)	207	Case–control and family study	2 coding polymorphisms	No association overall. Both SNPs showed association in subgroups, but results were not consistent between case–control and family based analysis	Possible role of IL4 receptor variants. Subgroup analysis may need to be interpreted with caution
IL5	Choi et al (2002)	105		1 promoter SNP	Negative result	Non-functional SNP and small sample size make drawing firm conclusions difficult
IL13	Choi et al (2002)	105		2 promoter and one exonic SNP	Negative result	The exonic SNP may be a functional marker, but again small sample size makes interpretation difficult
TLR4	Tal et al. (2003)	99	Case control	2 coding SNPs associated with LPS hypo-responsiveness	Positive association with both SNPs. OR 4.5, $p = 0.01$	The OR is unusually high for a genetic association study and the sample size is too small to be confident that the result will be replicated
CD14	Tal et al. (2003)	99	Case control	Single promoter SNP associated with serum CD14 levels	No association	Negative result. Although only 1 SNP was typed, there is good evidence that this is a functional marker. The small sample size makes it hard to be confident in the result
CCR5	Hull et al. (2003)	580	Case–control and family	5 SNPs assorted into haplotypes	Positive association with 2 promoter SNPs. OR 1.3, $p = 0.01$	Functional significance of associated SNPs unknown. Nevertheless, the result supports a role for CC chemokines in pathogenesis of severe disease
TNFa	Hoebee et al. (2004)	207	Case–control and family	One promoter SNP	No association	TNF-308 may be functional. Negative result decreases likelihood of role of TNF in explaining variation in RSV disease outcome

from 86 infants less than 12 months of age, admitted to hospital with a clinical diagnosis of RSV bronchiolitis. In all, 95 age- and sex-matched controls with no history of respiratory infections requiring hospitalisation during infancy were also enrolled. Nine SNPs were assayed in SPA1 and SPA2. These occur together in different combinations resulting in 19 alleles for SPA1 (denoted by $6A^{n}$) and 15 alleles for SPA2 (denoted by $1A^{m}$). The authors found a different distribution of both SPA1 and SPA2 alleles in cases compared to controls. Several of the SPA polymorphisms affect amino acid content of the protein. When alleles that resulted in the same amino acid change were clustered together, significantly different frequencies of allele types were found in the RSV-infection group compared to the controls ($p = 0.001$). The amino acid changes identified by Lofgren et al. are predicted to affect RSV binding to SPA or SPA aggregation.

The same group has published findings on surfactant protein D (SPD) variants (Lahti et al., 2002). SPD is also a collectin thought to be important in innate host defence. Three coding polymorphisms that alter amino acids in the SPD protein were studied in the same group of cases and controls as the SPA study. One of the 3 studied polymorphisms showed a difference between cases and controls (OR 1.6, $p = 0.03$). This amino acid change is proposed to affect the multimerisation of SPD and its ability to bind viruses. These findings support a role for SPA and SPD in RSV bronchiolitis pathogenesis.

Mannose-binding lectin

Mannose-binding lectin (MBL), like SPA and SPD is a collectin, and may also be involved in innate host defence. Commonly occurring genetic variants of MBL are associated with low levels of serum MBL and have been associated with several infectious diseases (Summerfield et al., 1997; Koch et al., 2001). Kristensen and colleagues from Soweto in South Africa (Kristensen et al., 2004), sought to determine if the same MBL variants influenced RSV disease risk. This was a hospital-based study of 55 infants with severe RSV infection compared to 113 sex- and age- matched controls. No statistically significant effect was found. This is consistent with a study showing neonatal MBL levels do not associate with RSV disease risk (Nielsen et al., 2003). Nevertheless infants with genotypes associated with low-serum MBL levels were slightly over-represented in the RSV group (OR 1.4, CI 0.4–4.6). A larger sample size may have identified a significant effect of these genotypes.

Interleukin-8

The predominant cell type in the respiratory secretions of infants with RSV bronchiolitis is the neutrophil. Interleukin-8 (IL8) is a potent neutrophil attractant and activator. It is present in high levels in airway secretions of infected infants, and IL8 levels correlate with disease severity (Smyth et al., 2002). Hull and colleagues in the UK (Hull et al., 2004) collected DNA from 580 infants with severe

RSV bronchiolitis identified prospectively and from an equal number of population controls derived from cord blood samples. DNA was also collected from the parents of the cases allowing a family based as well as a case–control analysis. The authors identified 8 SNPs in the IL8 gene plus 55 others in the flanking regions. Single SNP and haplotype analysis indicated that genetic variation in this region affects RSV disease risk, using both the case–control and the family-based analysis. The most consistent single SNP effect was found with the promoter SNP IL8-251 (OR 1.3, $p = 0.005$). This SNP has been correlated with IL8 production in vitro using whole blood stimulated with LPS (Hull et al., 2000). Haplotype analysis suggested the true functional element might lie upstream of IL8, although the analysis was not able to localise this effect precisely. These data suggest that infants who have more pronounced IL8 response to RSV infection are likely to suffer more severe disease.

Interleukin-9

It has been suggested that an imbalance between the Th1 and Th2 directed immune responses to RSV infection may be important in determining RSV disease severity. Interleukin-9 (IL9) promotes proliferation of Th2 cells and activates bronchial epithelial cells to produce mucin and chemokines. Hoebee and colleagues from The Netherlands (Hoebee et al., 2004) collected DNA from 207 children admitted to hospital with RSV bronchiolitis. There was no specified upper age limit, but the mean age was 4 months. Of the 207 children, 148 were considered to be native Dutch and used in the case–control study. DNA was collected from both parents. DNA was also collected from 447 adult Dutch controls. The investigators studied a single promoter SNP in IL9. Promoter regions are enriched for elements that control gene expression and SNPs in these regions have a higher than average chance of being functional. There are no experimental data, which indicate that the IL9 SNP selected (IL9-345) has any functional consequences. No association was found. The SNP occurs at low frequency (0.06). The combination of the relatively small sample size, the low frequency of the SNP and the lack of functional data make it difficult to draw any firm conclusions about the role of IL9 in RSV disease based on these data.

Interleukin-10

IL10 is a multifunctional cytokine that promotes Th2 immunity. It diminishes the cell-mediated immune response through a combination of cytokine, chemokine and antigen presentation inhibition and enhances humoral immunity by stimulating the proliferation of B cells and T cells. IL10 promoter haplotypes have been associated with altered levels of IL10 gene expression. Hoebee et al. (Hoebee et al., 2004) studied one of the SNPs that comprise the functional haplotype and found no association with RSV bronchiolitis. In a subgroup analysis, there appeared to be an effect in infants under 6 months of age. It is possible that this group was enriched for those more likely to have primary RSV infection. Wilson et al. (2005), using the Oxford RSV cohort, also studied this marker, along with 3 other IL10 haplotype tagging SNPs, and once again found no association in all cases of RSV bronchiolitis. They failed to replicate the Dutch group's finding of an effect in infants under 6 months. In a subgroup analysis, Wilson et al. found an association between a different IL10 promoter SNP and infants with severe RSV needing mechanical ventilation.

Interleukin-4, interleukin-5 and interleukin-13

Interleukin-4 (IL4), interleukin-13 (IL13) and interleukin-5 (IL5) have been identified as critical molecules in the Th2 response. The genes for these mediators are clustered on chromosome 5 and are obvious candidates for an RSV genetic association study.

Choi et al. (2002) from Korea collected DNA from 105 children with RSV LRI. The children were up to 24 months of age and lacked known risk factors. The control subjects consisted of 315 anonymous healthy Korean blood donors recruited at the Seoul National University Hospital. The authors studied 6 SNPs in IL4, 3 SNPs in IL13 and 1 SNP in IL5. The IL4 promoter SNP IL4-589 has been associated with altered IL4 transcriptional activity using reporter gene assays (the T allele is associated with higher rates of transcription), suggesting it is a marker for functional variation of IL4 gene activity. One of the SNPs in IL13 was in the coding region and in European populations has been associated with asthma and IgE levels. The promoter SNP in IL5 has no known function. The authors found that IL4-589T was commoner in cases than controls (OR 1.6, $p = 0.02$). Haplotype analysis did not strengthen this effect. The SNPs in IL5 and IL13 showed no association with severe disease. This study suggests that IL4, one of the Th2 signature cytokines, plays a role in RSV disease severity. It is important to note that the upper age limit in this study was 2 years, and it is possible that children with wheezing illness were included. Greater detail of the cases was not provided in the paper. Also the choice of blood donors as controls can introduce bias since this particular group of individuals may not be representative of the population.

Hoebee et al. studied the same SNP (IL4-589) in 207 Dutch infants with severe RSV (see IL9) (Hoebee et al., 2003). They also found that the IL4-589T polymorphism was commoner in cases and controls (OR 1.4, $p = 0.04$) with a trend in the same direction using a family-based analysis. (OR 1.3, $p = 0.1$).

The combination of the positive association of IL4-589T in 2 independent studies on 2 populations increases the likelihood that this result represents a genuine genetic association with severe RSV disease.

IL4 receptor alpha

Hoebee et al. (2003) also studied 2 polymorphisms in IL4Ra using the same group of 207 Dutch infants. Both SNPs result in amino acid changes and may have effects on receptor function, although this has not been tested experimentally. Neither SNP showed association with RSV bronchiolitis in this study. Although there were weak associations in 2 subgroups these were not consistent between the case-control and family-based analysis.

Toll-like receptor 4 and CD14

TLR4 and CD14 have been shown to be major lipopolysaccharide (LPS) receptors. The TLR4/CD14 receptor complex also interacts with other exogenous and endogenous proteins, such as RSV and fibrinogen (Kurt-Jones et al., 2000; Smiley et al., 2001). TLR4-deficient mice have a delayed clearance of RSV (Haynes et al., 2001). Tal et al. (2004) studied polymorphisms in CD14 and TLR4 in an Israeli Jewish population. Ninety-nine infants under 12 months, without known risk factors, with severe RSV needing hospital treatment were enrolled. An additional 82 ambulatory infants with mild RSV bronchiolitis and 90 healthy adults were also enrolled. Two SNPs in TLR4 were studied. These SNPs (Asp299Gly and Thr399Ile) are associated with hyporesponsiveness to inhaled LPS and an increased incidence of Gram-negative sepsis in human subjects (Arbour et al., 2000; Lorenz et al., 2002). Tal et al. found that both SNPs were more frequently found in severe cases compared to mild cases or controls (OR 4.5, $p = 0.01$). The odds ratio found is unusually high for a genetic association study and the sample size is small, particularly for a SNP that occurs at only 5% in the population. This combination increases that possibility that the observed association has arisen by chance.

The authors also studied one promoter SNP in CD14. This SNP (CD14-159) appears to correlate with soluble CD14 levels (Baldini et al., 1999; Kabesch et al., 2004). No effect of this SNP was seen on RSV disease risk. Although this study has the advantage of studying a polymorphism that appears to be associated with a functional effect, the sample size is too small to exclude a role for this gene variant.

CC chemokine receptor 5

The CC chemokines, regulated on activation, normal T cell expressed and secreted (RANTES) and macrophage inflammatory protein (MIP)-1a are important pro-inflammatory cytokines produced by RSV-infected airway epithelial cells. These chemokines are strongly chemotactic for T cells, monocytes, basophils, eosinophils, and, to a lesser degree, neutrophils. RANTES and MIP-1a are present at high levels in the respiratory secretion of infants with severe RSV disease and MIP-1a levels correlate with disease severity (Garofalo et al., 2001). RANTES and MIP-1a are the major ligands for CC chemokine receptor 5 (CCR5). Genetic variants of CCR5 have been linked to a number of diseases, most notably progression to AIDS after infection with human immunodeficiency virus (McDermott et al., 1998). Hull and colleagues, using the Oxford RSV cohort, studied 5 common SNPs in CCR5, which together describe all the common European CCR5 haplotypes (Hull et al., 2003). A family-based and case–control analysis found that a promoter SNP of CCR5 was associated with severe RSV bronchiolitis (OR 1.25, $p = 0.01$). The null variant CCR5d32 was not associated with disease. The authors suggest that the promoter SNP may increase expression of CCR5 resulting in more severe airways inflammation.

Tumour necrosis factor alpha

TNF is a major pro-inflammatory gene. A promoter polymorphism, TNF-308, has been reported to influence TNF transcription, and has been associated with several complex diseases, including asthma. Hoebee et al. (2004) studied this SNP in their Dutch cohort and found no association.

Other studies

In addition to the studies described above, Gentile et al. (2003), from the US, has studied the frequency of single SNPs in IL10, TNFa, TGFb, IFNg and IL6 in a population of 77 infants with severe RSV. There were no controls in this study. The authors attempted to determine if any of the SNPs affected outcomes of the severe illness using logistic regression analysis. SNPs in IL10, IFNg and IL6 predicted more severe disease. The study design is unusual and the sample size is too small to be confident of the results. Nevertheless, it supports a model of disease whereby genetic variation of the host inflammatory response is an important predictor of disease severity.

General comments

Taken together, these studies have investigated over 50 SNPs in 14 genes. SNPs in 6 genes have given positive associations with severe RSV. Only one SNP, IL4-589T, has given consistent results when studied by two different groups. The sample sizes used in all these studies are too small to be confident about positive or negative results. On their own, these results have contributed little to our understanding of RSV disease pathogenesis. This is an inevitable consequence of studying genes that we already believe to be important in the disease process. These studies have demonstrated that genetic association analysis of RSV bronchiolitis is possible. When applied to larger sample sets and more extensive lists of candidate genes it is likely that important patterns will emerge.

The future

Understanding how naturally occurring genetic variation affects individual risk to complex human disease and individual responses to drugs is now big business, not only for academic institutions but also for the biotechnical and pharmaceutical industry. It is likely that this field will provide the next big steps forward in our knowledge of diseases and how we treat them. Massive investments are being made to improve the technology needed to carry out large-scale genotyping work. It is already possible to type over 500,000 SNPs in large numbers of samples in a matter of a few weeks. Increasingly dense SNP maps describing the genetic variability across the genome are now publicly available and methods of determining the most efficient sets of tagging SNPs are being derived. Large-scale studies looking for functional variants, such as those that affect gene transcription are underway. I believe that RSV disease needs to be well placed to make the most of these advances. This can only be achieved by having large well documented collections of DNA samples from infants with RSV disease along with appropriate controls. International agreement on phenotype definition will assist in the important task of replicating results. It is likely that the first genome-wide association studies of complex diseases will be published in the next 3 years. While these are inevitably going to be a relatively crude first pass, it is possible that even at this level, novel and previously unexpected disease processes will be discovered. RSV bronchiolitis is a common disease everywhere in the world. It is readily recognised and the infants are treated in hospital. This combination makes it feasible to collect large sample sizes in a relatively short time scale. We should be aiming to have sample collections of 5000 cases and controls to make the best use of the technologies that will provide a much-needed boost in our understanding of how RSV causes severe disease.

References

Arbour NC, Lorenz E, Schutte BC, Zabner J, Kline JN, Jones M, Frees K, Watt JL, Schwartz DA. TLR4 mutations are associated with endotoxin hyporesponsiveness in humans. Nat Genet 2000; 25(2): 187–191.

Baldini M, Lohman IC, Halonen M, Erickson RP, Holt PG, Martinez FD. A Polymorphism in the 5′ flanking region of the CD14 gene is associated with circulating soluble CD14 levels and with total serum immunoglobulin E. Am J Respir Cell Mol Biol 1999; 20(5): 976–983.

Barr FE, Pedigo H, Johnson TR, Shepherd VL. Surfactant protein—a enhances uptake of respiratory syncytial virus by monocytes and U937 macrophages. Am J Respir Cell Mol Biol 2000; 23(5): 586–592.

Bont L, Heijnen CJ, Kavelaars A, van Aalderen WM, Brus F, Draaisma JM, Pekelharing-Berghuis M, van Diemen-Steenvoorde RA, Kimpen JL. Local interferon-gamma levels during respiratory syncytial virus lower respiratory tract infection are associated with disease severity. J Infect Dis 2001; 184(3): 355–358.

Bosken CH, Hunt WC, Lambert WE, Samet JM. A parental history of asthma is a risk factor for wheezing and nonwheezing respiratory illnesses in infants younger than 18 months of age. Am J Respir Crit Care Med 2000; 161(6): 1810–1815.

Botstein D, Risch N. Discovering genotypes underlying human phenotypes: past successes for mendelian disease, future approaches for complex disease. Nat Genet 2003; 33(Suppl): 228–237.

Bradley JP, Bacharier LB, Bonfiglio J, Schechtman KB, Strunk R, Storch G, Castro M. Severity of respiratory syncytial virus bronchiolitis is affected by cigarette smoke exposure and atopy. Pediatrics 2005; 115(1): e7–e14.

Brandenburg AH, Kleinjan A, van Het Land B, Moll HA, Timmerman HH, de Swart RL, Neijens HJ, Fokkens W, Osterhaus AD. Type 1-like immune response is found in children with respiratory syncytial virus infection regardless of clinical severity. J Med Virol 2000; 62(2): 267–277.

Burrows B, Lebowitz MD, Knudson RJ. Epidemiologic evidence that childhood problems predispose to airways disease in the adult (an association between adult and pediatric respiratory disorders). Pediatr Res 1977; 11(3 Pt 2): 218–220.

Camilli AE, Holberg CJ, Wright AL, Taussig LM. Parental childhood respiratory illness and respiratory illness in their infants. Group health medical associates. Pediatr Pulmonol 1993; 16(5): 275–280.

Chavez-Bueno S, Mejias A, Gomez AM, Olsen KD, Rios AM, Fonseca-Aten M, Ramilo O, Jafri HS. Respiratory syncytial virus-induced acute and chronic airway disease is independent of genetic background: an experimental murine model. Virol J 2005; 2: 46.

Choi EH, Lee HJ, Yoo T, Chanock SJ. A common haplotype of interleukin-4 gene IL4 is associated with severe respiratory syncytial virus disease in Korean children. J Infect Dis 2002; 186(9): 1207–1211.

Comstock GW. Tuberculosis in twins: a re-analysis of the Prophit survey. Am Rev Respir Dis 1978; 117(4): 621–624.

DeVincenzo JP, El Saleeby CM, Bush AJ. Respiratory syncytial virus load predicts disease severity in previously healthy infants. J Infect Dis 2005; 191(11): 1861–1868.

Ellsworth DL, Manolio TA. The emerging importance of genetics in epidemiologic research II. Issues in study design and gene mapping. Ann Epidemiol 1999; 9(2): 75–90.

Ewens WJ, Spielman RS. The transmission/disequilibrium test: history, subdivision, and admixture. Am J Hum Genet 1995; 57(2): 455–464.

Garofalo RP, Patti J, Hintz KA, Hill V, Ogra PL, Welliver RC. Macrophage inflammatory protein-1alpha (not T helper type 2 cytokines) is associated with severe forms of respiratory syncytial virus bronchiolitis. J Infect Dis 2001; 184(4): 393–399.

Gedda L, Berard-Magistretti S, Brenci G. Miscellaneous clinical case reports in twins. Acta Genet Med Gemellol (Roma) 1984; 33(3): 505–508.

Gentile DA, Doyle WJ, Zeevi A, Howe-Adams J, Kapadia S, Trecki J, Skoner DP. Cytokine gene polymorphisms moderate illness severity in infants with respiratory syncytial virus infection. Hum Immunol 2003; 64(3): 338–344.

Ghildyal R, Hartley C, Varrasso A, Meanger J, Voelker DR, Anders EM, Mills J. Surfactant protein A binds to the fusion glycoprotein of respiratory syncytial virus and neutralizes virion infectivity. J Infect Dis 1999; 180(6): 2009–2013.

Goetghebuer T, Kwiatkowski D, Thomson A, Hull J. Familial susceptibility to severe respiratory infection in early life. Pediatr Pulmonol 2004; 38(4): 321–328.

Graham BS, Johnson TR, Peebles RS. Immune-mediated disease pathogenesis in respiratory syncytial virus infection. Immunopharmacology 2000; 48(3): 237–247.

Hall CB, Douglas Jr. RG, Geiman JM. Quantitative shedding patterns of respiratory syncytial virus in infants. J Infect Dis 1975; 132(2): 151–156.

Haynes LM, Moore DD, Kurt-Jones EA, Finberg RW, Anderson LJ, Tripp RA. Involvement of toll-like receptor 4 in innate immunity to respiratory syncytial virus. J Virol 2001; 75(22): 10,730–10,737.

Hirschhorn JN, Altshuler D. Once and again-issues surrounding replication in genetic association studies. J Clin Endocrinol Metab 2002; 87(10): 4438–4441.

Hocbee B, Bont L, Rietveld E, van Oosten M, Hodemaekers HM, Nagelkerke NJ, Neijens HJ, Kimpen JL, Kimman TG. Influence of promoter variants of interleukin-10, interleukin-9, and tumor necrosis factor-alpha genes on respiratory syncytial virus bronchiolitis. J Infect Dis 2004; 189(2): 239–247.

Hoebee B, Rietveld E, Bont L, Oosten M, Hodemaekers HM, Nagelkerke NJ, Neijens HJ, Kimpen JL, Kimman TG. Association of severe respiratory syncytial virus bronchiolitis with interleukin-4 and interleukin-4 receptor alpha polymorphisms. J Infect Dis 2003; 187(1): 2–11.

Holman RC, Curns AT, Cheek JE, Bresee JS, Singleton RJ, Carver K, Anderson LJ. Respiratory syncytial virus hospitalizations among American Indian and Alaska native infants and the general United States infant population. Pediatrics 2004; 114(4): e437–e444.

Hull J, Rowlands K, Lockhart E, Moore C, Sharland M, Kwiatkowski D. Variants of the chemokine receptor CCR5 are associated with severe bronchiolitis caused by respiratory syncytial virus. J Infect Dis 2003; 188(6): 904–907.

Hull J, Rowlands K, Lockhart E, Sharland M, Moore C, Hanchard N, Kwiatkowski DP. Haplotype mapping of the bronchiolitis susceptibility locus near IL8. Hum Genet 2004; 114(3): 272–279.

Hull J, Thomson A, Kwiatkowski D. Association of respiratory syncytial virus bronchiolitis with the interleukin 8 gene region in UK families. Thorax 2000; 55(12): 1023–1027.

Ioannidis JP. Genetic associations: false or true? Trends Mol Med 2003; 9(4): 135–138.

Ioannidis JP, Trikalinos TA, Ntzani EE, Contopoulos-Ioannidis DG. Genetic associations in large versus small studies: an empirical assessment. Lancet 2003; 361(9357): 567–571.

Jepson AP, Banya WA, Sisay-Joof F, Hassan-King M, Bennett S, Whittle HC. Genetic regulation of fever in *Plasmodium falciparum* malaria in Gambian twin children. J Infect Dis 1995; 172(1): 316–319.

Kabesch M, Hasemann K, Schickinger V, Tzotcheva I, Bohnert A, Carr D, Baldini M, Hackstein H, Leupold W, Weiland SK, Martinez FD, Mutius E, Bein G. A promoter polymorphism in the CD14 gene is associated with elevated levels of soluble CD14 but not with IgE or atopic diseases. Allergy 2004; 59(5): 520–525.

Kim HW, Arrobio JO, Brandt CD, Jeffries BC, Pyles G, Reid JL, Chanock RM, Parrott RH. Epidemiology of respiratory syncytial virus infection in Washington, D.C. I. Importance of the virus in different respiratory tract disease syndromes and temporal distribution of infection. Am J Epidemiol 1973; 98(3): 216–225.

Kim HW, Canchola JG, Brandt CD, Pyles G, Chanock RM, Jensen K, Parrott RH. Respiratory syncytial virus disease in infants despite prior administration of antigenic inactivated vaccine. Am J Epidemiol 1969; 89(4): 422–434.

Kimura M. The Neutral Theory of Molecular Evolution. Cambridge: Cambridge University Press; 1983.

Kirkwood BR. Cohort and Case–Control Studies. Essentials of Medical Statistics. Oxford: Blackwell Scientific Publications; 1988; pp. 173–183.

Koch A, Melbye M, Sorensen P, Homoe P, Madsen HO, Molbak K, Hansen CH, Andersen LH, Hahn GW, Garred P. Acute respiratory tract infections and mannose-binding lectin insufficiency during early childhood. JAMA 2001; 285(10): 1316–1321.

Koopman LP, Smit HA, Heijnen ML, Wijga A, van Strien RT, Kerkhof M, Gerritsen J, Brunekreef B, de Jongste JC, Neijens HJ. Respiratory infections in infants: interaction of parental allergy, child care, and siblings—the PIAMA study. Pediatrics 2001; 108(4): 943–948.

Kristensen IA, Thiel S, Steffensen R, Madhi S, Sorour G, Olsen J. Mannan-binding lectin and RSV lower respiratory tract infection leading to hospitalization in children: a case–control study from Soweto, South Africa. Scand J Immunol 2004; 60(1-2): 184–188.

Kurt-Jones EA, Popova L, Kwinn L, Haynes LM, Jones LP, Tripp RA, Walsh EE, Freeman MW, Golenbock DT, Anderson LJ, Finberg RW. Pattern recognition receptors TLR4 and CD14 mediate response to respiratory syncytial virus. Nat Immunol 2000; 1(5): 398–401.

Lahti M, Lofgren J, Marttila R, Renko M, Klaavuniemi T, Haataja R, Ramet M, Hallman M. Surfactant protein D gene polymorphism associated with severe respiratory syncytial virus infection. Pediatr Res 2002; 51(6): 696–699.

Leeder SR, Corkhill R, Irwig LM, Holland WW, Colley JR. Influence of family factors on the incidence of lower respiratory illness during the first year of life. Br J Prev Soc Med 1976; 30(4): 203–212.

Legg JP, Hussain IR, Warner JA, Johnston SL, Warner JO. Type 1 and type 2 cytokine imbalance in acute respiratory syncytial virus bronchiolitis. Am J Respir Crit Care Med 2003; 168(6): 633–639.

Lofgren J, Ramet M, Renko M, Marttila R, Hallman M. Association between surfactant protein A gene locus and severe respiratory syncytial virus infection in infants. J Infect Dis 2002; 185(3): 283–289.

Lohmueller KE, Pearce CL, Pike M, Lander ES, Hirschhorn JN. Meta-analysis of genetic association studies supports a contribution of common variants to susceptibility to common disease. Nat Genet 2003; 33(2): 177–182.

Lorenz E, Mira JP, Frees KL, Schwartz DA. Relevance of mutations in the TLR4 receptor in patients with gram-negative septic shock. Arch Intern Med 2002; 162(9): 1028–1032.

Malaty HM, Engstrand L, Pedersen NL, Graham DY. *Helicobacter pylori* infection: genetic and environmental influences. A study of twins. Ann Intern Med 1994; 120(12): 982–986.

McConnochie KM, Roghmann KJ. Parental smoking, presence of older siblings, and family history of asthma increase risk of bronchiolitis. Am J Dis Child 1986; 140(8): 806–812.

McDermott DH, Zimmerman PA, Guignard F, Kleeberger CA, Leitman SF, Murphy PM. CCR5 promoter polymorphism and HIV-1 disease progression. Multicenter AIDS cohort study (MACS). Lancet 1998; 352(9131): 866–870.

Nielsen HE, Siersma V, Andersen S, Gahrn-Hansen B, Mordhorst CH, Norgaard-Pedersen B, Roder B, Sorensen TL, Temme R, Vestergaard BF. Respiratory syncytial virus infection—risk factors for hospital admission: a case–control study. Acta Paediatr 2003; 92(11): 1314–1321.

Openshaw PJ. Immunity and immunopathology to respiratory syncytial virus. The mouse model. Am J Respir Crit Care Med 1995; 152(4 Pt 2): S59–S62.

Page GP, George V, Go RC, Page PZ, Allison DB. Are we there yet? Deciding when one has demonstrated specific genetic causation in complex diseases and quantitative traits. Am J Hum Genet 2003; 73(4): 711–719.

Risch NJ. Searching for genetic determinants in the new millennium. Nature 2000; 405(6788): 847–856.

Risch N, Teng J. The relative power of family based and case–control designs for linkage disequilibrium studies of complex human diseases I. DNA pooling. Genome Res 1998; 8(12): 1273–1288.

Roman M, Calhoun WJ, Hinton KL, Avendano LF, Simon V, Escobar AM, Gaggero A, Diaz PV. Respiratory syncytial virus infection in infants is associated with predominant Th-2-like response. Am J Respir Crit Care Med 1997; 156(1): 190–195.

Smiley ST, King JA, Hancock WW. Fibrinogen stimulates macrophage chemokine secretion through toll-like receptor 4. J Immunol 2001; 167(5): 2887–2894.

Smyth RL, Mobbs KJ, O'Hea U, Ashby D, Hart CA. Respiratory syncytial virus bronchiolitis: disease severity, interleukin-8, and virus genotype. Pediatr Pulmonol 2002; 33(5): 339–346.

Sorensen TI, Nielsen GG, Andersen PK, Teasdale TW. Genetic and environmental influences on premature death in adult adoptees. N Engl J Med 1988; 318(12): 727–732.

Spielman RS, McGinnis RE, Ewens WJ. Transmission test for linkage disequilibrium: the insulin gene region and insulin-dependent diabetes mellitus (IDDM). Am J Hum Genet 1993; 52(3): 506–516.

Stark JM, McDowell SA, Koenigsknecht V, Prows DR, Leikauf JE, Le Vine AM, Leikauf D. Genetic susceptibility to respiratory syncytial virus infection in inbred mice. J Med Virol 2002; 67(1): 92–100.

Summerfield JA, Sumiya M, Levin M, Turner MW. Association of mutations in mannose binding protein gene with childhood infection in consecutive hospital series. BMJ 1997; 314(7089): 1229–1232.

Tal G, Mandelberg A, Dalal I, Cesar K, Somekh E, Tal A, Oron A, Itskovich S, Ballin A, Houri S, Beigelman A, Lider O, Rechavi G, Amariglio N. Association between common Toll-like receptor 4 mutations and severe respiratory syncytial virus disease. J Infect Dis 2004; 189(11): 2057–2063.

Terwilliger JD, Goring HH. Gene mapping in the 20th and 21st centuries: statistical methods, data analysis, and experimental design. Hum Biol 2000; 72(1): 63–132.

Trefny P, Stricker T, Baerlocher C, Sennhauser FH. Family history of atopy and clinical course of RSV infection in ambulatory and hospitalized infants. Pediatr Pulmonol 2000; 30(4): 302–306.

Welliver RC, Garofalo RP, Ogra PL. Beta-chemokines, but neither T helper type 1 nor T helper type 2 cytokines, correlate with severity of illness during respiratory syncytial virus infection. Pediatr Infect Dis J 2002; 21(5): 457–461.

Wilson J, Rowlands K, Rockett K, Moore C, Lockhart E, Sharland M, Kwiatkowski D, Hull J. Genetic variation at the IL10 gene locus is associated with severity of respiratory syncytial virus bronchiolitis. J Infect Dis 2005; 191(10): 1705–1709.

Wright PF, Gruber WC, Peters M, Reed G, Zhu Y, Robinson F, Coleman-Dockery S, Graham BS. Illness severity, viral shedding, and antibody responses in infants hospitalized with bronchiolitis caused by respiratory syncytial virus. J Infect Dis 2002; 185(8): 1011–1018.

Zhang L, Peeples ME, Boucher RC, Collins PL, Pickles RJ. Respiratory syncytial virus infection of human airway epithelial cells is polarized, specific to ciliated cells, and without obvious cytopathology. J Virol 2002; 76(11): 5654–5666.

Respiratory Syncytial Virus
Patricia Cane (Editor)

DOI 10.1016/S0168-7069(06)14005-7

Pathogenesis of RSV in Children

Stephen P. Brearey, Rosalind L. Smyth
Division of Child Health, School of Reproductive and Developmental Medicine, University of Liverpool, Alder Hey Children's Hospital, Liverpool, L12 2AP, UK

Introduction

Bronchiolitis, meaning inflammation of the bronchioles, is a clinical complex usually affecting children less than two years old. It is characterised by wheezing, dyspnoea, tachypnoea and poor feeding. The clinical characteristics, originally termed 'congestive catarrhal fever', have been recognised for over 150 years. It was not until the late 1950s that the epidemiology and viral aetiology of the illness were first described (Chanock and Finberg, 1957).

Respiratory syncytial virus (RSV) is the most common cause of bronchiolitis and is among the most important pathogens causing respiratory infection in infants worldwide. Epidemics occur during winter months, in temperate climates, and during the rainy season, in tropical climates. In the US, more than 120,000 infants are hospitalised annually with RSV infection, with more than 200 deaths attributed to RSV lower respiratory tract disease (Simoes, 2003). Total hospital charges for RSV-coded primary diagnoses during four years, from 1997 to 2000, were estimated to have been $2.6 billion (Leader and Kohlhase, 2003). Within hospitals, there is a high risk of nosocomial spread of RSV during epidemics, which can put vulnerable infants at risk of severe disease. Infection in infancy also predisposes children to the development of recurrent wheeze, thus increasing the long-term health care burden of this disease.

Prophylaxis is available as a recombinant monoclonal antibody, but is expensive and currently limited to infants at highest risk of severe disease (1998). Development of an effective vaccine would have a dramatic effect on morbidity and healthcare costs, but this is unlikely to occur soon. Treatment is generally supportive until the infection runs its natural course.

Viral infection and cytotoxicity

RSV first infects the epithelial cells of the upper respiratory tract. The incubation period is estimated to be between two and eight days (Domachowske and Rosenberg

1999). Viral replication in the nasopharynx has been shown to produce very large titres of RSV on tissue culture (Hall et al., 1976). Viral load in the upper airways peaks early, one to two days after onset of symptoms, and continues to decline even if lower respiratory tract symptoms subsequently develop (DeVincenzo et al., 2005).Infection will spread to the lower respiratory tract in 30–50% of infants, one–three days after the onset of the illness (Hall, 2001). The mechanism by which RSV spreads to the lower respiratory tract is thought to be by both direct spread along the respiratory epithelium and by aspiration of nasopharyngeal secretions (Richardson et al., 1978).

Following the infection of ciliated epithelial cells, the manifestations of bronchiolitis are caused by a combination of viral cytotoxicity and the immune response to infection.

Epithelial cell sloughing and mucous secretion cause airway obstruction and air trapping (McNamara and Smyth, 2002). This obstruction of the small airways has greater significance in infants, than older children and adults. Infants with pre-existing illnesses, such as congenital heart disease and chronic lung disease of prematurity are at further risk of severe RSV disease (Simoes and Groothuis, 2002).

The immune response to infection

The immune response to RSV infection includes innate and adaptive components. The innate immune response is rapid and recruits effector molecules and phagocytic cells to the site of infection through the release of cytokines. Adaptive immunity to RSV is generally composed of protective humoral immunity and the cellular response for viral clearance. Individual differences in these responses may explain the broad range in severity of disease. Recent research has highlighted that innate immunity in RSV disease is more important than previously thought. However, the differentiation between innate and adaptive immunity is becoming less distinct. Innate immune cells are capable of influencing the subsequent adaptive immune response and key components of the immune response to RSV infection, such as dendritic cells and macrophages, have an effect on both innate and adaptive cells (Iwasaki and Medzhitov, 2004). It is, therefore, important to recognise the interplay between innate and adaptive immune responses to RSV infection, rather than consider them as separate entities. The immune response to RSV infection is summarised in Fig. 1.

Humoral immunity

The humoral response to RSV infection results in the production of IgG, IgM and IgA antibodies in both blood and airway secretions. Indirect evidence that these antibodies have protective benefits are demonstrated by the reduced incidence of bronchiolitis in term babies in the first month of life, compared to the second and third months, and the increased risk of severe bronchiolitis in pre-term infants (de Sierra et al., 1993).

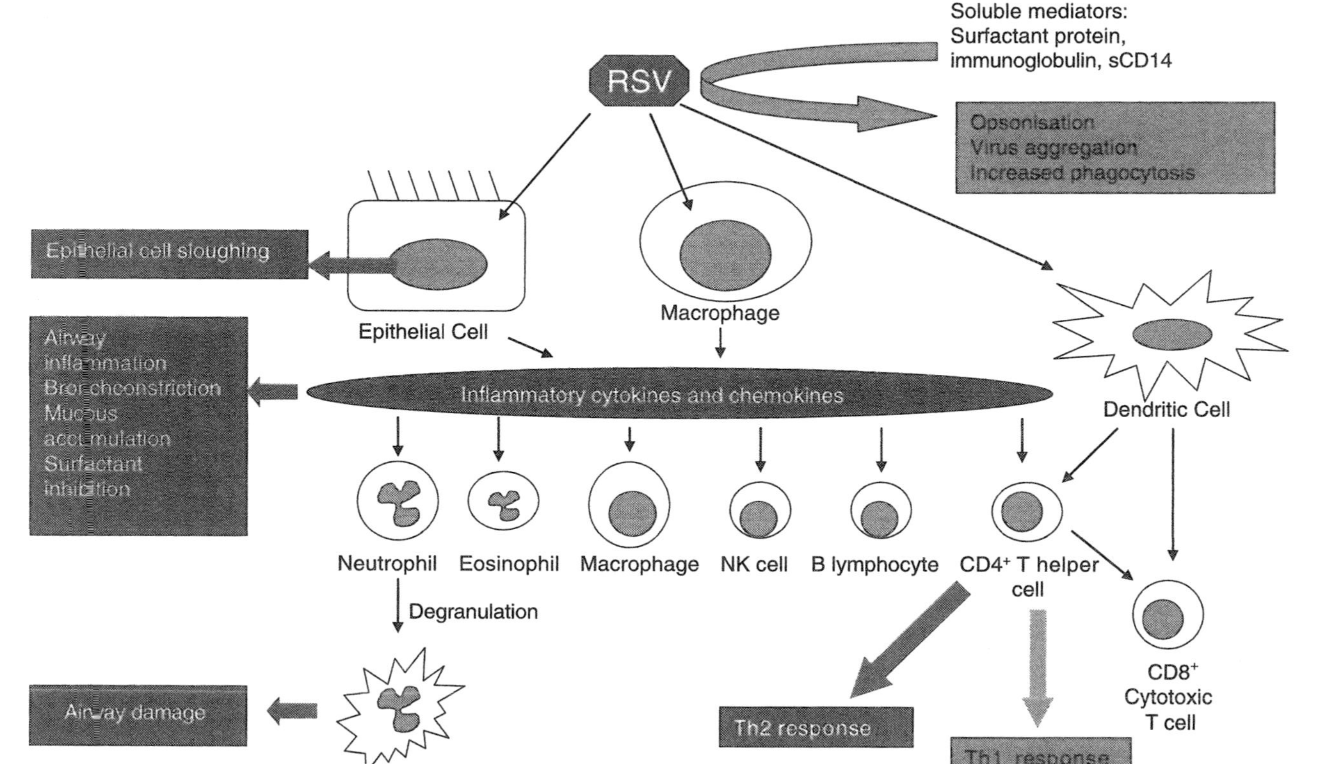

Fig. 1 Pathogenesis of RSV bronchiolitis. RSV first infects ciliated epithelial cells of the respiratory tract. Inflammatory cytokines and chemokines, secreted by infected epithelial cells and macrophages, attract inflammatory cells and cause inflammation and bronchoconstriction in the airway. The predominant inflammatory cells in the airway are neutrophils and alveolar macrophages. Dendritic cells are the main antigen-presenting cells that stimulate T-lymphocyte function. Neutrophil survival is prolonged and IL-9 secretion promotes mucus production. CD4+ T-helper lymphocytes may be skewed to produce proinflammatory (Th2) cytokines. The combination of epithelial cell sloughing, mucus plugging and airway inflammation leads to the clinical presentation of acute bronchiolitis (for colour version: see colour section on page 328).

Transplacental transfer ensures that RSV neutralising antibodies are present in the blood of all full-term newborns, after which levels decline (Beem et al., 1964). RSV-infected infants with higher levels of maternal anti-RSV antibodies have been shown to have a lower risk of hospitalisation and reduced severity of disease (Glezen et al., 1981). Although, even very young infants can produce serum and secretory antibodies, the antibody titres they produce are usually very low (McIntosh et al., 1978). IgG antibody is predominant in the lungs, while IgA predominates in the upper airways (1998). Several trials have demonstrated the efficacy of RSV neutralising antibodies, as a preventative treatment, in reducing the severity of disease (1998). Palivizumab is a humanised murine monoclonal IgG_1 antibody against the RSV F glycoprotein (Impact-RSV Study Group, 1998). It has been shown to reduce RSV viral load in the secretions of infants with bronchiolitis and is, therefore, thought to act by reducing viral replication in the lower airways (Devincenzo et al., 2003).

Epithelial cell response to infection

Epithelial cells are the primary target of RSV and infection proceeds by cell-to-cell spread of the virus. Two main defence mechanisms are employed by epithelial cells in response to infection: first, the production of molecules and proteins which have a direct antimicrobial effect, and second the recruitment of inflammatory cells and phagocytic cells to further augment the inflammatory response and contain the infection (Diamond et al., 2000).

Secreted defensins, collectins and mucus may all provide some antimicrobial properties against RSV. α and β defensins have some antiviral activity (Diamond et al., 2000) but their role in RSV infection has not been clarified. Mucous is secreted by goblet cells and can trap microorganisms before clearance by ciliary movement. RSV infection results in excessive mucous production which is inadequately cleared, thus contributing to airway obstruction in bronchiolitis (Miller et al., 2003).

Collectins are a group of structurally related proteins, which bind to pathogens and can mediate complement activation and opsonisation. Key members of the collectin family are surfactant proteins. Pulmonary surfactant provides early defence of viral infection. Surfactant proteins A (SP-A) and D (SP-D) can bind to the surface of a number of pathogens including RSV (Wright, 2005). The virus is thus opsonised and capable of binding to complement and receptors on phagocytic cells (neutrophils and macrophages), eosinophils and natural killer cells. SP-A has been shown to enhance opsonisation and receptor-mediated uptake of RSV by alveolar macrophages and monocytes (Barr et al., 2000). SP-A can also bind to the F protein of RSV, thus preventing viral entry to the cell and syncytia formation (Ghildyal et al., 1999). Polymorphisms in both SP-A and SP-D genes are associated with an increased risk of severe RSV disease (Lahti et al., 2002; Lofgren et al., 2002). During severe infection SP-A and SP-D levels in bronchoalveolar lavage (BAL) decrease (Kerr and Paton, 1999). A number of surfactant receptors have been identified (Tenner, 1999), including toll-like receptors 2 (TLR2) and 4 (TLR4) (Guillot et al., 2002).

Cytokine responses to RSV infection

Cytokines are secreted proteins that function as mediators of immune and inflammatory reactions. Chemokines are a sub-group of cytokines that stimulate leucocyte migration from the blood into tissues. Infected epithelial cells release proinflammatory substances and cytokines that increase capillary permeability and attract inflammatory cells. Table 1 summarises what is currently known from *in vitro* and clinical studies about important cytokines secreted by cells involved in the initial response to infection and the cytokines found in the airways of infants with bronchiolitis. From this body of evidence it is becoming increasingly apparent that the innate immune response to RSV infection is important to the pathogenesis of bronchiolitis.

In vitro, RSV-infected respiratory epithelial cells secrete interleukin-8 (IL-8), regulated on activation normal T cell expressed and secreted (RANTES),

Table 1

Summary of cytokines secreted by innate immune cells in response to RSV and corresponding cytokines isolated from the airways of RSV infected infants

Invitro studies	Clinical studies of RSV infected infants
Cytokines secreted by epithelial cells in response to RSV infection	*Cytokines isolated from the upper airways*
MCP-1, RANTES and IP-10 (Miller et al., 2004)	MIP-1α and RANTES (Bonville et al., 1999)
MIP-1α and RANTES (Becker and Soukup, 1999)	IL-β, IL-8, IL-6 and TNF-α (Noah et al., 2002)
IL-8 and RANTES (Mellow et al., 2004)	MIP-1α and MCP-1 (Garofalo et al., 2001)
MCP-1, RANTES and MIP-1α (Olszewska-Pazdrak et al., 1998)	IL-1, IL-8 and TNF-α (Hornsleth et al., 2001)
MIP-1α, RANTES and IL-8 (Harrison et al., 1999)	RANTES, MIP-1α, IL-6, IL-8 and IL-10 (Sheeran et al., 1999)
Cytokines secreted by macrophages in response to RSV infection	*Cytokines isolated from the lower airways*
RANTES and MIP-2 (Miller et al., 2004)	IL-8, IP-10, MCP-1 and MIP-1α (McNamara et al., 2005)
IL-10 (Panuska et al., 1990)	IL-6 and TNF-α (McNamara et al., 2004b)
IL-6, IL-8 and TNF-α (Becker et al., 1991)	RANTES, MIP-1-alpha, IL-6, IL-8 and IL-10 (Sheeran et al., 1999)
IL-1 (Salkind et al., 1991)	RANTES, MIP-1α and IL-8 (Harrison et al.,1999)
	IL-9 (McNamara et al., 2004a)
Cytokines secreted by neutrophils in response to RSV stimulation	
IL-8, MIP-1α and MIP-1β (Jaovisidha et al., 1999)	
IL-8 (Konig et al., 1993)	

macrophage inflammatory protein 1α (MIP-1α), monocyte chemoattractant protein 1 (MCP-1), interferon-inducible protein of 10 kDa (IP-10) and IL-6 (Becker and Soukup, 1999; Mellow et al., 2004; Miller et al., 2004). Chemokine production has also been shown to be dependent on infection with replicating RSV, which suggests viral replication is coupled with chemokine upregulation (Miller et al., 2004).

Other cells produce cytokines and chemokines in response to RSV infection. There is some *in vitro* evidence that RSV infects and replicates in alveolar macrophages (Panuska et al., 1990; Dakhama et al., 1998) and infected macrophages upregulate production of chemokines RANTES and MIP-2 (Miller et al., 2004). Other *in vitro* studies of alveolar macrophages have shown to secrete proinflammatory mediators IL-1, IL-6, IL-8, IL-10 and tumour necrosis factor-α (TNF-α) in response to RSV infection (Becker et al., 1991; Panuska et al., 1995). This results in further activation of macrophages and the recruitment and activation of inflammatory cells. *In vitro* work is supported by clinical studies that have found elevated concentrations of IL-8, RANTES, MIP-1α, MCP-1, IP-10 and IL-6 in the lower and upper respiratory tract of infants with RSV bronchiolitis (Bonville et al., 1999; Garofalo et al., 2001; McNamara et al., 2002b; Miller et al., 2004).

In vitro studies have demonstrated that neutrophils are also capable of secreting IL-8, MIP-1α and MIP-1β in response to RSV stimulation (Jaovisidha et al., 1999). A clinical study of 35 infants with severe RSV bronchiolitis also found large quantities of IL-9 in the lungs of infected infants compared to control infants and importantly discovered that neutrophils secreted the IL-9 (McNamara et al., 2002a). IL-9 is a Th2 lymphocyte-derived cytokine that has been shown to induce the production of proinflammatory cytokines and chemokines, as well as potently inducing mucus secretion in the lungs (Louahed et al., 2000).

Epithelial cells and dendritic cells will also secrete type I interferon (IFN-α and IFN-β) in response to RSV infection (Domachowske et al., 2001; Zhang et al., 2001). IFN-α and IFN-β have potent antiviral activity and can also induce expression of further chemokines attracting Th1-type lymphocytes such as IP-10 (Sauty et al., 1999). Studies of knockout mice, lacking genes for the IFN receptors, showed they generated Th2 responses to RSV infection (Johnson et al., 2005).

The role of macrophages in RSV infection

Alveolar macrophages mature when circulating monocytes migrate to the lung parenchyma. Macrophages, along with epithelial cells and resident dendritic cells, are the first to encounter RSV in the airways (Kimpen, 2001) and have an important role in orchestrating various immune responses to RSV infection. Alveolar macrophages do this by direct interaction with helper T (Th) cells and cytotoxic T cells (Janeway, 1999), the production of cytokines (Becker et al., 1991), phagocytosis of infected cells and antigen presentation (Kimpen, 2001). As described earlier, alveolar macrophages have shown to secrete proinflammatory mediators IL-1β, IL-6, IL-8, IL-10 and TNF-α in response to RSV infection (Becker et al., 1991; Panuska et al., 1995). These cytokines further upregulate the immune response by increasing vascular permeability and causing activation and recruitment of Th2-type lymphocytes, neutrophils, NK cells and eosinophils to the site of infection (McNamara and Smyth, 2002). This response to RSV infection is less significant in monocytes from neonatal cord blood than from adult blood, which may help explain why more severe disease is seen in younger infants (Matsuda et al., 1996). Macrophages also secrete the antiviral cytokine, IL-12. A study of children ventilated for RSV bronchiolitis found an inverse relationship between macrophage IL-12 production and duration of ventilation (Bont et al., 2000). It is possible, therefore, that a low macrophage IL-12 response to RSV infection may adversely affect the severity of RSV bronchiolitis.

Macrophages may be able to respond to RSV directly through direct interaction with TLRs. Ten TLRs have been identified in humans, each one recognising a distinctive non-human pathogen-associated molecular pattern (PAMP). Although their precise role is still being elucidated, there is increasing evidence that TLRs are important receptors of the innate and adaptive immune responses to RSV. TLR4 and its co-receptor, CD14, has been shown to recognise the RSV F protein and initiate cytokine and chemokine responses to the virus (Kurt-Jones et al., 2000). Human mononuclear cells exposed to RSV F protein showed induction of pro-inflammatory cytokines (IL-6, IL-8 and TNFα). This effect was dose dependent and blocked by anti-CD14 and anti-F protein antibodies. In murine alveolar macrophages, RSV-mediated activation of nuclear factor-κB (NF-κB) (an essential transcription factor for cytokine production) has been shown to be dependent on the functional expression of TLR4 (Haeberle et al., 2002). A clinical study of infants with RSV bronchiolitis found TLR4 was upregulated in blood monocytes of infected infants compared with controls (Gagro et al., 2004). Genetic susceptibility studies have identified two TLR4 gene mutations, Asp299Gly and Thr399lle, found to be associated with a significantly increased risk of severe RSV bronchiolitis (Tal et al., 2004).

Dendritic cells

Monocytes may also differentiate into dendritic cells, which have an important dual role of first stimulating the innate immune response to RSV infection and second, antigen presentation, activating naïve T cells to become RSV-specific effector T cells. Immature dendritic cells are present underneath the epithelial cell layer lining bronchioles and alveoli (Lambrecht and Hammad, 2003). Circulating plasmacytoid dendritic cells (pDCs) and myeloid dendritic cells (mDCs) are also recruited to sites of viral replication in the lungs (Gill et al., 2005). Mice infected with RSV demonstrated sustained increases in numbers of mature dendritic cells in the lungs (Beyer et al., 2004). Dendritic cells present antigen, with MHC II molecules, to naïve T cells, but this alone is not enough to induce their differentiation into effector T cells. Co-stimulatory molecules, such as CD-40, and proinflammatory cytokines are required to stimulate pathogen-specific T cells efficiently (Caux et al., 1994). Dendritic cells are capable of influencing T-cell responses to the type of pathogen that is encountered (Kapsenberg, 2003). For example, in response to intracellular bacteria, dendritic cells produce IL-12 to instruct Th1 polarisation, whereas extracellular parasites induce dendritic cells to instruct a Th2 polarisation (Kapsenberg, 2003). Immature cord blood dendritic cells that were infected with RSV resulted in reduced production of IFN-γ from co-cultured naïve T cells (Bartz et al., 2003).

Dendritic cells sense the presence of infection directly utilising pattern recognition receptors, of which TLRs are the most important (Schlender et al., 2005). TLR7 and TLR8 recognise viral single-stranded RNA in the endosomes of infected cells (Heil et al., 2004). TLR3 recognises double-stranded RNA in endosomes of the cell and initiates an immune response to RSV. In response to TLR stimulation, pDCs produce large amounts of type I interferon (IFN α and β) (Le and Tough, 2002). Type 1 interferon secreted locally recruits and activates innate immune cells to inhibit the spread of infection (Guerrero-Plata et al., 2005).

Many viruses have developed ways of evading innate and adaptive immune responses (Netea et al., 2004). RSV has been demonstrated to interfere with TLR7 and TLR9 signalling pathways in pDCs, resulting in significant reductions in type 1 IFN production (Schlender et al., 2005). In addition, mDCs infected with RSV demonstrate impaired CD4 T-cell proliferation and reduced production of Th1 cytokines (de Graaff et al., 2005). RSV non-structural proteins NS1 and NS2 have been implicated in virus induced inhibition of type 1 IFN production (Spann et al., 2004, 2005). Mice treated with intranasal siRNA targeted against NS1 showed substantially reduced viral titres in the lung and reduced airway inflammation and reactivity compared to controls (Zhang et al., 2005). RSV interference of dendritic cell function and type 1 IFN production may, therefore, contribute to the characteristic inflammatory response in the airways of infants with bronchiolitis.

T-helper lymphocyte response

In response to activated dendritic cells, naïve CD4+ Th0 lymphocytes have traditionally been considered to mature into two groups, according to the cytokine profiles they secrete. Th1 cells produce IFN-γ, IL-2 and other antiviral cytokines. Th2 cells produce cytokines, such as IL-4, that induce eosinophil proliferation, release of leucotrienes and IgE antibodies leading to an enhanced inflammatory response.

Interest in the role of CD4+ T-helper (Th) lymphocytes in the pathogenesis of bronchiolitis emerged following the unsuccessful trial of the formalin-inactivated RSV vaccine and subsequent animal studies. Infants that received the formalininactivated vaccine later developed more severe naturally acquired RSV bronchiolitis than unvaccinated infants (Kim et al., 1969b). When natural RSV infection occurred in children given the vaccine, 80% of these children were hospitalised and two died. This occurred despite the infants developing complement fixing and neutralizing antibodies after vaccination (Kim et al., 1969a). After immunizations in the trial were completed, it was observed that blood lymphocytes from vaccinated infants exhibited an exaggerated response to RSV antigens *in vitro* (Kim et al., 1976). On histological examination of their lungs, the two vaccinees who died had an excess of eosinophils, thus suggesting they suffered from a predominantly Th2 response (Kim et al.,1969b). Further studies on mice demonstrated that the formalin-inactivated vaccine induced high levels of RSV-specific memory CD4+ lymphocytes. Subsequent infection with the wild-type virus, resulted in a predominantly Th2-lymphocyte response (Graham et al., 1993). It has been hypothesised therefore that, RSV infection in human infants, induces an exuberant and predominantly Th2 inflammatory response, which is responsible for the immunopathogenic effects that cause clinical bronchiolitis (Domachowske and Rosenberg, 1999).

The idea that RSV bronchiolitis might be a Th2 disease is only supported to a limited extent by clinical studies. Genetic linkage studies have demonstrated an increased risk of severe RSV disease (Odds ratio 1.6) in infants with a polymorphism of the Th2 cytokine, IL-4 (Choi et al., 2002; Hoebee et al., 2003). A number of groups studying cytokine patterns in the blood and upper and lower airways of infected infants have given differing results. Studies of the blood of infected infants observed reductions in both IFNγ and IL-4 levels, but an increase in the IL-4/IFNγ ratio compared to control infants (Renzi et al., 1997; Roman et al., 1997). This was supported by studies of the nasal lavage fluid of infants with bronchiolitis, which also observed increased IL-4/IFNγ ratios compared with infants with only upper-airway symptoms (Legg et al., 2003). Another group, however, measured very high levels of IFNγ in the nasal lavage fluid of infected infants, but lower levels in ventilated infants than non-ventilated infants (Bont et al., 2001). A study investigating the immune response to RSV in blood and nasal washings from infected infants found that the immune response was dominated by the production of IFN-γ, and that only low levels of IL-4 and IL-10 were detectable (Brandenburg et al., 2000). Another study observed a mixed Th1 and Th2 cytokine response, with neither lymphocyte response dominant in infants with milder disease (de et al., 2003). Infants with severe disease have demonstrated a similar mixed response. BAL from ventilated infants with bronchiolitis revealed an IFNγ polarised response in 6 of 24 infants sampled, whereas 12 showed an IL-4 polarised response (Mobbs et al., 2002). The implication of this study is that more than one mechanism is likely to be responsible for the immune-mediated disease seen in severe bronchiolitis. BAL samples taken from less severely affected infants in another study found increased levels of IL-5 and increased IL-5/IFN-γ ratios compared to control infants (Kim et al., 2003). This study also identified two sub-groups with bronchiolitis: those with and without eosinophils in their BAL fluid. Those with eosinophils in their lungs had increased IL-5 levels, whereas those without eosinophils did not.

There is some evidence that the cellular immune response is more likely to produce a Th2-type response in early infancy. A study of the nasopharyngeal secretions of RSV-infected infants, discovered that those under three months of age had considerably higher levels of IL-4 than those over three months of age

(Kristjansson et al., 2005). Analysis of nasopharyngeal secretions from a large number of infants with bronchiolitis revealed that severe bronchiolitis was characterised by a more balanced Th1–Th2 response, whereas MIP-1α was markedly increased in infants with severe bronchiolitis (Garofalo et al., 2001). Thus, the severity of RSV bronchiolitis appeared to be related more to chemokine release by epithelial cells and neutrophils, than to Th2 cytokine production by lymphocytes. It is likely that multiple factors influence the T-lymphocyte response to RSV infection.

Neutrophil recruitment, activation and survival

Neutrophils are the predominant airway leucocytes in RSV bronchiolitis (Everard et al., 1994). They have been found to represent 93% of cells in the upper airway and up to 85% in the lower airway (Everard et al., 1994; Smith et al., 2001; McNamara et al., 2003). Studies of neutrophil chemotaxis, adhesion and cytotoxicity suggest that neutrophils play an important role in the pathological changes that occur in RSV bronchiolitis (Wang and Forsyth, 2000b).

Infected respiratory epithelial cells produce large quantities of the potent neutrophil chemoattractant, IL-8 (Kunkel et al., 1991). Serum and bronchoalveolar lavage samples from infants with severe RSV bronchiolitis have elevated IL-8 levels (Bont et al., 1999; Harrison et al., 1999). In addition, there is a strong correlation between the amounts of nasopharyngeal IL-8 mRNA and disease severity in RSV bronchiolitis (Smyth et al., 2002). A genetic susceptibility study found a two-fold increased risk of severe bronchiolitis for infants carrying the 251A allele of the IL-8 gene and this allele is associated with increased IL-8 production (Hull et al., 2000). *In vitro* studies demonstrate a biphasic pattern IL-8 gene expression in respiratory epithelial cells infected with RSV (Fiedler et al.,1995). The first peak occurs at 2 h and is independent of viral replication. This enables a rapid inflammatory response to occur before RSV infection can be established. Late expression, at 24 h, is dependent on viral replication. More recent studies have shown that IL-8 synthesis and protein secretion are continuously upregulated by persistently infected epithelial cells (Tirado et al., 2005).

The process of neutrophil recruitment from the blood into the infected airways can be divided into four steps: rolling, adhesion, extravasation and migration (McNamara and Smyth, 2002). Neutrophil adhesion of the vascular endothelium is mediated by two families of adhesion molecules: selectins and integrins. In RSV infection, L-selectin binds weakly to neutrophils, allowing them to roll along the endothelium (Wang and Forsyth, 2000). Neutrophils become anchored to the epithelium by intercellular adhesion molecule 1 (ICAM-1) binding to its receptors: the lymphocyte function-associated molecule 1 (LFA-1; CD11a/CD18) and Mac-1 (CD11b/CD18) (Wang et al., 1998a). Expression of these integrins and ICAM-1 are both increased in peripheral blood neutrophils of RSV-infected infants (Wang and Forsyth, 2000c). Neutrophils then pass between endothelial cells and migrate along a chemoattractant concentration gradient to the site of infection (Janeway, 1999).

Once in the airways, neutrophils are activated in response to RSV infection. It is likely that neutrophil activation occurs in response to inflammatory cytokines released by infected epithelial cells. Some *invitro* studies have demonstrated that RSV can directly activate neutrophils (Konig et al., 1996; Jaovisidha et al., 1999), but the purity of the viral preparations used was not demonstrated and more recent work has shown that purified RSV is a weak activator of neutrophils (Bataki et al., 2005). Activation by RSV may depend on the presence of other molecules, such as surfactant proteins. Activated neutrophils release products such as myeloperoxidase and neutrophil elastase into the airways that amplify viral cytotoxicity (bu-Harb et al., 1999). Respiratory epithelial cells, infected with RSV *invitro*, showed significantly increased cell damage in the presence of neutrophils (Wang et al., 1998b). In addition to this effect on epithelial cells, neutrophils have been shown to secrete IL-9 in large quantities in the lungs of severely infected infants (McNamara et al., 2004a). IL-9 is a potent proinflammatory cytokine that is known to cause eosinophilic inflammation, bronchial hyperresponsiveness and increased mucous production (Dong et al., 1999; Louahed et al., 2000).

The cytotoxic effect of neutrophils is enhanced by their retention at the site of infection. Neutrophil adhesion to epithelial cells uses similar molecular interactions used for adhesion to endothelial cells. In RSV-infected epithelial cells, expression of adhesion molecules, ICAM-1 and vascular cell adhesion molecule 1 (VCAM-1), is increased (Atsuta et al., 1997). Antibodies to integrins and ICAM-1 have also been shown to reduce the quantity of neutrophils in the airways of rats infected with RSV (Sorkness et al., 2000). Increased neutrophil adhesion to epithelial cells in RSV disease is both time and dose dependent (Stark et al., 1996).

Apoptosis of neutrophils is an important innate regulatory process, which limits neutrophil-induced inflammation in the airways. Apoptotic neutrophils are phagocytosed by macrophages via the vitronectin or phosphatidylserine receptors, thus preventing the release of harmful neutrophil products (Fadok et al., 1992). Neutrophil survival is thought to be prolonged in RSV bronchiolitis (Jones et al., 2002). A recent study demonstrated that isolated peripheral blood neutrophils, exposed to nasal lavage fluid from infants with RSV bronchiolitis, had a reduced rate of apoptosis (Jones et al., 2002). This observation may relate to the presence of IL-8, leucotriene-B_4 (LTB_4) and granulocyte–monocyte colony-stimulating factor (GM-CSF) in the airways of infants with RSV bronchiolitis, which have been shown to inhibit neutrophil apoptosis (Lee et al., 1993; Sampson, 2000).

Eosinophils

As described earlier, the possible importance of eosinophils in the pathogenesis of RSV bronchiolitis was demonstrated after the unsuccessful trial of the formalin-inactivated RSV vaccine in the 1960s (Kim et al., 1969b). Post-mortem examination revealed peribronchiolar monocytic infiltration with an excess of eosinophils. Further *invitro* studies showed RSV-infected respiratory epithelial cells secrete the eosinophil chemoattractants RANTES and MIP-1α (Harrison et al., 1999). Eosinophil-secretory proteins have also been isolated from the upper and lower airways of infants with RSV bronchiolitis (Harrison et al., 1999). The secretory ribonucleases, eosinophil cationic protein (ECP) and eosinophil-derived neurotoxin (EDN) have been detected in the lower airways of infected infants and ECP concentrations found to correlate with MIP-1α levels (Harrison et al., 1999). In addition, a study of blood samples taken from infants with RSV bronchiolitis found reduced levels of ECP compared to ECP levels in blood from convalescent and control infants, suggesting that peripheral blood eosinophils may have been recruited to the lungs (Smyth et al., 1997).

However, clinical studies have demonstrated eosinophils constitute less than 1% of the inflammatory cells in the lungs of infants with severe RSV disease (McNamara et al., 2003). This may be due to failure of the immune response to attract and activate eosinophils, a restriction in eosinophil migration in the airways or that the life span of eosinophils is very short after they have been recruited to the lungs, activated, released their granulation products and become necrotic or apoptotic.

Natural killer cells

Natural killer (NK) cells recognise and kill virus-infected cells by recognising the virus-induced changes in MHC class I expression and presentation on the cell surface. NK cells in mice have been shown to migrate to the lungs in the first 48 h after RSV infection (Hussell and Openshaw, 1998). In infants, admitted to hospital with RSV bronchiolitis, lower concentrations of blood NK cells were found compared to controls, suggesting probable NK cell recruitment to the lungs (De Weerd et al., 1998). TLR4-deficient mice challenged with RSV exhibit impaired NK cell pulmonary trafficking, deficient NK cell function, impaired IL-12 expression and impaired virus clearance (Haynes et al., 2001). This suggests that NK cells and TLR4 have an important role in viral clearance in this animal model. Along with alveolar macrophages, NK cells produce large amounts of IFN-γ (Hussell and Openshaw, 1998) in response to cytokines (IFN-β, IL-12 and TNF-α) secreted by infected epithelial cells (Hussell and Openshaw, 1998, 2000; Hussell et al., 2001). Studies of mice with depleted NK cells have shown an increased viral load five days after infection (Anderson et al., 1989). Further studies of mice infected with the RSV deletion mutant, expressing no G or SH protein, led to increased numbers of NK cells in BAL fluid compared to mice infected with the wild-type virus (Tripp et al., 1999). This implies that RSV modifies this part of the innate immune response to infection.

Cell-mediated immunity

The cellular immune response has a role in both viral clearance and may be involved in the pathogenesis of RSV bronchiolitis. The cell-mediated response comprises

CD4+ T-helper lymphocytes, described above, and CD8+ cytotoxic T lymphocytes. The role of cell-mediated immunity is demonstrated in children with deficient cellular immunity who shed the virus for many months after initial infection, compared to two weeks for immunocompetent infants (Fishaut et al., 1980). Mice studies confirm this clinical observation. Mice depleted of either CD4+ or CD8+ lymphocytes still eradicated the virus, but RSV infection was markedly prolonged (Graham et al., 1991). Passive transfer of RSV-specific CD4+ or CD8+ lymphocytes resulted in increased pulmonary shedding of the virus along with increased pulmonary damage (Munoz et al., 1991).

Cytotoxic T-lymphocyte response

CD8+ Cytotoxic T-lymphocytes (CTLs) promote clearance of RSV from the lungs but has also been shown to cause pulmonary injury in mouse models by inducing an inflammatory response (Cannon et al., 1988). In addition, reduced blood CTL concentrations in infants admitted with RSV bronchiolitis have been observed, compared to samples taken one week after infection (De Weerd et al., 1998). It has been suggested that this is due to a redistribution of CTLs from the peripheral blood to the lungs. However, other studies do not support the hypothesis that CTL cytotoxicity is responsible for the pathogenic features of RSV bronchiolitis. RSV-specific CTLs are recruited to the airways within 10 days of infection and peak well after the most severe manifestations of the disease have past (Chiba et al., 1989). Although most RSV bronchiolitis occurs in infants two to five months old, CTL cytotoxicity to RSV infected cells increases with age (Hall, 1998). Less than 40% of infants under five months of age demonstrated CTL cytotoxicity to RSV compared to 65% for the six month to two-year-old children (Chiba et al., 1989). CTLs specific for a number of RSV proteins (SH, F, M and NS2) have been identified, but the inability of the G protein to induce a CTL response may enable the virus to subvert the cellular immune response (Srikiatkhachorn and Braciale, 1997).

Neurogenic-mediated inflammation

Substance P is a bronchoconstrictor and potent proinflammatory mediator secreted by nocioceptive fibres in response to physical and chemical changes in the lower respiratory tract (Piedimonte et al., 1999). RSV infection has been shown to sensitise the airways to substance P by upregulating its neurokinin-1 (NK-1) receptor on a number of target cells (Piedimonte, 2001). These cells include lymphocytes, macrophages and mast cells that secrete inflammatory cytokines such as TNFα in response to substance P stimulation. The resultant inflammation and hyperreactivity may persist after RSV infection has resolved and may explain the post-bronchiolitic symptoms seen in some children (Piedimonte, 2002).

Apnoea is a common complication of RSV bronchiolitis and a study of weanling rats found that chemically induced apnoea was significantly prolonged in RSV-infected rats compared to uninfected controls (Sabogal et al., 2005). Apnoea-related mortality only occurred in the RSV-infected rats. A reduction in the duration of apnoea was observed after inhibition of neurokinin receptors for substance P, as well as central gamma-aminobutyric acid (GABA) receptors. This provides a possible mechanism for RSV-induced apnoea in early life.

Conclusion

The pathogenesis of RSV bronchiolitis is largely related to the immune response to infection. Reasons for the great variability in clinical severity of the illness can be summarised as either differences in infants' immune response to RSV infection or susceptibility to viral interference in immune function. Better understanding of the early response to RSV infection and how this influences later inflammatory reactions has been outlined. Cytokines and chemokines secreted by epithelial cells, macrophages, neutrophils and dendritic cells have an important role in recruiting and activating further inflammatory cells. Persistence of neutrophils in the lungs of infected infants and their prolonged survival amplify parenchymal damage, mucus production and inflammation in the lungs. Although the importance of innate immunity has come to light in recent years, further work is required to elucidate the interplay between the innate and adaptive components of the immune response to RSV infection.

References

Anderson JJ, Serin M, Harrop J, Amin S, Toms GL, Scott R. Natural killer cell response to respiratory syncytial virus in the Balb/c mouse model. Adv Exp Med Biol 1989; 257: 211–220.

Atsuta J, Sterbinsky SA, Plitt J, Schwiebert LM, Bochner BS, Schleimer RP. Phenotyping and cytokine regulation of the BEAS-2B human bronchial epithelial cell: demonstration of inducible expression of the adhesion molecules VCAM-1 and ICAM-1. Am J Respir Cell Mol Biol 1997; 17(5): 571–582.

Barr FE, Pedigo H, Johnson TR, Shepherd VL. Surfactant protein-A enhances uptake of respiratory syncytial virus by monocytes and U937 macrophages. Am J Respir Cell Mol. Biol 2000; 23(5): 586–592.

Bartz H, Turkel O, Hoffjan S, Rothoeft T, Gonschorek A, Schauer U. Respiratory syncytial virus decreases the capacity of myeloid dendritic cells to induce interferon-gamma in naive T cells. Immunology 2003; 10(1): 49–57.

Bataki EL, Evans GS, Everard ML. Respiratory syncytial virus and neutrophil activation. Clin. Exp. Immunol 2005; 140(3): 470–477.

Becker S, Quay J, Soukup J. Cytokine (tumor necrosis factor, IL-6, and IL-8) production by respiratory syncytial virus-infected human alveolar macrophages. J Immunol 1991; 147(12): 4307–4312.

Becker S, Soukup JM. Airway epithelial cell-induced activation of monocytes and eosinophils in respiratory syncytial viral infection. Immunobiology 1999; 201(1): 88–106.

Beem M, Egerer R, Anderson J. Respiratory syncytial virus neutralizing antibodies in persons residing in Chicago, Illinois. Pediatrics 1964; 34: 761–770.

Beyer M, Bartz H, Horner K, Doths S, Koerner-Rettberg C, Schwarze J. Sustained increases in numbers of pulmonary dendritic cells after respiratory syncytial virus infection. J Allergy Clin Immunol 2004; 113(1): 127–133.

Bont L, Heijnen CJ, Kavelaars A, van Aalderen WM, Brus F, Draaisma JM, Pekelharing-Berghuis M, Diemen-Steenvoorde RA, Kimpen JL. Local interferon-gamma levels during respiratory syncytial virus lower respiratory tract infection are associated with disease severity. J Infect Dis 2001; 184(3): 355–358.

Bont L, Heijnen CJ, Kavelaars A, van Aalderen WM, Brus F, Draaisma JT, Geelen SM, van Vught HJ, Kimpen JL. Peripheral blood cytokine responses and disease severity in respiratory syncytial virus bronchiolitis. Eur Respir J 1999; 14(1): 144–149.

Bont L, Kavelaars A, Heijnen CJ, van Vught AJ, Kimpen JL. Monocyte interleukin-12 production is inversely related to duration of respiratory failure in respiratory syncytial virus bronchiolitis. J Infect Dis 2000; 181(5): 1772–1775.

Bonville CA, Rosenberg HF, Domachowske JB. Macrophage inflammatory protein-1alpha and RANTES are present in nasal secretions during ongoing upper respiratory tract infection. Pediatr Allergy Immunol 1999; 10(1): 39–44.

Brandenburg AH, Kleinjan A, van Het LB, Moll HA, Timmerman HH, de Swart RL, Neijens HJ, Fokkens W, Osterhaus AD. Type 1-like immune response is found in children with respiratory syncytial virus infection regardless of clinical severity. J Med Virol 2000; 62(2): 267–277.

bu-Harb M, Bell F, Finn A, Rao WH, Nixon L, Shale D, Everard ML. IL-8 and neutrophil elastase levels in the respiratory tract of infants with RSV bronchiolitis. Eur Respir J 1999; 14(1): 139–143.

Cannon MJ, Openshaw PJ, Askonas BA. Cytotoxic T cells clear virus but augment lung pathology in mice infected with respiratory syncytial virus. J Exp Med 1988; 168(3): 1163–1168.

Caux C, Massacrier C, Vanbervliet B, Dubois B, Van KC, Durand I, Banchereau J. Activation of human dendritic cells through CD40 cross-linking. J Exp Med 1994; 180(4): 1263–1272.

Chanock RM, Finberg L. Recovery from infants with respiratory illness of a virus related to chimpanzee coryza agent (CCA) Epidemiological aspects of infection in infants and young children. Am J Hyg 1957; 66: 291–300.

Chiba Y, Higashidate Y, Suga K, Honjo K, Tsutsumi H, Ogra PL. Development of cell-mediated cytotoxic immunity to respiratory syncytial virus in human infants following naturally acquired infection. J Med Virol 1989; 28(3): 133–139.

Choi EH, Lee HJ, Yoo T, Chanock SJ. A common haplotype of interleukin-4 gene IL4 is associated with severe respiratory syncytial virus disease in Korean children. J Infect Dis 2002; 186(9): 1207–1211.

Dakhama A, Kaan PM, Hegele RG. Permissiveness of guinea pig alveolar macrophage subpopulations to acute respiratory syncytial virus infection *in vitro*. Chest 1998; 114(6): 1681–1688.

de WL, Koopman LP, van BI, Brandenburg AH, Mulder PG, de Swart RL, Fokkens WJ, Neijens HJ, Osterhaus AD. Moderate local and systemic respiratory syncytial virus-specific T-cell responses upon mild or subclinical RSV infection. J Med Virol 2003; 70(2): 309–318.

de Graaff PM, de Jong EC, van Capel TM, van Dijk ME, Roholl PJ, Boes J, Luytjes W, Kimpen JL, van Bleek GM. Respiratory syncytial virus infection of monocyte-derived dendritic cells decreases their capacity to activate CD4 T cells. J Immunol 2005; 175(9): 5904–5911.

de Sierra TM, Kumar ML, Wasser TE, Murphy BR, Subbarao EK. Respiratory syncytial virus-specific immunoglobulins in preterm infants. J Pediatr 1993; 122(5 Pt 1): 787–791.

De Weerd W, Twilhaar WN, Kimpen JL. T cell subset analysis in peripheral blood of children with RSV bronchiolitis. Scand J Infect Dis 1998; 30(1): 77–80.

Devincenzo JP, Aitken J, Harrison L. Respiratory syncytial virus (RSV) loads in premature infants with and without prophylactic RSV fusion protein monoclonal antibody. J Pediatr 2003; 143(1): 123–126.

DeVincenzo JP, El Saleeby CM, Bush AJ. Respiratory syncytial virus load predicts disease severity in previously healthy infants. J Infect Dis 2005; 191(11): 1861–1868.

Diamond G, Legarda D, Ryan LK. The innate immune response of the respiratory epithelium. Immunol Rev 2000; 173: 27–38.

Domachowske JB, Bonville CA, Rosenberg HF. Gene expression in epithelial cells in response to pneumovirus infection. Respir Res 2001; 2(4): 225–233.

Domachowske JB, Rosenberg HF. Respiratory syncytial virus infection: immune response, immunopathogenesis, and treatment. Clin Microbiol Rev 1999; 12(2): 298–309.

Dong Q, Louahed J, Vink A, Sullivan CD, Messler CJ, Zhou Y, Haczku A, Huaux F, Arras M, Holroyd KJ, Renauld JC, Levitt RC, Nicolaides NC. IL-9 induces chemokine expression in lung epithelial cells and baseline airway eosinophilia in transgenic mice. Eur J Immunol 1999; 29(7): 2130–2139.

Everard ML, Swarbrick A, Wrightham M, McIntyre J, Dunkley C, James PD, Sewell HF, Milner AD. Analysis of cells obtained by bronchial lavage of infants with respiratory syncytial virus infection. Arch Dis Child 1994; 71(5): 428–432.

Fadok VA, Savill JS, Haslett C, Bratton DL, Doherty DE, Campbell PA, Henson PM. Different populations of macrophages use either the vitronectin receptor or the phosphatidylserine receptor to recognize and remove apoptotic cells. J. Immunol 1992; 149(12): 4029–4035.

Fiedler MA, Wernke-Dollries K, Stark JM. Respiratory syncytial virus increases IL-8 gene expression and protein release in A549 cells. Am J Physiol 1995; 269(6 Pt 1): L865–L872.

Fishaut M, Tubergen D, McIntosh K. Cellular response to respiratory viruses with particular reference to children with disorders of cell-mediated immunity. J Pediatr 1980; 96(2): 179–186.

Gagro A, Tominac M, Krsulovic-Hresic V, Bace A, Matic M, Drazenovic V, Mlinaric-Galinovic G, Kosor E, Gotovac K, Bolanca I, Batinica S, Rabatic S. Increased Toll-like receptor 4 expression in infants with respiratory syncytial virus bronchiolitis. Clin Exp Immunol 2004; 135(2): 267–272.

Garofalo RP, Patti J, Hintz KA, Hill V, Ogra PL, Welliver RC. Macrophage inflammatory protein-1alpha (not t helper type 2 cytokines) is associated with severe forms of respiratory syncytial virus bronchiolitis. J Infect Dis 2001; 184(4): 393–399.

Ghildyal R, Hartley C, Varrasso A, Meanger J, Voelker DR, Anders EM, Mills J. Surfactant protein A binds to the fusion glycoprotein of respiratory syncytial virus and neutralizes virion infectivity. J Infect Dis 1999; 180(6): 2009–2013.

Gill MA, Palucka AK, Barton T, Ghaffar F, Jafri H, Banchereau J, Ramilo O. Mobilization of plasmacytoid and myeloid dendritic cells to mucosal sites in children with respiratory syncytial virus and other viral respiratory infections. J Infect Dis 2005; 191(7): 1105–1115.

Glezen WP, Paredes A, Allison JE, Taber LH, Frank AL. Risk of respiratory syncytial virus infection for infants from low-income families in relationship to age, sex, ethnic group, and maternal antibody level. J Pediatr 1981; 98(5): 708–715.

Graham BS, Bunton LA, Wright PF, Karzon DT. Role of T lymphocyte subsets in the pathogenesis of primary infection and rechallenge with respiratory syncytial virus in mice. J Clin Invest 1991; 88(3): 1026–1033.

Graham BS, Henderson GS, Tang YW, Lu X, Neuzil KM, Colley DG. Priming immunization determines T helper cytokine mRNA expression patterns in lungs of mice challenged with respiratory syncytial virus. J Immunol 1993; 151(4): 2032–2040.

Guerrero-Plata A, Baron S, Poast JS, Adegboyega PA, Casola A, Garofalo RP. Activity and regulation of alpha interferon in respiratory syncytial virus and human metapneumovirus experimental infections. J Virol 2005; 79(16): 10190–10199.

Guillot L, Balloy V, McCormack FX, Golenbock DT, Chignard M, Si-Tahar M. Cutting edge: the immunostimulatory activity of the lung surfactant protein-A involves Toll-like receptor 4. J Immunol 2002; 168(12): 5989–5992.

Haeberle HA, Takizawa R, Casola A, Brasier AR, Dieterich HJ, Van RN, Gatalica Z, Garofalo RP. Respiratory syncytial virus-induced activation of nuclear factor-kappaB in the lung involves alveolar macrophages and toll-like receptor 4-dependent pathways. J Infect Dis 2002; 186(9): 1199–1206.

Hall CB. Respiratory syncytial virus. In: Textbook of Paediatric Infectious Diseases (Feigin RD, Cherry JD, editors). Philadelphia: W.B. Saunders; 1998; pp. 2084–2111.

Hall CB. Respiratory syncytial virus and parainfluenza virus. N Engl J Med 2001; 344(25): 1917–1928.

Hall CB, Douglas Jr. RG, Geiman JM. Respiratory syncytial virus infections in infants: quantitation and duration of shedding. J Pediatr 1976; 89(1): 11–15.

Harrison AM, Bonville CA, Rosenberg HF, Domachowske JB. Respiratory syncytical virus-induced chemokine expression in the lower airways: eosinophil recruitment and degranulation. Am J Respir Crit Care Med 1999; 159(6): 1918–1924.

Haynes LM, Moore DD, Kurt-Jones EA, Finberg RW, Anderson LJ, Tripp RA. Involvement of toll-like receptor 4 in innate immunity to respiratory syncytial virus. J Virol 2001; 75(22): 10730–10737.

Heil F, Hemmi H, Hochrein H, Ampenberger F, Kirschning C, Akira S, Lipford G, Wagner H, Bauer S. Species-specific recognition of single-stranded RNA via toll-like receptor 7 and 8. Science 2004; 303(5663): 1526–1529.

Hoebee B, Rietveld E, Bont L, Oosten M, Hodemaekers HM, Nagelkerke NJ, Neijens HJ, Kimpen JL, Kimman TG. Association of severe respiratory syncytial virus bronchiolitis with interleukin-4 and interleukin-4 receptor alpha polymorphisms. J Infect Dis 2003; 187(1): 2–11.

Hornsleth A, Loland L, Larsen LB. Cytokines and chemokines in respiratory secretion and severity of disease in infants with respiratory syncytial virus (RSV) infection. J Clin Virol 2001; 21(2): 163–170.

Hull J, Thomson A, Kwiatkowski D. Association of respiratory syncytial virus bronchiolitis with the interleukin 8 gene region in UK families. Thorax 2000; 55(12): 1023–1027.

Hussell T, Openshaw PJ. Intracellular IFN-gamma expression in natural killer cells precedes lung CD8+ T cell recruitment during respiratory syncytial virus infection. J Gen Virol 1998; 79(Pt 11): 2593–2601.

Hussell T, Openshaw PJ. IL-12-activated NK cells reduce lung eosinophilia to the attachment protein of respiratory syncytial virus but do not enhance the severity of illness in CD8 T cell-immunodeficient conditions. J Immunol 2000; 165(12): 7109–7115.

Hussell T, Pennycook A, Openshaw PJ. Inhibition of tumor necrosis factor reduces the severity of virus-specific lung immunopathology. Eur J Immunol 2001; 31(9): 2566–2573.

Impact-RSV Study Group. Palivizumab, a humanized respiratory syncytial virus monoclonal antibody, reduces hospitalization from respiratory syncytial virus infection in high-risk infants. Pediatrics 1998; 102(3): 531–537.

Iwasaki A, Medzhitov R. Toll-like receptor control of the adaptive immune responses. Nat Immunol 2004; 5(10): 987–995.

Janeway CA. Host defence against infection. In: Immunobiology (Janeway CA, Travers P, Walport M, Capra JD, editors). 4th ed. Edinburgh: Churchill Livingstone; 1999; pp. 363–415.

Jaovisidha P, Peeples ME, Brees AA, Carpenter LR, Moy JN. Respiratory syncytial virus stimulates neutrophil degranulation and chemokine release. J Immunol 1999; 163(5): 2816–2820.

Johnson TR, Mertz SE, Gitiban N, Hammond S, Legallo R, Durbin RK, Durbin JE. Role for innate IFNs in determining respiratory syncytial virus immunopathology. J Immunol 2005; 174(11): 7234–7241.

Jones A, Qui JM, Bataki E, Elphick H, Ritson S, Evans GS, Everard ML. Neutrophil survival is prolonged in the airways of healthy infants and infants with RSV bronchiolitis. Eur Respir J 2002; 20(3): 651–657.

Kapsenberg ML. Dendritic-cell control of pathogen-driven T-cell polarization. Nat Rev Immunol 2003; 3(12): 984–993.

Kerr MH, Paton JY. Surfactant protein levels in severe respiratory syncytial virus infection. Am J Respir Crit Care Med 1999; 159(4 Pt 1): 1115–1118.

Kim CK, Kim SW, Park CS, Kim BI, Kang H, Koh YY. Bronchoalveolar lavage cytokine profiles in acute asthma and acute bronchiolitis. J Allergy Clin Immunol 2003; 112(1): 64–71.

Kim HW, Bellanti JA, Arrobio JO, Mills J, Brandt CD, Chanock RM, Parrott RH. Respiratory syncytial virus neutralizing activity in nasal secretions following natural infection. Proc Soc Exp Biol Med 1969a; 131(2): 658–661.

Kim HW, Canchola JG, Brandt CD, Pyles G, Chanock RM, Jensen K, Parrott RH. Respiratory syncytial virus disease in infants despite prior administration of antigenic inactivated vaccine. Am J Epidemiol 1969b; 89(4): 422–434.

Kim HW, Leikin SL, Arrobio J, Brandt CD, Chanock RM, Parrott RH. Cell-mediated immunity to respiratory syncytial virus induced by inactivated vaccine or by infection. Pediatr Res 1976; 10(1): 75–78.

Kimpen JL. Respiratory syncytial virus and asthma The role of monocytes. Am J Respir Crit Care Med 2001; 163(3 Pt 2): S7–S9.

Konig B, Krusat T, Streckert HJ, Konig W. IL-8 release from human neutrophils by the respiratory syncytial virus is independent of viral replication. J Leukoc Biol 1996; 60(2): 253–260.

Kristjansson S, Bjarnarson SP, Wennergren G, Palsdottir AH, Arnadottir T, Haraldsson A, Jonsdottir I. Respiratory syncytial virus and other respiratory viruses during the first 3 months of life promote a local TH2-like response. J Allergy Clin Immunol 2005; 116(4): 805–811.

Kunkel SL, Standiford T, Kasahara K, Strieter RM. Interleukin-8 (IL-8): the major neutrophil chemotactic factor in the lung. Exp Lung Res 1991; 17(1): 17–23.

Kurt-Jones EA, Popova L, Kwinn L, Haynes LM, Jones LP, Tripp RA, Walsh EE, Freeman MW, Golenbock DT, Anderson LJ, Finberg RW. Pattern recognition receptors TLR4 and CD14 mediate response to respiratory syncytial virus. Nat Immunol 2000; 1(5): 398–401.

Lahti M, Lofgren J, Marttila R, Renko M, Klaavuniemi T, Haataja R, Ramet M, Hallman M. Surfactant protein D gene polymorphism associated with severe respiratory syncytial virus infection. Pediatr Res 2002; 51(6): 696–699.

Lambrecht BN, Hammad H. Taking our breath away: dendritic cells in the pathogenesis of asthma. Nat Rev Immunol 2003; 3(12): 994–1003.

Le BA, Tough DF. Links between innate and adaptive immunity via type I interferon. Curr Opin Immunol 2002; 14(4): 432–436.

Leader S, Kohlhase K. Recent trends in severe respiratory syncytial virus (RSV) among US infants, 1997 to 2000. J Pediatr 2003; 143(Suppl 5): S127–S132.

Lee A, Whyte MK, Haslett C. Inhibition of apoptosis and prolongation of neutrophil functional longevity by inflammatory mediators. J Leukoc Biol 1993; 54(4): 283–288.

Legg JP, Hussain IR, Warner JA, Johnston SL, Warner JO. Type 1 and type 2 cytokine imbalance in acute respiratory syncytial. Am J Respir Crit Care Med 2003; 168(6): 633–639.

Lofgren J, Ramet M, Renko M, Marttila R, Hallman M. Association between surfactant protein A gene locus and severe respiratory syncytial virus infection in infants. J Infect Dis 2002; 185(3): 283–289.

Louahed J, Toda M, Jen J, Hamid Q, Renauld JC, Levitt RC, Nicolaides NC. Interleukin-9 upregulates mucus expression in the airways. Am J Respir Cell Mol Biol 2000; 22(6): 649–656.

Matsuda K, Tsutsumi H, Sone S, Yoto Y, Oya K, Okamoto Y, Ogra PL, Chiba S. Characteristics of IL-6 and TNF-alpha production by respiratory syncytial virus-infected macrophages in the neonate. J Med Virol 1996; 48(2): 199–203.

McIntosh K, Masters HB, Orr I, Chao RK, Barkin RM. The immunologic response to infection with respiratory syncytial virus in infants. J Infect Dis 1978; 138(1): 24–32.

McNamara PS, Flanagan BF, Baldwin LM, Newland P, Hart CA, Smyth RL. Interleukin 9 production in the lungs of infants with severe respiratory syncytial virus bronchiolitis. Lancet 2004a; 363(9414): 1031–1037.

McNamara PS, Flanagan BF, Selby AM, Hart CA, Smyth RL. Pro- and anti-inflammatory responses in respiratory syncytial virus bronchiolitis. Eur Respir J 2004b; 23(1): 106–112.

McNamara PS, Flanagan BF, Hart CA, Smyth RL. Production of chemokines in the lungs of infants with severe respiratory syncytial virus bronchiolitis. J Infect Dis 2005; 191(8): 1225–1232.

McNamara PS, Ritson PC, Flanagan BF, Hart CA, Smyth RL. Interleukin-9 in severe RSV bronchiolitis. Eur Respir J 2002a; 20(38): 17 s.

McNamara PS, Ritson P, Selby A, Hart CA, Smyth RL. Bronchoalveolar lavage cellularity in infants with severe respiratory syncytial virus bronchiolitis. Arch Dis Child 2003; 88(10): 922–926.

McNamara PS, Smyth RL. The pathogenesis of respiratory syncytial virus disease in childhood. Br Med Bull 2002; 61(1): 13–28.

Mellow TE, Murphy PC, Carson JL, Noah TL, Zhang L, Pickles RJ. The effect of respiratory synctial virus on chemokine release by differentiated airway epithelium. Exp Lung Res 2004; 30(1): 43–57.

Miller AL, Bowlin TL, Lukacs NW. Respiratory syncytial virus-induced chemokine production: linking viral replication to chemokine production *in vitro* and *in vivo*. J Infect Dis 2004; 189(8): 1419–1430.

Miller AL, Strieter RM, Gruber AD, Ho SB, Lukacs NW. CXCR2 regulates respiratory syncytial virus-induced airway hyperreactivity and mucus overproduction. J Immunol 2003; 170(6): 3348–3356.

Mobbs KJ, Smyth RL, O'Hea U, Ashby D, Ritson P, Hart CA. Cytokines in severe respiratory syncytial virus bronchiolitis. Pediatr Pulmonol 2002; 33(no. 6): 449–452.

Munoz JL, McCarthy CA, Clark ME, Hall CB. Respiratory syncytial virus infection in C57BL/6 mice: clearance of virus from the lungs with virus-specific cytotoxic T cells. J Virol 1991; 65(8): 4494–4497.

Netea MG, Van der Meer JW, Kullberg BJ. Toll-like receptors as an escape mechanism from the host defense. Trends Microbiol 2004; 12(11): 484–488.

Noah TL, Ivins SS, Murphy P, Kazachkova I, Moats-Staats B, Henderson FW. Chemokines and inflammation in the nasal passages of infants with respiratory syncytial virus bronchiolitis. Clin Immunol 2002; 104(1): 86–95.

Olszewska-Pazdrak B, Casola A, Saito T, Alam R, Crowe SE, Mei F, Ogra PL, Garofalo RP. Cell-specific expression of RANTES, MCP-1, and MIP-1alpha by lower airway epithelial cells and eosinophils infected with respiratory syncytial virus. J Virol 1998; 72(6): 4756–4764.

Panuska JR, Cirino NM, Midulla F, Despot JE, McFadden Jr. ER, Huang YT. Productive infection of isolated human alveolar macrophages by respiratory syncytial virus. J Clin Invest 1990; 86(1): 113–119.

Panuska JR, Merolla R, Rebert NA, Hoffmann SP, Tsivitse P, Cirino NM, Silverman RH, Rankin JA. Respiratory syncytial virus induces interleukin-10 by human alveolar macrophages. Supression of early cytokine production and implications for incomplete immunity. J Clin Invest 1995; 96(5): 2445–2453.

Piedimonte G. Neural mechanisms of respiratory syncytial virus-induced inflammation and prevention of respiratory syncytial virus sequelae. Am J Respir Crit Care Med 2001; 163(3 Pt 2): S18–S21.

Piedimonte G. Origins of reactive airways disease in early life: do viral infections play a role? Acta Paediatr Suppl 2002; 91(437): 6–11.

Piedimonte G, Rodriguez MM, King KA, McLean S, Jiang X. Respiratory syncytial virus upregulates expression of the substance P receptor in rat lungs. Am J Physiol 1999; 277(4 Pt 1): L831–L840.

Renzi PM, Turgeon JP, Yang JP, Drblik SP, Marcotte JE, Pedneault L, Spier S. Cellular immunity is activated and a TH-2 response is associated with early wheezing in infants after bronchiolitis. J Pediatr 1997; 130(4): 584–593.

Richardson LS, Belshe RB, Sly DL, London WT, Prevar DA, Camargo E, Chanock RM. Experimental respiratory syncytial virus pneumonia in cebus monkeys. J Med Virol 1978; 2(1): 45–59.

Roman M, Calhoun WJ, Hinton KL, Avendano LF, Simon V, Escobar AM, Gaggero A, Diaz PV. Respiratory syncytial virus infection in infants is associated with predominant Th-2-like response. Am J Respir Crit Care Med 1997; 156(1): 190–195.

Sabogal C, Auais A, Napchan G, Mager E, Zhou BG, Suguihara C, Bancalari E, Piedimonte G. Effect of respiratory syncytial virus on apnea in weanling rats. Pediatr Res 2005; 57(6): 819–825.

Salkind AR, McCarthy DO, Nichols JE, Domurat FM, Walsh EE, Roberts Jr. NJ. Interleukin-1-inhibitor activity induced by respiratory syncytial virus: abrogation of virus-specific and alternate human lymphocyte proliferative responses. J Infect Dis 1991; 163(1): 71–77.

Sampson AP. The role of eosinophils and neutrophils in inflammation. Clin Exp Allergy 2000; 30(Suppl 1): 22–27.

Sauty A, Dziejman M, Taha RA, Iarossi AS, Neote K, Garcia-Zepeda EA, Hamid Q, Luster AD. The T cell-specific CXC chemokines IP-10, Mig, and I-TAC are expressed by activated human bronchial epithelial cells. J Immunol 1999; 162(6): 3549–3558.

Schlender J, Hornung V, Finke S, Gunthner-Biller M, Marozin S, Brzozka K, Moghim S, Endres S, Hartmann G, Conzelmann KK. Inhibition of toll-like receptor 7- and 9-mediated alpha/beta interferon production in human plasmacytoid dendritic cells by respiratory syncytial virus and measles virus. J Virol 2005; 79(9): 5507–5515.

Sheeran P, Jafri H, Carubelli C, Saavedra J, Johnson C, Krisher K, Sanchez PJ, Ramilo O. Elevated cytokine concentrations in the nasopharyngeal and tracheal secretions of children with respiratory syncytial virus disease. Pediatr Infect Dis J 1999; 18(2): 115–122.

Simoes EA. Environmental and demographic risk factors for respiratory syncytial virus lower respiratory tract disease. J Pediatr 2003; 143(Suppl 5): S118–S126.

Simoes EA, Groothuis JR. Respiratory syncytial virus prophylaxis—the story so far. Respir Med 2002; 96(Suppl B): S15–S24.

Smith PK, Wang SZ, Dowling KD, Forsyth KD. Leucocyte populations in respiratory syncytial virus-induced bronchiolitis. J Paediatr Child Health 2001; 37(2): 146–151.

Smyth RL, Fletcher JN, Thomas HM, Hart CA. Immunological responses to respiratory syncytial virus infection in infancy. Arch Dis Child 1997; 76(3): 210–214.

Smyth RL, Mobbs KJ, O'Hea U, Ashby D, Hart CA. Respiratory syncytial virus bronchiolitis: disease severity, interleukin-8, and virus genotype. Pediatr Pulmonol 2002; 33(5): 339–346.

Sorkness RL, Mehta H, Kaplan MR, Miyasaka M, Hefle SL, Lemanske RF. Effect of ICAM-1 blockade on lung inflammation and physiology during acute viral bronchiolitis in rats. Pediatr Res 2000; 47(6): 819–824.

Spann KM, Tran KC, Chi B, Rabin RL, Collins PL. Suppression of the induction of alpha, beta, and lambda interferons by the NS1 and NS2 proteins of human respiratory syncytial virus in human epithelial cells and macrophages. J Virol 2004; 78(8): 4363–4369.

Spann KM, Tran KC, Collins PL. Effects of nonstructural proteins NS1 and NS2 of human respiratory syncytial virus on interferon regulatory factor 3, NF-kappaB, and proinflammatory cytokines. J Virol 2005; 79(9): 5353–5362.

Srikiatkhachorn A, Braciale TJ. Virus-specific CD8+ T lymphocytes downregulate T helper cell type 2 cytokine secretion and pulmonary eosinophilia during experimental murine respiratory syncytial virus infection. J Exp Med 1997; 186(3): 421–432.

Stark JM, Godding V, Sedgwick JB, Busse WW. Respiratory syncytial virus infection enhances neutrophil and eosinophil adhesion to cultured respiratory epithelial cells. Roles of CD18 and intercellular adhesion molecule-1. J Immunol 1996; 156(12): 4774–4782.

Tal G, Mandelberg A, Dalal I, Cesar K, Somekh E, Tal A, Oron A, Itskovich S, Ballin A, Houri S, Beigelman A, Lider O, Rechavi G, Amariglio N. Association between common Toll-like receptor 4 mutations and severe respiratory syncytial virus disease. J Infect Dis 2004; 189(11): 2057–2063.

Tenner AJ. Membrane receptors for soluble defense collagens. Curr Opin Immunol 1999; 11(1): 34–41.

Tirado R, Ortega A, Sarmiento RE, Gomez B. Interleukin-8 mRNA synthesis and protein secretion are continuously up-regulated by respiratory syncytial virus persistently infected cells. Cell Immunol 2005; 233(1): 61–71.

Tripp RA, Moore D, Jones L, Sullender W, Winter J, Anderson LJ. Respiratory syncytial virus G and/or SH protein alters Th1 cytokines, natural killer cells, and neutrophils responding to pulmonary infection in BALB/c mice. J Virol 1999; 73(9): 7099–7107.

Wang SZ, Forsyth KD. The interaction of neutrophils with respiratory epithelial cells in viral infection. Respirology 2000; 5(1): 1–10.

Wang SZ, Smith PK, Lovejoy M, Bowden JJ, Alpers JH, Forsyth KD. Shedding of L-selectin and PECAM-1 and upregulation of Mac-1 and ICAM-1 on neutrophils in RSV bronchiolitis. Am J Physiol 1998a; 275(5 Pt 1): L983–L989.

Wang SZ, Xu H, Wraith A, Bowden JJ, Alpers JH, Forsyth KD. Neutrophils induce damage to respiratory epithelial cells infected with respiratory syncytial virus. Eur Respir J 1998b; 12(3): 612–618.

Wright JR. Immunoregulatory functions of surfactant proteins. Nat Rev Immunol 2005; 5(1): 58–68.

Zhang Y, Luxon BA, Casola A, Garofalo RP, Jamaluddin M, Brasier AR. Expression of respiratory syncytial virus-induced chemokine gene networks in lower airway epithelial cells revealed by cDNA microarrays. J Virol 2001; 75(19): 9044–9058.

Zhang W, Yang H, Kong X, Mohapatra S, San Juan-Vergara H, Hellermann G, Behera S, Singam R, Lockey RF, Mohapatra SS. Inhibition of respiratory syncytial virus infection with intranasal siRNA nanoparticles targeting the viral NS1 gene. Nat Med 2005; 11(1): 56–62.

Respiratory Syncytial Virus
Patricia Cane (Editor)

DOI 10.1016/S0168-7069(06)14006-9

RSV Infection in Elderly Adults

Yoshihiko Murata, Ann R. Falsey
Department of Medicine, University of Rochester School of Medicine and Dentistry and Department of Medicine, Rochester General Hospital, 1425 Portland Avenue, Rochester, NY 14621, USA

Introduction

Nearly 50 years ago, respiratory syncytial virus (RSV) was first isolated from a child with bronchiolitis. Since its discovery, RSV is now widely appreciated as a predictable cause of wintertime respiratory tract infections in persons of all ages and the most common cause of lower respiratory tract infections in the pediatric population (Hall, 2001). Thus, among many clinicians, the prevalent perception is that infants and young children are the only populations which are affected by RSV. However, clinical and epidemiological data collected during the last three decades have shown that RSV is a clinically significant cause of respiratory tract infections in elderly adults. RSV causes a substantial disease burden among older adults who reside in the community or in long-term care facilities (Falsey and Walsh, 2000; Falsey et al., 2005). Adults with underlying cardiopulmonary disorders and/or immunosuppressive conditions appear to be at highest risk for severe RSV disease. In this chapter, we will review the epidemiology, clinical manifestations, methods of diagnosis, treatment, and prevention options for RSV in elderly adults.

Epidemiology

Three types of studies have examined the role of RSV as a significant pathogen of elderly adults: (1) mathematical modeling and estimates of disease burden; (2) outbreak and prospective studies in long term care facilities; and (3) epidemiological studies involving community-residing elderly adults. Taken together, these studies provide strong evidence that RSV is an important cause of morbidity and mortality in this patient population.

Mathematical modeling and estimates of disease burden

As depicted in Table 1, mathematical modeling linking viral isolate databases with hospitalization and deaths was used in two studies to estimate the effect of RSV on mortality rates. For these studies, it should be noted that viral isolates were generally obtained from pediatric populations, while events such as hospitalizations

Table 1

Estimates of disease burden attributable to RSV among elderly adults

Mathematical modeling studies				
Study (year published)	Data used from study years	Population	Method	# Annual deaths of elderly adults attributable to RSV
Nicholson (1996)	1975–1990	England and Wales	Regression analysis	22,000–23,000 each winter
Thompson et al. (2003)	1976–1999	United States	Poisson regression modeling	Approximately 10,000
Retrospective studies				
	Data used from study years	Population	# Annual hospitalizations of elderly adults attributable to RSV	# Annual deaths of elderly adults attributable to RSV
Fleming and Cross (1993)	1989–1993	Clinical surveillance data from sentinel general practitioners, England[a]	RSV ≈ Influenza[a]	RSV ≈ Influenza[a]
Griffin et al. (2002)	1995–1999	Persons with chronic lung disease in the Tennessee Medicaid program, USA	18 per 1000 persons	5 per 1000 persons

[a]Correlation between viral isolation reports (influenza, RSV) and incidence of acute respiratory disease and deaths suggest that RSV is as important as influenza viruses in causing morbidity and excess deaths in this patient population (Fleming and Cross, 1993).

and deaths were found in elderly populations. The first study used regression analysis to examine the effects of RSV and influenza viruses A and B on the mortality rates in England and Wales (Nicholson, 1996). Based on morbidity and mortality data from sentinel general practices during the period 1975 to 1990, the estimated mortality associated with RSV was calculated to be at least that of influenza. The second study used similar mathematical techniques to analyze data from the United States to again compare the RSV- and influenza-associated mortalities (Thompson, et al., 2003). In this study, influenza was associated with up to three times as many deaths as RSV. However, for all underlying respiratory or circulatory deaths during the period of 1990–1991 to 1998–1999 RSV seasons, 78% of RSV-associated deaths occurred among persons aged 65 years or older. The two estimates of RSV-associated mortality rates are similar in magnitude across two different population-derived datasets and are in accord with results from epidemiological studies in elderly adults (see below).

Also shown in Table 1 are the results of two retrospective studies of estimates of disease burden. One study focused on cases of acute respiratory disease in elderly adults and deaths in the United Kingdom over four consecutive winters from 1989 to 1993 (Fleming and Cross, 1993). The investigators correlated peaks of viral activity with those of acute respiratory diseases. During most winters, the peak activities of RSV and influenza coincided and the contribution of each virus to the overall incidence in respiratory diseases was difficult to sort out. However, when the peak activities of RSV and influenza were temporally separated, a clearly distinct spike in death rates among the elderly was observed for each virus. Thus, the authors conclude that RSV is as important as influenza viruses as a cause of excess deaths among elderly adults. Another population-based retrospective study examined the relationship from 1995 to 1999 between viral surveillance data from a pediatric clinic and hospitalizations and deaths among persons with chronic lung disease in Tennessee (Griffin et al., 2002). In this study, based on circulation rates of RSV and influenza viruses, the investigators found that the rates of RSV-associated hospitalizations and deaths in elderly adults were similar to those associated with influenza virus (Griffin et al., 2002).

RSV in residents of long-term care facilities and adult day care

RSV was first appreciated as a substantial problem in older adults residing in long-term care facilities. As summarized in Table 2, a number of RSV outbreaks among long-term care residents have been reported. In outbreak situations, attack rates are highly variable (2–89%). This variability may be due to differences in case definitions, diagnostic tests used, and the populations studied in each outbreak analysis. Nosocomial spread of RSV infection is primarily responsible for outbreaks in these closed populations and also contributes to the widely variable rates of infection.

Prospective studies of RSV infection in this patient population provide a more accurate assessment of infection rates (Table 2). Typically, such prospective studies

Table 2

RSV Infection in elderly adults residing in long-term care facilities

Study (year)	Method[a]	Number of RSV cases	Attack rate (%)	Pneumonia (% of cases)	Death (% of cases)
Hornsleth et al. (1975)	P	10	7	0	0
CDC (1977)[b]	O	15	19	47	40
Garvie and Gray (1980)	O	40	43		3
Mathur et al. (1980)	P	8	1.4	25	0
BCDSC (1983)[c]	O	15	N/A		53
	O	24	89		10
	O	16	40		0
Morales et al. (1983)	P	12	10	16	5
Hart (1984)	O	20	40		20
Sorvillo et al. (1984)	O	40	40	55	20
Mandal et al. (1985)	O	8	30	13	13
Arroyo et al. (1988)	P	5	9	0	0
Gross et al. (1988)	P	8	3.4		0
Aguis et al. (1990)	O	52	12	42	12
Nicholson et al. (1990)	O	9	2		0
Falsey et al. (1990)[d]	P	2	2.3		
	P	11	18		
Osterweil and Norman (1990)	P	34	15	3	2
Falsey et al. (1992)	P	40	7	10	5
Wald et al. (1995)	P	9	3.5	22	0
Orr et al. (1996)	P	3	2	33	[e]

Note: N/A, not available.

Source: Adapted from Falsey and Walsh (2000).

[a]O, outbreak; P, prospective.

[b]CDC, Centers for Disease Control.

[c]BCDSC: Public Health Laboratory Service Communicable Disease Surveillance Centre, England (1983).

[d]More than one outbreak reported in a single publication.

[e]Only evaluated febrile illnesses.

have evaluated all respiratory infections, and thus provide a comprehensive view of the spectrum of disease. In addition, RSV cases are based on specific laboratory criteria (e.g. viral culture, serologies, and/or molecular diagnostic procedures). RSV infection rates in prospective studies of adults in long-term care facilities have ranged from 1.4% to 18% (Table 2).

Attendees of senior day care programs can also be at risk for RSV infection. A study that examined viral infections among staff and elderly participants of an adult day care program revealed that RSV was a commonly identified pathogen in both groups (Falsey et al., 1995). Over a 15-month period, approximately 10% of the elderly and 5% of the staff developed RSV infections. In this study, children from a nearby center visited the elderly daycare participants once a week, although a direct causal link between such visits and RSV disease was not established.

Similar to widely variable rates of infection, previous epidemiological studies have yielded varying data on the rates of morbidity and mortality associated with RSV infection. For example, the incidence of pneumonia and death rates has ranged between 0–55% and 0–53%, respectively (Table 2; Ellis et al., 2003). Again, these differences likely reflect study methodology but also may have been influenced by the including the virulence of RSV strains and the frailty of study participants. The true incidence of pneumonia among RSV-infected elderly adults in long-term care facilities may be underestimated since chest radiographic studies are frequently not obtained.

Community-dwelling elderly adults

Several studies have examined the role of RSV among patients with community-acquired pneumonia. In one study, Dowell et al. (1996) found that RSV was the third most commonly identified pathogen among 1195 adults of all ages with community-acquired pneumonia. In this study, RSV was found in 4.4% of study patients, while *Streptococcus pneumoniae* and influenza were noted in 6.2% and 5.4% of the patient population, respectively. Of the 57 RSV-infected patients, the majority (68%) was 65 years of age or older, while eight patients were younger than 40 years old. Other studies of adults with community-acquired pneumonia have identified RSV as an etiological agent but again with varying infection rates (Table 3). Based on studies conducted over the last 30 years, it is reasonable to estimate that RSV accounts for 2–5% of community-acquired pneumonias throughout the year and 5–15% of cases during the winter months (Table 3; Falsey and Walsh, 2000).

Most studies of RSV in elderly adults in the community have focused on hospitalized patients (Table 3). In two separate studies of community-dwelling elderly adults who were hospitalized with acute cardiopulmonary disease, RSV was identified in 9–10% of such patients, while influenza was found in 9–13% (Falsey et al., 1995, 2005). In both studies, the morbidity and mortality rates among RSV-infected patients were significant with respect to ICU care (15–18%), ventilatory support (10–13%), and deaths (8–10%); these numbers are similar to those associated with influenza A infections in the two studies. With regard to hospitalizations in the second study, RSV accounted for up to 10% of admissions for pneumonia, 11% of COPD exacerbations, 7% of congestive heart failure, and 5% of asthma during the five consecutive winter months during the four study years (Falsey, et al., 2005).

The rate of RSV infection among prospective cohorts of healthy elderly adults has been examined in several studies (Nicholson et al., 1990; Falsey et al., 2005). In

Table 3

RSV pneumonia in adults

Study (year published)	Location	Years of study	Winter season only	# Positive/# tested (% positive)
Fransen et al. (1969)	Sweden	1963–1966		31/598 (5.2)
Hers et al. (1969)	Netherlands	1967–1968		10/207 (4.3)
Vikerfors et al. (1987)	Sweden	1971–1980		57/2,400 (2.0)
Kimball et al. (1983)	USA	1980–1981	W	2/100 (2.0)
Stanek and Heinz (1988)	Czechoslovakia	1983–1985		2/74 (2.7)
Zaroukian and Leader (1988)	USA	1987–1988	W	3/55 (5.4)
Melbye et al. (1992)	Norway	1988–1989	W	5/36 (13.9)
Falsey et al. (1995)	USA	1989–1992	W	69/483 (14.3)
Marrie (1994)	Canada	1991–1994		0/149 (0)
Dowell et al. (1996)	USA	1990–1992		53/1,195 (4.4)
Ruiz et al. (1999)	Spain	1996–1997		5/204 (2.4)
Lerida et al. (2000)	Spain	1995–1997		17/250 (6.8)
Falsey et al. (2005)	USA	1999–2003	W	44/414 (10.6)

Note: W, Study was conducted during the winter seasons.
Source: Adapted from Falsey and Walsh (2000).

the United Kingdom, Nicholson et al. followed 533 elderly adults and documented annual RSV infection in approximately 3% per year. In a recently published study of 608 healthy elderly and 540 high-risk adults (i.e. those with chronic heart or lung disease), RSV infection was found in 3–7% of healthy elderly patients and in 4–10% of adults with high-risk conditions each year (Falsey et al., 2005). The higher infection rates in the second study likely reflect the use of RT-PCR-based diagnostic methods. These studies confirm that RSV is an important pathogen in adults of advanced age or with underlying high-risk conditions.

Lastly, RSV also contributes to the annual surge of elderly adults seeking outpatient care for respiratory illnesses each winter. Using specimens obtained during outpatient visits to sentinel physicians over three consecutive winters and utilizing viral culture and RT-PCR as diagnostic methods, these investigators identified influenza A and RSV from nasopharyngeal swabs from patients of all ages (Zambon et al., 2001). Of note, among adults over age 65, 13–42% were identified to have influenza A and 10–19% had RSV.

Based on these data, it is not surprising that the economic burden of RSV in elderly adults in the United States is high. One study estimated this figure to be \$150–680 million annually for RSV pneumonia alone (Han, et al., 1999). This estimate would likely be much higher if the costs of chronic cardiopulmonary conditions (e.g. asthma, COPD, and chronic cardiac disease) were included.

Clinical manifestations and complications of RSV infection in elderly adults

RSV infection can cause a variety of signs and symptoms in elderly adults. The clinical manifestations of RSV may range from a mild common cold syndrome to severe respiratory distress and failure (Table 4). Rhinorrhea, nasal congestion, and cough are frequently reported in RSV infections, while sore throat has been noted in approximately 25% of cases. Gastrointestinal symptoms are quite uncommon and fever is 38°C or less in about half of the reported RSV infections. On physical examination, rales are noted in about a third of cases and wheezing is common, even in patients without underlying lung disease. Radiographic abnormalities may be found in patients with signs and symptoms of lower respiratory tract disease. Typically, uni- or bilateral patchy subsegmental alveolar infiltrates are observed on chest radiographs. On rare instances, lobar consolidation has been reported in adults with RSV (Dowell et al., 1995).

Table 4

Clinical manifestations of RSV infection in elderly adults

Reference	Falsey and Walsh (2000)	Falsey et al. (2005)		
	% of patients	Prospective cohort		
		Healthy	High risk	Hospitalized
		% of patients		
Symptoms				
Rhinorrhea/nasal congestion	67–92	84	65	66
Sore throat	20–33	42	35	28
Headache	3	N/A	N/A	N/A
Hoarseness	22–27	44	31	27
Cough	90–97	80	77	95
Sputum	22–67	65	65	76
Dyspnea	11–20	7	60	94
Systemic/constitutional	44–80	54	58	41
Gastrointestinal	0	N/A	N/A	N/A
Signs				
Fever >38°C	20–56	N/A	N/A	53
Rales	33–40	3	8	63
Wheezing	6–35	6	27	23
Laboratory findings				
Chest X-ray infiltrates	0–22	N/A	N/A	30

Note: N/A, not available.
Source: Falsey and Walsh (2000) and Falsey et al. (2005).

In general, RSV infection is indistinguishable from illness associated with the commonly circulating respiratory viruses, such as influenza. However, there are some clues to differentiate RSV from influenza. Rhinorrhea, wheezing, and dyspnea are more common with RSV, whereas influenza is more commonly associated with fever, gastrointestinal complaints, and myalgias (Mathur et al., 1980; Wald et al., 1995; Walsh et al., 2004).

Bacterial superinfection with RSV in children is considered uncommon (Hall, 2001). This issue has not been well studied in adults and potential pathogens have been found in up to 30% of adult patients with RSV. Unfortunately, the quality of sputum samples was not addressed in most studies. We recently observed a rate of 11.6% for bacterial infections in patients hospitalized with documented RSV infection when only documented bacteremia or positive cultures from sputum samples of adequate quality were accepted for diagnosis (Falsey A.R. and Walsh E.E., unpublished observations).

In a recent prospective study, almost all RSV infections were symptomatic and frequently led to acute changes in level of function and increased use of health care services (Falsey et al., 2005). In a large prospective study, the duration of illness caused by RSV was approximately two weeks and was similar to that caused by influenza A (Falsey et al., 2005). These observations are not unexpected, especially given the study population and its advanced age and/or concomitant medical conditions. Thus, practicing clinicians should keep in mind that RSV infections in elderly adults can cause short- and possibly long-term changes in functional status.

Diagnosis of RSV infection

Since the clinical manifestations are variable and are similar to those caused by other common respiratory viruses, diagnosis of RSV infection in elderly adults requires laboratory confirmation. This may be accomplished by serology, viral culture, or qualitative or semi-quantitative detection of viral antigens or nucleic acid sequences.

Collection of clinical samples

For detection of RSV, respiratory tract secretions may be obtained from patients using one or more sampling methods, including nasopharyngeal swabs, nasal washes, or collection of sputum or bronchial alveolar lavage fluids. In our clinical experience, nasal washes, which are commonly used to collect respiratory secretions in the pediatric patients, are poorly tolerated in elderly adults. Thus, it is acceptable to use nasopharyngeal swabs to collect secretions despite the somewhat lower viral titers associated with this method (Walsh and Falsey, 1999). This limitation may not be clinically significant, especially if molecular diagnostic methods are used to detect RSV infection (see below). If available, sputum samples may have higher titers than nasal swabs and may offer a higher diagnostic yield (Falsey and Walsh, unpublished data).

Viral culture

For detection of RSV infection in the pediatric patient population, viral culture is reasonably sensitive and highly specific (Hall, 1975). However, the general applicability of viral culture methods to detect RSV infection in adults is limited by the following: (1) the relative thermolability of RSV (Hall, 2001); (2) significantly less viral shedding occurs in the respiratory tract of adults as compared to that in pediatric patients ($\leqslant 10^3$ PFU/mL vs. $\leqslant 10^6$ PFU/mL, respectively) (Hall et al., 1976; Englund et al., 1996); and (3) the shorter duration of viral shedding in adults as compared to pediatric patients (approximately 3–4 days (Hall et al., 1976) vs. 7–14 days (Falsey et al., 2003), respectively). Taken together, these observations have limited the value of viral culture to identify RSV infection in adults.

Several studies of RSV infection in adults indicate that viral culture is less sensitive than serology as evidence of recent RSV infection. In a study utilizing optimal culture techniques and transport times, viral cultures were positive in only 45% of elderly nursing home residents with serologically documented RSV (Falsey et al., 1992). Even when bedside inoculation of patient samples was used, viral culture was positive in only 67% of serologically confirmed RSV infections among seniors attending daycare. When samples were transported to the laboratory for culture inoculations, the yield fell to 45%, thus confirming the difficulties of culture.

Since viral culture is frequently the only option for the acute diagnosis of RSV that is available to clinicians, two points should be noted. First, for optimal yield, specimens should be placed on ice and rapidly transported to the clinical laboratory. Second, a negative culture should not be interpreted as absence of RSV infection.

Antigen detection

Enzyme immunoassay (EIA) and indirect immunofluorescence assay (IFA) methods to detect RSV-derived viral antigens have been used successfully in children (Kellogg, 1991). These methods were found to be 75–95% sensitive for the detection of RSV antigens in pediatric populations. However, antigen detection methods are not nearly as sensitive when used in elderly adults. In a study of 60 elderly patients with RSV infection documented by viral culture, serology, or molecular techniques, commercially available IFA and EIA tests identified 23% and 10% of RSV infections, respectively (Casiano-Colon et al., 2003). Since the positive predictive value of these tests is poor, we do not recommend the routine use of antigen detection tests in the adult populations. Rapid antigen testing may be appropriate in specific clinical situations such as an immunocompromised elderly patient in whom the viral load may be greater (Englund et al., 1996).

Serology

Methods to identify RSV-specific IgM and IgG via complement fixation (CF) or EIA have been described. Previous studies have defined acute RSV infection as one of the following: (1) a single laboratory value of elevated CF titer; (2) detection of RSV-specific IgM in acute sera; or (3) at least a four-fold increase in anti-RSV titer from paired serum samples. Although CF assays are generally commercially available, the utility of a single elevated CF result to diagnose RSV infections has not been rigorously validated in epidemiological studies. A ⩾4-fold rise in RSV-specific antibody either by CF or EIA is an acceptable method of diagnosis. A fourfold rise in antibody by CF serology appears to be about 50% sensitive as compared to EIA serology when purified viral proteins are used in assays (Marrie et al., 2001). Most older people with RSV infection (83–95%) demonstrate a ⩾4-fold rise in RSV-specific IgG as measured by EIA (Falsey et al., 1995, 2005).

One of the limitations of serologies to detect RSV infections is that false-negative results may occur in hospitalized patients in whom acute sera may not be available until many days following the onset of illness. Although the retrospective nature of serology limits the clinical utility of this type of assay, it may be useful in certain circumstances such as outbreak investigations in long-term care facilities.

RT-PCR

To circumvent the limitations of diagnostic methods described above, RT-PCR methods have been developed to detect the presence of RSV-derived RNA sequences (Walsh et al., 2001; Borg et al., 2003; Falsey et al., 2003). As compared to other diagnostic methods, RT-PCR can detect minute quantities of RSV and also can rapidly identify acute infections in patients whose other diagnostic tests for RSV may be negative. In most RSV RT-PCR assays, primers are used to amplify conserved portions of the F and N genes of RSV (Walsh et al., 2001). Depending of the primers used in the amplification process, strain-specific RT-PCR can differentiate between RSV groups A and B (Fan, et al. 1998; Stockton, et al. 1998).

Several studies in pediatric and adult patient populations have used RT-PCR to identify RSV infections. In a large study in adults in which over 1000 respiratory illnesses were evaluated by three methods (viral culture, serology, and RT-PCR), RT-PCR was found to be 75% sensitive and 99% specific for diagnosing RSV infection, whereas viral culture was 39% sensitive and 100% specific (Falsey et al., 2002). Quantitative RT-PCR appears to correlate relatively well with culture-derived RSV titers and also appears to correlate with active or recent RSV infection (Falsey et al., 2003). In the RSV challenge model and studies of natural infection in adults, RSV sequences were not detected after about 10 days (Falsey et al., 2003; Lee et al., 2004). These results are consistent with surveillance studies among asymptomatic community-dwelling adults in which RSV RNA sequences were detected infrequently (0.6% asymptomatic patients) even at times in which RSV is prevalent in the community (Falsey et al., 2006).

Relevance of diagnostic methods to clinical care and epidemiological studies

The method by which RSV infection is identified is important not only for the management of patients but also for the evaluation of epidemiological studies. Earlier epidemiological studies vastly underestimated the incidence of RSV infections because only viral culture and/or antigen detection methods were used to identify illnesses. In contrast, studies using RT-PCR as one of the diagnostic methods provide a more accurate assessment of the incidence of RSV infection in the adult population. This concept has been validated by recently published epidemiological studies. A study using viral culture and IFA methods identified RSV in 2% of elderly adults with respiratory illness in Sweden (Ostlund et al., 2004). In contrast, a French study that used RT-PCR showed that 4.8–11% of respiratory illnesses in a similar adult population were caused by RSV (Freymuth et al., 2004). Thus, there is significant evidence to support the notion that RSV is a significant pathogen in elderly adults.

Immunity and pathogenesis of RSV in elderly adults

Reinfection with RSV occurs throughout life, suggesting that acquired immunity following each infection is incomplete (Hall, 2001). However, the presence of neutralizing serum antibodies is at least partially protective and the risk of re-infection in children and adults is inversely correlated with the serum levels of these antibodies (Glezen et al., 1986; Walsh et al., 2004). The severity of RSV infection in the elderly appears to be multifactorial, including the frail medical condition of these patients and the increased incidence of underlying cardiopulmonary disease (Walsh et al., 2004). However, there is no specific defect among the elderly with respect to serum antibody levels (Falsey et al., 1999a, 1999b). Paradoxically, elderly adults have a more robust antibody response to RSV infection as compared to younger persons (Walsh and Falsey, 2004a, b). Taken together, these data raise the issue of immunosenescence, i.e. an age-related diminished immune response to RSV, possibly due to defects in T-cell function or an imbalance between the Th1 and Th2 responses (Miller, 1996; Mbawuike et al., 1997; Gardner and Murasko, 2002).

There are limited animal and human studies on age-related changes in RSV-specific immune responses. As compared to young mice, old mice infected with RSV have diminished CD8+ CTL responses and γ-interferon production, increased IL-4 production by splenic lymphocytes, and higher RSV titers in lungs (Zhang et al., 2002). In human studies, we have found that older subjects at baseline produced significantly fewer γ-interferon ELISPOTs in response to RSV as compared to young adults (Looney et al., 2002). In contrast, in another study, the frequencies of CD4 IL-10- and CD4/CD8 γ-interferon-secreting memory T cells specific for RSV were not significantly different between young and elderly subjects (Lee et al., 2005). However, in the latter study, the ratio of IL-10/γ-interferon was significantly reduced among elderly study participants, suggesting an imbalance of the immune response. Overall, given the paucity of currently available data, age-related immune response against RSV merits further research and remains as one of the major hurdles in the development of vaccines against RSV.

Treatment of RSV infection

Current treatment strategies for elderly adults with RSV infection are primarily supportive in nature. Administration of antipyretics, intravenous fluids, and/or oxygen may be appropriate as clinically warranted. In elderly RSV-infected patients who are acutely wheezing, it may not be unreasonable to administer corticosteroids and/or bronchodilators, particularly since the diagnosis is often delayed, if made at all. However, it should be noted that no formal controlled trials to use such agents for treatment of RSV-related wheezing or respiratory distress in this patient population have been performed to date. Lastly, if clinical suspicion for co-existing bacterial infection is high, e.g. fevers, productive sputum and/or infiltrates seen on a chest radiographs, it may be appropriate to initiate antibiotic therapy since the presence of concomitant bacterial infection may be difficult to determine.

Ribavirin

As of this writing, aerosolized ribavirin is the only antiviral agent that has been approved in the United States for the treatment of hospitalized infants and young children with severe lower respiratory tract RSV infections. Placebo-controlled, randomized clinical studies using ribavirin to treat RSV have not consistently shown a statistically significant beneficial effect (Hall et al., 1983, 1985; Rodriguez et al., 1999). However, taken together, studies of ribavirin to treat RSV infections appear to show a trend toward clinical benefit.

Data on the safety and efficacy of ribavirin in elderly adults with RSV are limited to anecdotal reports. Aerosolized ribavirin was well tolerated in eight RSV-uninfected elderly volunteers, including those with COPD (Liss and Bernstein, 1988). In one of the few publications on the treatment of adults with RSV, one of two adult patients with hospital-acquired RSV died despite treatment with ribavirin (Feldman et al., 1994). The traditional method of ribavirin administration to young children, a prolonged dosing period of 20 mg/mL for 18 h/day via face mask, may be poorly tolerated by elderly patients with cognitive or physical limitations. An intermittent course of high-dose aerosolized ribavirin (60 mg/mL via face mask for 2 h, administered thrice daily) has been used in some pediatric patients (Englund et al., 1990) and may be better tolerated in the elderly adult population. This regimen has been used under extenuating circumstances in RSV-infected immunocompromized patients (Englund et al., 1990). Given the lack of data on the use of ribavirin in the elderly, no general recommendation on its use may be made.

Immunoglobulin preparations

At this time, two immunoglobulin preparations are licensed for the prevention of RSV infections: a polyclonal, high-titered anti-RSV IgG (RSVIGIV) (Groothuis et al., 1993, 1995) and a humanized monoclonal antibody against an epitope of the RSV F protein (palivizumab) (The IMpact RSV Study Group, 1998). As of this writing, RSVIVIG is not currently available in the United States. Both products are indicated for use as prophylactic use in high-risk children. There are no data on the use of immunoglobulin preparations in the elderly adults with RSV.

Use of antiviral agents in immunocompromised adult patients

Immunocompromised patients with lower respiratory tract symptoms and in whom the clinical suspicion for RSV infection is high should be considered for antiviral treatment prior to the onset of respiratory failure since mortality is very high once mechanical ventilation is required (Hertz et al., 1989; Harrington et al., 1992; Whimbey et al., 1995a, b). In bone marrow transplant recipients, the combination of immunoglobulins and ribavirin lowered the mortality associated with RSV pneumonia as compared to historical controls (50% vs. 70%, respectively; Whimbey et al., 1996). Although bone marrow and organ transplants are relatively uncommon in elderly adults, the clinical experience on the use of antiviral agents in immunocompromised patients can be extrapolated to severely ill elderly adults with primary (e.g. malignancies, prolonged steroid use) or secondary (e.g. post-chemotherapy) causes of immunosuppression.

Prevention of RSV infection

RSV is transmitted via fomites and large droplet aerosols (Hall et al., 1980; Hall and Douglas, 1981). Thus, RSV transmission requires autoinoculation from close contact with an infected patient or contaminated environmental surfaces (Hall et al., 1975). In long-term care facilities, RSV tends to spread slowly over several days to weeks. This manner of transmission and pattern of spread is in contrast to those of the influenza virus, which spreads rapidly via small particle aerosols and can cause explosive outbreaks in the community and in health care facilities.

Although various infection control strategies to prevent the transmission of RSV have been described, the cornerstone of such policies is strict hand washing. The use of gowns and gloves has also been advocated in pediatric wards (Madge et al., 1992). Masks are not required, but cohorting and subsequent contact isolation of infected patients is strongly advocated if possible. Education of medical and ancillary personnel regarding the mode of transmission of respiratory viruses and the value of vigilant handwashing led to a significant decrease in the rates of acute respiratory tract infections in adult day care centers (Falsey et al., 1999a, b).

As with many other infectious diseases, immunization may be the most effective method of preventing severe RSV disease in adults with advanced age or with underlying cardiopulmonary conditions. Efforts to develop a vaccine against RSV for children and adults are ongoing (Dudas and Karron, 1998). Low serum levels of neutralizing antibody against RSV have been shown to be a risk factor for RSV infection and associated illness (Walsh et al., 2004; Walsh and Falsey, 2004a, b). Thus, a vaccine to increase neutralizing antibody titer may offer some benefit. Both subunit and live attenuated vaccines have been tried with varying success. Following immunization with a purified RSV F protein subunit vaccine, a four-fold rise in anti-RSV antibody was detected in 61% of healthy community-dwelling elderly adults and in 47% of healthy adults in long-term care facilities (Falsey and Walsh, 1996, 1997). An experimental recombinant vaccine comprised of a portion of the RSV G protein has also been shown to elicit antibody response in Phase 2 clinical trials (Power et al., 2001). Passive transfer of human antibodies generated by this vaccine protected SCID mouse lungs against experimental RSV challenge (Plotnicky-Gilquin et al., 2002). In another study, administration of a live attenuated RSV vaccine in healthy young and elderly adults led to the development of only modest immune response, presumably due to relatively low rates of infection (Gonzalez et al., 2000). However, despite ongoing efforts, a safe and effective vaccine against RSV is not available for any age group.

Conclusions

Epidemiological and clinical data that have accrued over the last three decades have firmly established that RSV is a significant pathogen among elderly adults. Advances in diagnostic methods, especially those using molecular techniques, have greatly aided recent retrospective and prospective studies on RSV infections in older adults. Given the vulnerability of elderly adults to RSV-associated morbidity and mortality, especially in those with underlying cardiopulmonary disease, new therapeutic drugs and preventive vaccines would be beneficial and likely cost-effective.

References

Agius G, Dindinaud G, Biggar RJ, et al. An epidemic of respiratory syncytial virus in elderly people: clinical and serological findings. J Med Virol 1990; 30: 117.

Arroyo JC, Jordan W, Milligan L. Upper respiratory tract infection and serum antibody responses in nursing home patients. Am J Infect Control 1988; 16: 152.

Borg I, Rohde G, Loseke S, et al. Evaluation of quantitative real-time PCR for the detection of respiratory syncytial virus in pulmonary diseases. Eur Respir J 2003; 21: 944.

Casiano-Colon AE, Hulbert BB, Mayer TK, et al. Lack of sensitivity of rapid antigen tests for the diagnosis of respiratory syncytial virus infection in adults. J Clin Virol 2003; 28: 169.

Centers for Disease Control (CDC). Epidemiologic notes and reports: respiratory syncytial virus—Missouri. MMWR 1977; 26: 351.

Dowell SF, Anderson LJ, Gary Jr. HE, et al. Respiratory syncytial virus is an important cause of community-acquired lower respiratory tract infection among hospitalized adults. J Infect Dis 1996; 174: 456.

Dudas R, Karron R. Respiratory syncytial virus vaccines. Clin Microbiol Rev 1998; 11: 430.

Englund JA, Piedra P, Jefferson LS, et al. High-dose, short-duration ribavirin aerosol therapy in children with suspected respiratory syncytial virus infection. J Pediatr 1990; 117: 313.

Englund JA, Piedra P, Jewell A, et al. Rapid diagnosis of respiratory syncytial virus infections in immunocompromised adults. J Clin Microbiol 1996; 34: 1649.

Ellis SE, Coffey CS, Mitchel Jr. EF, et al. Influenza- and respiratory syncytial virus-associated morbidity and mortality in the nursing home population. J Am Geriatr Soc 2003; 51: 761.

Falsey AR, Criddle MM, Kolassa JE, et al. Evaluation of a handwashing intervention to reduce respiratory illness rates in senior day-care centers. Infect Control Hosp Epidemiol 1999a; 20: 200.

Falsey AR, Criddle MC, Walsh EE. Detection of respiratory syncytial virus and human metapneumovirus by reverse transcription polymerase chain reaction in adults with and without respiratory illness. J Clin Virol 2006; 35: 46.

Falsey AR, Cunningham CK, Barker WH, et al. Respiratory syncytial virus and influenza A infections in the hospitalized elderly. J Infect Dis 1995; 172: 389.

Falsey AR, Formica MA, Treanor JJ, et al. Comparison of quantitative reverse transcription-PCR to viral culture for assessment of respiratory syncytial virus shedding. J Clin Micro 2003; 41: 4160.

Falsey AR, Formica MA, Walsh EE. Diagnosis of respiratory syncytial virus infection: comparison of reverse transcription-PCR to viral culture and serology in adults with respiratory illness. J Clin Micro 2002; 40: 817.

Falsey AR, Hennessey PA, Formica MA, et al. Respiratory syncytial virus infection in elderly and high-risk adults. N Engl J Med 2005; 352: 1749.

Falsey AR, Treanor JJ, Betts RF, et al. Viral respiratory infections in the institutionalized elderly: clinical and epidemiological findings. J Am Geriatr Soc 1992; 40: 115.

Falsey AR, Walsh EE. Safety and immunogenicity of a respiratory syncytial virus subunit vaccine (PFP-2) in ambulatory adults over age 60. Vaccine 1996; 14: 1214.

Falsey AR, Walsh EE. Safety and immunogenicity of a respiratory syncytial virus subunit vaccine (PFP-2) in the institutionalized elderly. Vaccine 1997; 15: 1130.

Falsey AR, Walsh EE. Respiratory syncytial virus infection in adults. Clin Microbiol Rev 2000; 13: 371.

Falsey AR, Walsh EE, Betts RF. Serologic evidence of respiratory syncytial virus infection in nursing home patients. J Infect Dis 1990; 162: 568.

Falsey AR, Walsh EE, Looney RJ, et al. Comparison of respiratory syncytial virus humoral immunity and response to infection in young and elderly adults. J Med Virol 1999b; 59: 221.

Fan J, Henrickson KJ, Savatski LL. Rapid simultaneous diagnosis of infections with respiratory syncytial viruses A and B, influenza viruses A and B, and human parainfluenza virus types 1, 2, and 3 by multiplex quantitative reverse transcription: polymerase chain reaction-enzyme hybridization [hexaplex] assay. Clin Infect Dis 1998; 26: 1.

Feldman RJ, Fidalgo HC, John Jr. JF. Respiratory syncytial virus in a cardiac surgery intensive care unit. J Thorac Cardiovasc Surg 1994; 108: 1152.

Fleming DM, Cross KW. Respiratory syncytial virus or influenza? Lancet 1993; 342: 1507.

Fransen H, Heigl Z, Wolontis S, et al. Infections with viruses in patients hospitalized with acute respiratory illness, Stockholm, 1963–1967. Scand J Infect Dis 1969; 1: 127.

Freymuth F, Vabret A, Gouarin S, et al. Epidemiology and diagnosis of respiratory syncytial virus in adults. Rev Mal Respir 2004; 21: 13.

Gardner EM, Murasko DM. Age-related changes in type 1 and type 2 cytokine production in humans. Biogerontology 2002; 3: 271.

Garvie DG, Gray J. Outbreak of respiratory syncytial virus infection in the elderly. Br Med J 1980; 281: 1253.

Glezen WP, Taber LH, Frank AL, et al. Risk of primary infection and reinfection with respiratory syncytial virus. Am J Dis Child 1986; 140: 543.

Gonzalez IM, Karron RA, Elchelberger M, et al. Evaluation of the live attenuated *cpts* 248/404 RSV vaccine in combination with a subunit RSV vaccine (PFP-2) in healthy young and older adults. Vaccine 2000; 18: 1763.

Griffin MR, Coffey CS, Neuzil KM, et al. Winter viruses: influenza- and respiratory syncytial virus-related morbidity in chronic lung disease. Arch Intern Med 2002; 162: 1229.

Groothuis JR, Simoes EAF, Hemming VG, the Respiratory Syncytial Virus Immune Globulin Study Group. Respiratory syncytial virus (RSV) infection in preterm infants and the protective effects of RSV immune globulin (RSVIG). Pediatrics 1995; 95: 463.

Groothuis JR, Simoes E, Levin MJ. et al., for the Respiratory Syncytial Virus Immune Globulin Study Group. Prophylactic administration of respiratory syncytial virus immune globulin to high-risk infants and young children. N Engl J Med 1993; 329: 1524.

Gross PA, Rodsteinm M, LaMontagne JR, et al. Epidemiology of acute respiratory illness during an influenza outbreak in a nursing home: a prospective study. Arch Intern Med 1988; 148: 559.

Hall CB. Clinically useful method for the isolation of respiratory syncytial virus. J Infect Dis 1975; 131: 1.

Hall CB. Respiratory syncitial virus and parainfluenza virus. N Engl J Med 2001; 344: 1917.

Hall CB, Douglas RG. Modes of transmission of respiratory syncytial virus. J Pediatr 1981; 99: 100.

Hall CB, Douglas RG, Geiman JM, et al. Nosocomial respiratory syncytial virus infections. N Engl J Med 1975; 293: 1343.

Hall CB, Douglas RG, Geiman JM. Respiratory syncytial virus infections in infants: quantitation and duration of shedding. J Pediatr 1976; 131: 1.

Hall CB, Douglas RG, Geiman JM. Possible transmission by fomites of respiratory syncytial virus. J Infect Dis 1980; 141: 98.

Hall CB, McBride JT, Gala CL, et al. Ribavirin treatment of respiratory syncytial viral infection in infants with underlying cardiopulmonary disease. JAMA 1985; 254: 3047.

Hall CB, McBride JT, Walsh EE, et al. Aerosolized ribavirin treatment of infants with respiratory syncytial viral infection. N Engl J Med 1983; 308: 1443.

Han LL, Alexander JP, Anderson LJ. Respiratory syncytial virus pneumonia among the elderly: an assessment of disease burden. J Infect Dis 1999; 179: 25.

Harrington RD, Hooton TM, Hackman RC, et al. An outbreak of respiratory syncytial virus in a bone marrow transplant center. J Infect Dis 1992; 165: 987.

Hart RJC. An outbreak of respiratory syncytial virus infection in an old people's home. J Infect Dis 1984; 8: 259.

Hers JFP, Masurel N, Gans JC. Acute respiratory disease associated with pulmonary involvement in military servicemen in the Netherlands. Am Rev Respir Dis 1969; 100: 499.

Hertz MI, Englund JA, Snover D, et al. Respiratory syncytial virus-induced acute lung injury in adult patients with bone marrow transplants: a clinical approach and review of the literature. Medicine (Baltimore) 1989; 68: 269.

Hornsleth A, Siggarrd-Anderson J, Hjort L. Epidemiology of herpesvirus and respiratory virus infections. Part 1; serologic findings. Geriatrics 1975; 30: 61.

Kellogg JA. Culture vs. direct antigen assays for detection of microbial pathogens from lower respiratory tract specimens suspected of containing the respiratory syncytial virus. Arch Pathol Lab Med 1991; 115: 451.

Kimball AM, Foy HM, Cooney MK, et al. Isolation of respiratory syncytial and influenza viruses from the sputum of patients hospitalized with pneumonia. J Infect Dis 1983; 147: 181.

Lee FE-H, Walsh EE, Falsey AR, et al. Experimental infection of humans with A2 respiratory syncytial virus. Antiviral Res 2004; 63: 191.

Lee FE-H, Walsh EE, Falsey AR, et al. The balance between influenza- and RSV-specific CD4 T cells secreting IL-10 or IFNγ in young and healthy-elderly subjects. Mech Age Dev 2005; 126: 1223.

Lerida A, Marron A, Casanova A, et al. Respiratory syncytial virus infection in adult patients hospitalized with community-acquired pneumonia. Enferm Infecc Microbiol Clin 2000; 18: 177.

Liss HP, Bernstein J. Ribavirin aerosol in the elderly. Chest 1988; 93: 1239.

Looney RJ, Falsey AR, Walsh E, et al. Effect of aging on cytokine production in response to respiratory syncytial virus infection. J Infect Dis 2002; 185: 682.

Madge P, Paton JY, McColl JH, et al. Prospective controlled study of four infection-control procedures to prevent nosocomial infection with respiratory syncytial virus. Lancet 1992; 340: 1079.

Mandal SK, Joglekar VM, Khan AS. An outbreak of respiratory syncytial virus infection in a continuing-care geriatric ward. Age Aging 1985; 14: 184.

Marrie TJ. Community-acquired pneumonia. Clin Infect Dis 1994; 18: 501.

Marrie TJ, Falsey AR, Campbell NN et al. The complement fixation test is not sensitive for the diagnosis of respiratory syncytial virus in patients with community acquired pneumonia (CAP) [abstract]. The 41st Interscience Conference on Antimicrobial Agents and Chemotherapy, December 16–19; Chicago (IL); 2001.

Mathur U, Bentley DW, Hall CB. Concurrent respiratory syncytial virus and influenza A infections in the institutionalized elderly and chronically ill. Ann Int Med 1980; 93: 49.

Mbawuike IN, Acuna CL, Walz KC, et al. Cytokines and impaired CD8+ CTL activity among elderly persons and the enhancing effect of IL-12. Mech Ageing Devel 1997; 94: 25.

Melbye H, Berdal BP, Straume B, et al. Pneumonia—a clinical or radiographic diagnosis? Scand J Infect Dis 1992; 24: 647.

Miller RA. The aging immune system: primer and prospectus. Science 1996; 273: 70.

Morales F, Calder MA, Inglis JM, et al. A study of respiratory infection in the elderly to assess the role of respiratory syncytial virus. J Infect 1983; 7: 236.

Nicholson KG. Impact of influenza and respiratory syncytial virus on mortality in England and Wales from January 1975 to December 1990. Epidemiol Infect 1996; 116: 51.

Nicholson KG, Baker DJ, Farquhar A, et al. Acute upper respiratory tract viral illness and influenza immunization in homes for the elderly. Epidemiol Infect 1990; 105: 609.

Orr PH, Peeling RW, Fast M, et al. Serological study of responses to selected pathogens causing respiratory tract infection in the institutionalized elderly. Clin Infect Dis 1996; 23: 1240.

Osterweil D, Norman D. An outbreak of an influenza-like illness in a nursing home. J Am Geriatr Soc 1990; 38: 659.

Ostlund MR, Wirgart BZ, Linde A, et al. Respiratory virus infections in Stockholm during seven seasons: a retrospective study of laboratory diagnosis. Scand J Infect Dis 2004; 36: 460.

Plotnicky-Gilquin H, Cyblat-Chanal D, Goetsch L, et al. Passive transfer of serum antibodies induced by BBG2Na, a subunit vaccine, in the elderly protects SCID mouse lungs against respiratory syncytial virus challenge. Virology 2002; 303: 130.

Power UF, Nguyen TN, Rietveld E, et al. Safety and immunogenicity of a novel recombinant subunit respiratory syncytial virus vaccine (BBG2Na) in healthy young adults. J Infect Dis 2001; 184: 1456.

Public Health Laboratory Service Communicable Diseases Surveillance Centre. Respiratory syncytial virus infection in the elderly, 1976–1982. Br Med J 1983; 287: 1618.

Rodriguez WJ, Arrobio J, Fink R, et al. Prospective follow-up and pulmonary functions from a placebo-controlled randomized trial of ribavirin therapy in respiratory syncytial virus bronchiolitis. Arch Pediatr Adolesc Med 1999; 153: 469.

Ruiz M, Ewig S, Marcos MA, et al. Etiology of community-acquired pneumonia: impact on age, co-morbidity, and severity. Am J Respir Crit Care Med 1999; 160: 397.

Sorvillo FJ, Huie SF, Strassburg MD, et al. An outbreak of respiratory syncytial virus pneumonia in a nursing home for the elderly. J Infect Dis 1984; 9: 252.

Stanek J, Heinz F. On the epidemiology and etiology of pneumonia in adults. J Hyg Epidemiol Microbiol 1988; 1: 31.

Stockton J, Ellis JS, Saville M, et al. Multiplex PCR for typing and subtyping influenza and respiratory syncytial viruses. J Clin Microbiol 1998; 36: 2990.

The IMpact RSV Study Group. Palivizumab, a humanized respiratory syncytial virus monoclonal antibody, reduces hospitalization from respiratory syncytial virus infection in high-risk infants. Pediatrics 1998; 102: 531.

Thompson WW, Shay DK, Weintraub E, et al. Mortality associated with influenza and respiratory syncytial virus in the United States. JAMA 2003; 289: 179.

Vikerfors T, Grandien M, Olcen P. Respiratory syncytial virus in adults. Am Rev Respir Dis 1987; 136: 561.

Wald TG, Miller BA, Shult P, et al. Can respiratory syncytial virus and influenza A be distinguished clinically in institutionalized older persons? J Am Geriatr Soc 1995; 43: 170.

Walsh EE, Falsey AR. A simple and reproducible method for collecting nasal secretions in frail elderly adults for measurement of virus-specific IgA. J Infect Dis 1999; 179: 1268.

Walsh EE, Falsey AR. Age related differences in humoral immune response to respiratory syncytial virus infection in adults. J Med Virol 2004a; 73: 295.

Walsh EE, Falsey AR. Humoral and mucosal immunity in protection from natural respiratory syncytial virus infection in adults. J Infect Dis 2004b; 190: 373.

Walsh EE, Falsey AR, Swinburne IA, et al. Reverse transcription polymerase chain reaction (RT-PCR) for diagnosis of respiratory syncytial virus infection in adults: use of a single-tube "hanging droplet" nested PCR. J Med Virol 2001; 63: 259.

Walsh EE, Peterson DR, Falsey AR. Risk factors for severe respiratory syncytial virus infection in elderly adults. J Infect Dis 2004; 189: 233.

Whimbey E, Champlin RE, Couch RB, et al. Community respiratory virus infections among hospitalized adult bone marrow transplant recipients. Clin Infect Dis 1996; 22: 778.

Whimbey E, Champlin RE, Englund JA, et al. Combination therapy with aerosolized ribavirin and intravenous immunoglobulin for respiratory syncytial virus disease in adult bone marrow transplant recipients. Bone Marrow Transplant 1995a; 16: 393.

Whimbey E, Couch RB, Englund JA, et al. Respiratory syncytial virus pneumonia in hospitalized adult patients with leukemia. Clin Infect Dis 1995b; 21: 376.

Zambon MC, Stockton JD, Clewley JP, et al. Contribution of influenza and respiratory syncytial virus to community cases of influenza-like illness: an observational study. Lancet 2001; 358: 1410.

Zaroukian MH, Leader I. Community-acquired pneumonia and infection with respiratory syncytial virus. Ann Intern Med 1988; 109: 515.

Zhang Y, Wang Y, Gilmore X, et al. An aged mouse model for RSV infection and diminished CD8(+) CTL responses. Exp Biol Med (Maywood) 2002; 227: 133.

Patricia Cane (Editor)

DOI 10.1016/S0168-7069(06)14007-0

Respiratory Syncytial Virus Disease Burden in the Developing World

D. James Nokes[a,b]
[a]*Centre for Geographic Medicine Research—Coast (CGMRC), Kenya Medical Research Institute (KEMRI)/Wellcome Trust Research Programme, Kilifi, Kenya*
[b]*Department of Biological Sciences, University of Warwick, Coventry, UK*

Introduction

Why this review now? There are three key reasons. First, recent advances in RSV vaccines, second, increased opportunity for vaccine implementation in the most resource-poor nations, and third, growth, since the last key review (Weber et al., 1998b), in RSV research interest in countries in the developing world, and the related published literature. The recent report (Karron et al., 2005) of a trial of a recombinant live attenuated RSV vaccine is of key significance since it demonstrates, for the first time in the key target age group of 1–2 months, a vaccine which is sufficiently attenuated yet apparently remaining immunogenic. Further trials are needed and there is an argument that vaccine trials in the developing world should closely follow those in industrialised countries or be included in multi-country trials (Belshe et al., 2004). Funding available for the development and implementation of novel vaccines has never been greater and in particular the focus of support of the Global Alliance on Vaccines and Immunization (GAVI) on the poorer nations has created an environment in which advances in vaccine development may see rapid progress towards the goal of implementation (GAVI, 2006). Two related issues arise. First there is the requirement to establish the burden of disease caused by a particular infectious agent, by which comparison can be made with other infectious diseases competing for health resources, and second there is a need to establish suitable sites for vaccine trials which at least fulfil the criteria of having detailed baseline denominator-based data on RSV-related disease, with observed incidence of adequate magnitude to power trials, requisite infrastructure for case surveillance and expertise in clinical trials to ensure good clinical research practice (Mulholland et al., 1999b). Recent studies on RSV in the developing world which are denominator-based are beginning to establish the comparative burden of RSV, in particular relative to all-cause acute lower respiratory tract infection (LRTI).

The review article of Weber et al. (1998b) provides a suitable point of departure for this chapter—in fact, it is highly recommended that this paper is consulted in conjunction with the present review. A key aim here is to highlight important data from the developing world since the review of Weber et al, loosely identifable as related to disease burden, with emphasis on the characteristics of RSV in populations—incidence of disease by severity, age-distribution, associated-mortality, certain risk factors for transmisison and disease, co-morbidity, and seasonality. Importance is placed on identifying advances in those areas previously highlighted as deficient, and, as important, to uncover those aspects that remain poorly understood, with little published data, and where more empirical data and research is recommended. Finally, emphasis is also given to issues that relate to vaccine development, trials and implementation, e.g. age at delivery for greater effectiveness in relation to age-distribution of disease; burden of disease in relation to all cause ARI, as a means of comparing health intervention priorities; assessment of long-term effects of severe RSV infection which relates to vaccine efficacy assessment.

Methods, definitions, limitations

The phrase 'developing world' has been interpreted broadly. It might easily have been replaced with 'tropical and developing countries', or 'resource poor settings'. It has been taken to mean regions, countries, populations, or communities of the world not usually thought of as part of the recognised 'industrialised' world, which are on average or substantially of low income, in population transition, rural or undergoing urbanisation, and in which health care may be under-resourced. A literature search was carried out in Pubmed and Web of Science using 'respiratory syncytial viruses' as a medical subject heading (MeSH term), or 'respiratory syncytial virus' or 'RSV' as text words, together with either (a) key words for sub-Saharan Africa, Central and South America or Asia (excluding Japan) or (b) 'developing country' [MeSH] or 'developing countr*', or (c) each of the 75 countries which are identified as the most resource-poor by GAVI (GAVI, 2006). Articles were included if more recently published than Weber et al. (around 1996) and up to 31/10/2005. Where the review covered earlier dates included (i) studies from GAVI countries and (ii) certain aspects of disease burden not covered in the earlier review, e.g. within-hospital infection and controlled prevalence studies. It is useful to mention an area excluded from this review; notably the numerous studies now published on the molecular epidemiology of RSV as this is covered in the chapter by Patricia Cane in this book.

Denominator-based data on incidence

There is a large literature that testifies to the importance of RSV as a cause of both community and hospitalised childhood LRI in resource-poor settings. In the review of Weber et al. (1998b), the estimated proportion of community-acquired LRTI in children due to RSV was 10% (range 1–22%) from community-based studies and 18% (6–40%) from hospital out-patient or in-patient studies.[1] Furthermore of all viral LRTI, RSV was estimated to account for between 44% (range 7–73%) in community studies and 65% (range 27–96%) from hospital studies.[2] In a WHO review of 28 studies in the developing world (Rudan et al., 2004), the median estimate of the incidence of clinical pneumonia (using the WHO case definition of moderate and severe ARI) was 280 cases/1000 child years (cy) (IQR 210–710) and an estimated 6–12% severe enough for admission. Back-of-the-envelope calculations generate incidences of RSV-pneumonia in children under 5 years in the community of 28 cases/1000 cy (IQR 21-71) (i.e. 0.1×280), and in the hospital of 2–15 cases/1000 cy (i.e. $210 \times 0.06 \times 0.18$ to $710 \times 0.12 \times 0.18$). Wright and Cutts (2000) using a similar approach, assuming an incidence of childhood pneumonia in the community of 400 cases/1000 cy, 18% of LRTI due to RSV, and a scaling factor for the proportion of LRTI that is pneumonia of 40–74%, derived estimates of childhood RSV associated LRTI of 97–180 cases/1000 cy in the under fives. Such incidence estimates are useful starting points but are clearly crude, with compounding imprecision due to uncertainty of each component of the calculation.

The need for denominator-based studies

Surveillance of RSV-associated LRTI within well-characterised populations is likely to generate the most precise estimates of RSV incidence, suitable for determining local disease burden and comparison with incidence data from other locations and for other infectious diseases. Recognising the paucity of such data, and the urgency for its collection to assist government health officials and immunization programme managers to establish disease-control priorities, the WHO developed a generic protocol setting out a clear case for denominator-based studies to estimate the incidence of LRTI due to RSV in children under 5 years of age in developing countries (Wright and Cutts, 2000). WHO also commissioned four denominator-based studies, three in sub-Saharan Africa and one in Indonesia, the results of which were recently published (Robertson et al., 2004). At that time the key limitations of previous disease burden studies were perceived to be (i) in general, poorly defined population denominator for incidence estimation, (ii) inadequate information on the severity of disease by age, (iii) poor age-stratification and in particular too few infants and neonates by which to define incidence in these key vaccine target groups, (iv) absence of rural studies with potentially differing risk factors for transmission than urban poor, i.e. the generality of past data was

[1]Based on studies that used the immunofluorescent antibody test (IFAT) for antigen detection.

[2]The proportion of LRTI that is RSV positive or viral LRTI that is RSV, depends significantly upon the method of determination, particularly the use of IFAT. While overall viral isolation was unchanged between studies using and those not using IFAT, the proportion of viral LRTI due to RSV increased significantly, suggesting an increased sensitivity for RSV using IFAT at the expense of that for other viruses, especially adenovirus (Weber et al., 1998b).

uncertain, (v) information on the effects of seasonal variations, and (vi), in general, insufficiently standardised methods (Wright and Cutts, 2000). To what extent these shortcomings have been redressed is assessed below.

Estimates of disease burden and quality assessment

Tables 1 and 2 and Fig. 1 summarise the available denominator-based studies of RSV incidence. There are representatives from a wide geographical area, in particular, Latin America (3), sub-Saharan Africa (6), and Asia (5). The two remaining studies, one from Alaska, USA (Yukon-Kuskokwim Delta) (Karron et al., 1999) and one from Southern Israel (Negev region) (Dagan et al., 1993), are included as they report on native populations whose demographic characteristics are suggestive of a developing country (high growth rates and high proportion under 5 years).

The rates reported here for developing countries are not dissimilar to those recorded for the industrialised world. For example, the study of a birth cohort recruited from low-income urban families in the US (Glezen et al., 1986) under active surveillance reported a rate of RSV-LRTI of 224 cases/1000 cy in infants. Studies of similar design presented in Table 2 (Cali, Colombia and Kilifi, Kenya) reported infant rates between 154 and 220 cases /1000 cy. A longitudinal cohort study of OP presentations with LRTI in the US reported a rate of 44 cases/1000 cy in infants (Fisher et al., 1997), which compares with rates of 30 and 25 cases /1000 cy in infants from studies in Mozambique and Colombia, respectively. Rates of RSV-ARI hospitalisation in developed countries range from 1 to 20 cases/1000 infants (Collins et al., 2001; Robertson et al., 2004). These span the range shown in Table 2 (Fig. 1) other than for two studies which stand out as having rates of disease which appear high in comparison with the published literature. The relatively high rate of RSV-sLRTI in the Kilifi, Kenya study (100 cases/1000 cy) suggests there is considerable severe RSV within the community that does not present to health facilities. The rate of RSV hospitalisations in native Alaskans is among the very highest recorded, similar to rates from Native American Indians and commensurate with rates of hospitalisation of infants with high risk for RSV disease (e.g. children who are premature or with chronic lung or congenital lung disease) (Bockova et al., 2002).

Inclusion of a study in this review merely required some attempt by the authors to provide an estimate of the catchment population from which RSV cases were identified. For this reason, among others, they are not all equal in merit. For each study, factors which may have an influence on incidence estimates, and a significant bearing on the quality of data, have been identified (Table 1). These factors are explicitly defined in Table 3 with comment on their possible influence on data derived; these issues are of importance at the design stage of disease-burden studies (see also Wright and Cutts, 2000).

Ignoring practical and logistic constraints, the ideal (but expensive) study for estimating disease burden is (i) age-cross-sectional in design within a stable population with rolling recruitment and dropout, and denominator size based on

Table 1

Methods of studies reporting the incidence of respiratory syncytial virus associated LRTI in the developing world

Location, population (reference)	Period of study	Denominator	Case ascertainment	Severity definitions[a] (assessor)	Specimen details. Diagnostic tests
Rio de Janeiro, Brazil; Urban poor (Sutmoller et al., 1995)	1987–1989, 36 months, 3 epidemics	All children < 5y enrolled following baseline census of two low-income communities	Active weekly home visits by HCW	LRTI: one or more of RR > 50, chest retractions, wheezing, rales, stridor, cyanosis. (HCW at home)	NPA (shallow) at home by HCW. IFAT, culture
Cali, Colombia Urban poor (Berman et al., 1983)	1977–1979, 25 months, 2 epidemics	Children < 15y in baseline census, in closely monitored community	Passive surveillance through all (5) health clinics of community	LRTI: croup, tracheobronchitis, bronchiolitis, or pneumonia (physician in clinic)	NP Swabs (1977) in clinic, NW (1978–1979) in lab. Culture, serology (4-fold rise in CFT Ab)
Cali, Colombia Urban poor (Borrero et al., 1990)	1986–1988, 17 months,	Birth cohort selected within well-defined community and followed until 17m. 20% lost to follow up	Active weekly home visits (AN), regular clinic appointments, clinic referral for ARI (AN, RN), and passive referral encouraged to clinic serving community	LRTI: one or more of RR50/min, retractions, wheezing, rales, stridor, cyanosis (physician in clinic)	NPA in clinic. IFAT and culture
Alaska, USA; Rural (Karron et al., 1999)	1993–1996, 36 months, 3 epidemics	Recorded births in each year of study	Passive surveillance at hospitals (2) serving community	LRTI: admitted with ARI	NPA in ward. IFAT and culture
Western Region, The Gambia; Urban–rural (Weber et al., 2002)	1994–1996, 36 months, 3 epidemics	Estimated population at risk < 1y	Passive surveillance at main (3) hospitals serving community	LRTI: admission diagnosis of acute LRTI, or received oxygen	NPA in ward. IFAT

Table 1 (*continued*)

Location, population (reference)	Period of study	Denominator	Case ascertainment	Severity definitions[a] (assessor)	Specimen details. Diagnostic tests
Ibadan, Nigeria Peri-urban and rural (Robertson et al., 2004)	1999–2001, 24 months, 2 epidemics	All children <5y from two communities under demographic surveillance	Active weekly home visits by CN	LRTI: increased RR with or without cough, indrawing, fever. (CN, physician at home)	NW at home by CN. Rapid Ag ELISA
Kilifi District, Kenya; Rural (Nokes et al., 2004)	2002–2003, 15 months, 2 epidemics	Birth cohort within DSS followed through first year of life. Recruitment from maternity ward or MCHC at District Hospital. ~10% drop out	Active home visits (TFW) (weekly during RSV epidemic, monthly otherwise), referral for ARI, passive referral encouraged to District hospital	LRTI: c or db AND $\geqslant$1 of (1) increased RR (2) indrawing (3) $O_2<90\%$ or inability to feed if clinical dx LRTI/ bronchiolitis. sLRTI: LRTI with (2) or (3). (CO or MO in clinic or ward)	NW at home, clinic or ward by TFW or CO. IFAT
Manhica, Mozambique; Rural (Loscertales et al., 2002, Robertson et al., 2004)	1999–2000, 12 months, 1 epidemic	Estimated population at risk <1y	Passive surveillance at OP of District hospital (TMA)	LRTI: c or nd or db AND $\geqslant$1 of (1) increased RR (2) indrawing (3) stridor (4) wheezing (5) apnoea (TMA)	NW in OP. Rapid Ag ELISA
		Estimated population at risk <5y	Passive surveillance at IP of District hospital	LRTI: as above	NW in ward. Rapid Ag ELISA

Agincourt, South Africa; Rural villages (Robertson et al., 2004)	2000–2001, 12 months, 1+ epidemic	Estimated population at risk < 5y based on annual census and vital events update	Passive health clinic (6) surveillance by community nurses	sLRTI: ⩾3 of (1) increased RR, (2) indrawing (3) stridor (4) wheezing (5) apnoea (CN)	NW in clinic. Rapid Ag ELISA
Soweto, South Africa; Urban poor (Madhi et al , 2000)	1997–1998, 13 months, 1 epidemic	Deduced from estimated birth cohort in catchment area of hospital	Passive tertiary referral hospital IP surveillance 2–23 months	sLRTI: cough AND (1) tachypnea and indrawing OR (2) O_2 saturation <90%	NW in ward. IFAT, shell vial culture
Negev Region, Israel; Rural (Dagan et al., 1993)	1987, 4 months, 1 epidemic	Livebirths recorded during year of study. Data on Bedouin and Jews	Passive surveillance at main medical centre	LRTI: bronchiolitis	NW in ward. ELISA, culture, serology
Takhli District, Thailand; Rural (Suwanjutha et al., 2002)	1998–2001, 28 months, 2 epidemics	All children < 5y enrolled following baseline census, with continuous enrolment of newborn and censoring at age 5 years	Active surveillance for LRI signs with referral to District hospital.	LRTI: WHO protocol with CXR confirmation (hospital physician)	NPA at hospital. IFAT
Bandung, Indonesia Peri-urban + rural (Robertson et al., 2004)	1999–2001, 24 months, 2 epidemics	Baseline census and enrolment of children < 5y in two communities	Active weekly home visits (CHW with supervisors). Children with LRTI signs taken to clinic	LRTI: c or db AND ⩾1 of (1) increased RR, (2) indrawing, (3) stridor, (4) wheezing, (5) apnoea (physician)	NW at clinic by physician. Rapid Ag ELISA

Table 1 (*continued*)

Location, population (reference)	Period of study	Denominator	Case ascertainment	Severity definitions[a] (assessor)	Specimen details. Diagnostic tests
Lombok, Indonesia Rural (Djelantik et al., 2003a)	2000–2001, 24 months	Derived from annual survey of birth records in 83 study villages, with adjustment for deaths in children <2y	Passive surveillance by all health centres and hospitals of villages. Effective referral procedures	sLRTI: WHO protocol LRTI with (1) chest indrawing OR (2) RR $\geqslant 60$ and age <2 months (physician)	NW at hospital. Rapid Ag ELISA
Hong Kong, China Urban (Chan et al., 1999)	1993–1997, 60 months	Estimated population at risk <5y	Passive surveillance at tertiary hospital	LRTI: admitted with ARI	NPA, BL, EA, NS in ward. IFAT, culture
Metro manila, Phillipines; Urban poor (Tupasi et al., 1990)	1985–1987, 24 months	Baseline census, random multi-stage sample of households, recruitment of children <5y with continuous enrolment of newborn and censoring at age 5 years	Weekly home visits (nurses). Children with LRTI signs were referred to clinic to confirm (physician). Passive referral to main hospital	LRTI: cough AND $\geqslant 1$ of (1) cyanosis, (2) indrawing (without wheezing), (3) increased RR (hospital physician)	NPA at hospital. IFAT, culture

Abbreviations: dx, diagnosis; c, cough; nd, nasal discharge; db, difficulty in breathing; RR, respiratory rate; TMA, trained medical assistant; CO, clinical officer; MO, medical officer; DSS, Demographic Surveillance System.

[a]As listed in Table 2. In each case these also define criteria for collecting specimens with the exceptions of Kilifi, Kenya and Manhica, Mozambique (OP) studies in which the minimum criterion was signs of URTI.

Table 2

Incidence estimates of LRTI and RSV-associated LRTI per 1000 cy (95% CI) from studies in developing countries

Location	Severity type[a]	Age class (years)	Population	Child years (cy)[b]	Total incidence/1000 cy (95% CL)[c]	RSV incidence/1000 cy (95% CL)
CS America						
Rio de Janeiro, Brazil (Sutmoller et al., 1995)	LRTI com	<5	262	786	64 (46–81)	14 (6–22)
Cali, Colombia (Berman et al., 1983)[d]	LRTI OP	<15	8,748	18,225	67 (64–71)	6 (5–7)
		<5	4,958	10,329	107 (101–113)	9 (7–11)
		<1	992	2,066	250 (228–271)	25 (18–31)
Cali, Colombia (Borrero et al., 1990)	LRTI com	<1.5	340	413	1,715 (1,565–1,864)	200 (149–241)
		<1	205	399	1,946 (1,755–2,137)	220 (156–284)
N America						
Alaska, USA (Karron et al., 1999)	LRTI IP	<1	1,801	1,801	522 (489–555)	155 (137–173)
SS Africa						
Western Gambia (urban)(Weber et al., 2002)	LRTI IP	<1	20,338	–	53	9
Western Gambia (rural) (Weber et al., 2002)	LRTI IP	<1	–	–	160	18
Ibadan, Nigeria (Robertson et al., 2004)	LRTI com	<5	–	1,579	270 (244–296)	116 (78–154)
		<1	–	316	323 (260–386)	94 (79–109)
Kilifi, Kenya (Nokes et al., 2004)	LRTI com	<1	338	311	1,029 (916–1,042)	154 (111-198)
	sLRTI com	<1	338	311	463 (387–539)	100 (54-135)
	LRTI IP	<1	338	311	103 (67–139)	13 (0–25)
Manhica, Mozambique (Robertson et al., 2004)	LRTI OP	<1	–	1,342	509 (471–547)	30 (21–39)
	LRTI IP	<1	–	1,342	126 (107–145)	15 (8–22)
		<5	–	6,020	68 (61–75)	5 (3–7)
Agincourt, South Africa (Robertson et al., 2004)	sLRTI OP	<1	–	1,652	332 (304–360)	15 (9–21)
		<5	–	8,258	80 (74–86)	9 (7–11)
Soweto, South Africa (Madhi et al., 2000)[e]	sLRTI IP	<2	24,000	24,000	–	4 (3–4)
Middle East						
Negev, Israel (Bedouin) (Dagan et al., 1993)	LRTI IP	<1	2,991	2,991	–	18 (13–23)

Table 2 (*continued*)

Location	Severity type[a]	Age class (years)	Population	Child years (cy)[b]	Total incidence/1000 cy (95% CL)[c]	RSV incidence/1000 cy (95% CL)
SE Asia						
Takhli, Thailand (Suwanjutha et al., 2002)	LRTI com	<5	6,244	14,569	32 (29–35)	8 (7–10)
Bandung, Indonesia (Robertson et al., 2004)	LRTI com	<1	–	284	178 (129–227)	41 (17–65)
		<5	–	1,420	191 (168–214)	34 (24–44)
	sLRTI com	<1	–	284	25 (7–43)	16 (1–31)
		<5	–	1,420	22 (14–30)	10 (5–15)
Lombok, Indonesia (Djelantik et al., 2003a)	LRTI IP	<1	15,000	15,000	–	25 (22–28)
		<2	30,000	30,000	–	14 (13–15)
Hong Kong, China (Chan et al., 1999)	LRTI IP	<5	–	49,6000	19 (19–20)	3 (2–3)
Metro Manila, Phillipines (Tupasi et al., 1990)	LRTI com	<5	–	1,418	527 (489–565)	28 (19–37)

[a]Severity types: (s)LRTI com—(severe) LRTI identified through active surveillance of the community; (s)LRTI OP—(severe) LRTI identified through passive out-patient department/clinic surveillance; (s)LRTI IP—(severe) LRTI diagnosed on admission to hospital.
[b]Where not provided, crude estimates based on denominator data provided, and scaled as necessary. Does not account for infant or under 5 mortality.
[c]95% confidence limits (CL) = $rate\ +/-1.96\sqrt{rate/cy}.1000$.
[d]Assumes 48% of RSV cases <1 yr & 90% LRTI <5 yrs.
[e]Rate estimated from prevalence in HIV+ and HIV– scaled by population representation.

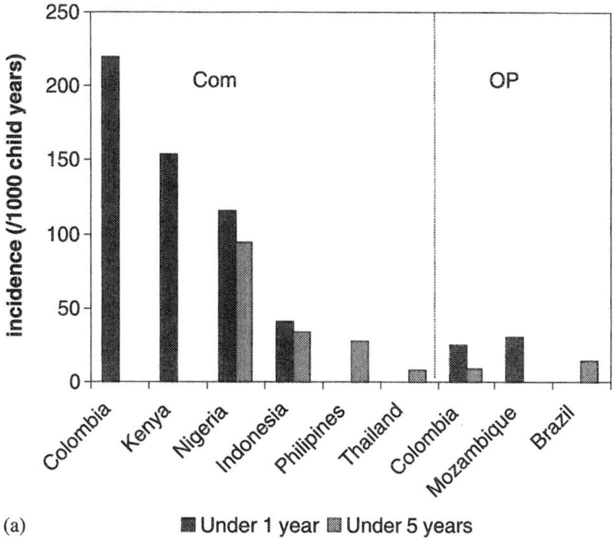

(a)

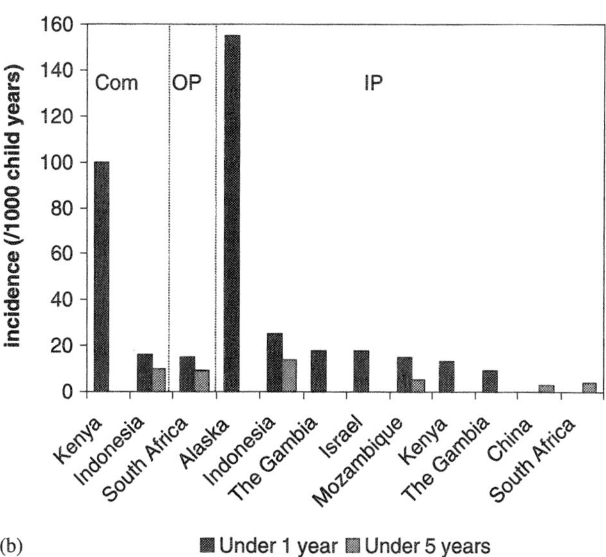

(b)

Fig. 1 Incidence of RSV-LRTI (panel a) and severe or hospitalised RSV-LRTI (panel b) stratified by age group and surveillance method for disease burden studies detailed in Tables 1 and 2. Community, out-patient or in-patient surveillance are abbreviated to com., OP, and IP, respectively.

expected incidence and required estimate precision, (ii) employs surveillance of ARI over a suitably long period to offset bias from temporal variation that couples frequent (e.g. weekly) active surveillance to efficient passive clinic referral, with (iii) samples collected by NPA or NW tested by a variety of assays preferably (or IFAT

Table 3

Factors that affect the interpretation and accuracy of disease burden data

Factor	Considerations
Design	• Cross-sectional (requires rolling recruitment of newborn and censoring at upper age limit) or cohort (vulnerable to bias in exposure time unless recruitment occurs throughout epidemic and non-epidemic period) • Age range—age-dependent risk hence need to be well stratified to enable comparison. Cohort studies vulnerable to bias in estimates by age • Sample size— attention to confidence intervals on estimates • Sampling bias—should be representative of defined population group • Population denominator—defined by specific census/inferred from national data/updated/not updated/cohort size followed up
Location	Rates may differ by location, e.g. rural, peri-urban, urban, and in relation to SES. Transmission related to socio-demography.
Years of case detection	• Duration—ideally over several years to average out year to year variation • Number of epidemics—influence magnitude of incidence estimate, unless scaled for average annual ratio within/between epidemic • Seasonality—can incur bias due to time-dependent incidence
Method of case ascertainment	• Active—Community visits. Frequency of visits. May or may not involve encouragement of parents to take children to clinic if ARI is observed • Passive—(i) OP presentations (ii) IP admissions—by definition severe. Influenced by care-seeking behaviour, also cost, distance and time issues
Assessor	Experience and training of assesors of severity. Clinician, nurse, trained field health worker, untrained operator
Collection of specimen	• Minimum criteria—sensitivity of case ascertainment. Severity—mild, severe, very severe. Defintion—WHO guidelines or other • Who collects: technical competence of staff. • Where collected: access to health facilities; quality of sample collection
Nasal sampling method	Sensitivity of method: NPA gold standard, NW comparable to NPA, swabs less sensitive
Laboratory diagnosis	• Rapid Ag assay: IFAT technical competence or EIA technically easy. But IFAT sensitivity >EIA • Other options culture/shell vial, and serum antibody (rising titre e.g. CFT, ELISA), PCR. Note that the more assays used, each with less than perfect specificity, the greater chance of false positives, although sensitivity should improve

if a single assay), and (iv) using suitably qualified and trained staff to undertake clinical and laboratory diagnosis and sample collection. Scrutiny of Tables 1 and 2 reveals that most studies (an exception is the early BOSTID study from the Philippines (Tupasi et al., 1990)) fall short of following these rigorous criteria in full. However, the key requirement is to record all cases of disease of specified severity within a community of known size. While the different study designs will have achieved this goal to different degrees, exactly to what extent this was achieved is largely unknown. It is likely that least confidence can be assigned to passive surveillance estimates where the catchment population was not clearly defined and there was little assurance of a high referral rate to the health facilities. In the study in Lombok, Indonesia (Djelantik et al., 2003a), villages were selected on the basis of proximity to a district hospital, good cooperation in previous surveillance projects, and prior successful referral practice. Importantly, they also monitored the effectiveness of the referral practices and determined that 90% of patients presenting with severe pneumonia were referred to a study hospital. In The Gambia, Weber et al. (2002) reported a decrease in reported incidence with an increase in cost of transport to the study hospital. It is probable that this provides a measure of referral efficiency (though spatial variation in incidence cannot be excluded), identifying variation in reporting rates across the study population that needs to be accounted for in incidence estimation. Measures of outcome of this nature should be an integral part of future disease burden studies, particularly those relying on passive referral methods.

Interpreting heterogeneity in incidence

Estimates of RSV associated disease incidence are highly variable (Table 2, Fig. 1). Similarly, study methodology (Table 1) varies considerably. It is difficult to deduce how much incidence variation is down to methodological differences and how much due to variation intrinsic to the study populations. Fig. 1 presents the incidence data of Table 2, stratified by three methodological factors with strong influence on estimates, namely, (i) the inclusion age range (ii) the method of case ascertainment, i.e. actively within the community or passively through clinic/hospital out-patients or in-patient presentation, and (iii) disease severity (the latter two being correlated). In general, rates are higher through active surveillance within a community, and for infants, and lower for increased upper age, passive surveillance and increased severity. These patterns arise from differences in the likelihood that a case arising in the community will present to a health facility and the known relationship between severity and age (highly correlated with primary infection vs. re-infection) (Glezen et al., 1981, 1986).

While the stratification in Fig. 1 explains a substantial part of the incidence variation, there remains considerable difference within these groups. Estimates of the incidence of RSV-associated LRTI range from 41 to 210 cases/1000 cy in under ones and 8 to 94 cases/1000 cy in the under fives from community studies, estimates from OP studies are at the lower end of community-based estimates (Fig. 1a). In general, incidence estimates for more severe disease fall quite tightly in the range 8–25 cases/1000 cy in under ones and 3–14 in the under fives, irrespective of the method of case ascertainment (Fig. 1b). The exceptions are a community study in Kenya, and admission data for Native Alaskans, with incidences of 100–155 cases of severe LRTI/1000 cy in the under ones. Some of this remaining variation will be accountable to differences in sensitivity of case ascertainment. For example, community studies in which diagnosis and nasal sampling was undertaken at the household (Borrero et al., 1990, Robertson et al., 2004), are likely to miss fewer cases than those requiring referral and confirmation of cases to a health facility (Tupasi et al., 1990; Suwanjutha et al., 2002; Robertson et al., 2004). However, in Kenya (Nokes et al., 2004) although NW were collected in the household, clinical diagnosis was dependent upon passive (parental) and active (field worker) referral to the clinic at the District Hospital (note however, that travel costs were reimbursed). The study in Western Gambia (Weber et al., 2002) clearly demonstrated that the cost of getting to a health centre (correlated to distance, time, and ease of access) influenced substantially the estimated rate of severe RSV disease in children under 1 year; the rate declining by an order of magnitude between those nearest ($\sim$10/1000 cy) and those farthest ($<$1/1000 cy). Studies also differ with respect to nasal sample methods and laboratory diagnostic assays. However, it is difficult to attribute the variation in incidence to these differences. With reference to urban–rural variation, 6 of the study populations could be described as urban (4 of which were specifically described as poor populations), 7 as rural and 3 as combined urban–rural. The more recent studies tend to be rural or combined urban–rural (redressing the imbalance cited earlier). Any relationship between RSV incidence and urban–rural population type is unclear when comparing between countries. Within country comparison would be more revealing; in the single within country comparison Weber et al. (2002) identified higher rates in a rural than a urban location (Table 2, Fig. 1).

It is reasonable to assume that the greater the severity of disease the more likely a child will present to a health facility, thus reducing the difference in incidence estimates between community and hospital methods of surveillance. The study from Kenya is thus a perplexing outlier, though it should be noted that there are few community studies of severe RSV disease. It follows also that the more severe the disease the less important a relationship between accessibility (cost, distance, time) and incidence. Interestingly however, the Gambia data (Weber et al., 2002) show a roughly equivalent slope (log scale) for the relationship between transport costs and incidence of ARI, RSV-sLRTI and RSV-very severe LRTI.

Among the highest reported incidences are those from the only two birth cohort studies (Table 1; Borrero et al., 1990, Nokes et al., 2004). Both studies were of short duration and with potential bias for increased at-risk observation time. Additionally, and probably of most significance, both involved active surveillance coupled to passive referral in which parents were encouraged to bring children to the study health facilities if respiratory symptoms were observed. Hence these high incidences may be in part methodological, but probably provide nearer the actual rates of RSV disease occurring in their study populations.

Finally, we are left with variation that is not methodological in origin. For example, it is difficult to ascribe differences in methods to variation in the incidence of RSV-LRTI between Kilifi and Cali (high) and Bandung, Takhul and Manila (low), all of which involved active surveillance of cases (Table 1, Fig. 1a). Similarly, for the difference between the estimates of RSV-sLRTI in Kilifi and Bandung (active surveillance) and in Alaska and all the other studies (passive surveillance) (Table 1, Fig. 1b). It seems probable that social-economic-cultural risk factors for infection and disease play a role, such as religious practices (Robertson et al., 2004), family size and structure, schooling age and characteristics, environmental pollution such as indoor smoke, co-infections (e.g. HIV (Madhi et al., 2000)), human metapneumovirus (Semple et al., 2005), nutritional status or host genetics. The studies of native Americans report the highest levels of hospitalised RSV-sLRTI, for which a genetic predisposing component seems very likely (Karron et al., 1999; Bockova et al., 2002). These risk factors are of considerable intrinsic interest, and a few will be considered in further detail later in the review.

At this stage it is worth considering to what degree the variation in RSV-related LRTI incidence varies in relation to changes in total LRTI within study populations (Fig. 2). There appears to be a clear linear relationship between the total incidence of LRTI and RSV associated LRTI (Fig. 2a), although perhaps less strong for more severe disease. Such a pattern argues for a relatively constant proportion of LRTI due to RSV, and while Fig. 2b shows the proportion to mostly lie within the range 5–25%, there are key outliers, particularly at the lower end of incidence estimates (i.e. the more severe disease estimates). These relationships might simply reflect a case of 'the harder you look the more you find'. Alternatively, if the differences are not due to sensitivity of case ascertainment, then it may be that risk factors which promote LRTI (e.g. nutritional, socio-economic status) also promote RSV transmission.

Age-related incidence

Much of the recent difficulties in vaccine development has arisen from the desire to target neonates aged 1–2 months as those deemed most at risk of severe disease. Hospital-based studies in developing countries show similar age-distribution as in industrialised countries: on average 39% of cases are under 6 months, and 63% under 1 year (Weber et al., 1998b). In the past, there has been a deficit in community-based studies reporting the age distribution of children with RSV infection, and studies reporting age-specific incidencce.

Unfortunately, to-date there remains a paucity of finely age-stratifed data on RSV incidence. The studies listed in Tables 1 and 2 clearly illustrate the importance of incidence in the first year of life over incidence in older age groups. The two birth cohort studies with active follow-up yield infant rates per 1000 cy of RSV-LRTI of

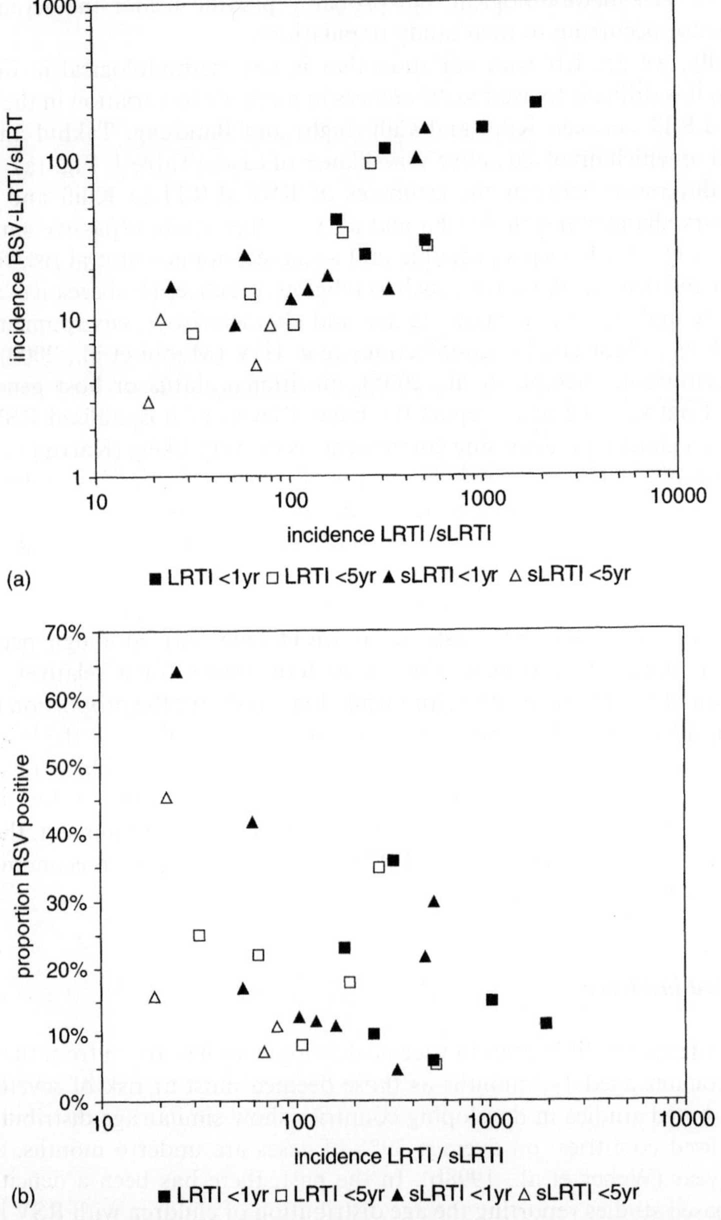

Fig. 2 Relationship between the incidence of LRTI disease and (panel a) RSV disease or (panel b) proportion RSV positive, stratified by disease severity and age class, for disease burden studies detailed in Tables 1 and 2. Disease severity is defined as lower respiratory tract infection (LRTI) or severe or hospitalised LRTI (sLRTI).

220 (Borrero et al., 1990) and 154 (Nokes et al., 2004), and of RSV-sLRTI of 100 (Nokes et al., 2004). Finer age stratification from cohort studies is problematic unless there is a rolling recruitment over one or more years to iron out age-related bias in observation time within epidemics (at risk) and between (not at risk). One interesting observation from the cohort study in rural Kenya, was that the risk of developing LRTI or severe LRTI following presumed primary RSV infection (37% and 25%, respectively), was independent of infant age (i.e., there was no evidence for an increased risk of disease following infection in 0–2-month-olds relative to 3–5, 6–8 or 9–11-month olds).

The only finely age-stratified incidence data that exist come from the recent WHO studies (Robertson et al., 2004) in Nigeria, Mozambique, South Africa, and Indonesia. These are age-cross-sectional in design; better for investigating age-stratified incidence. The key features of these data are (i) the incidience of RSV-LRTI and RSV-sLRTI in children 3–11 months is as high or usually higher than incidence in neonates 0–2 months olds, (ii) peak incidence (/1000 cy) in the first year of life was ~70–200 cases RSV-LRTI and ~20 cases RSV-sLRTI, (iii) while highest estimates occur in the first year of life, significant incidence occurs in the second year of life (e.g. > 100 cases RSV-LRTI and up to 7 cases RSV-sLRTI) and in some instances extends into the 2–4 years old group (e.g. > 50 cases RSV-LRTI and > 5 cases RSV-sLRTI), (iii) the levels and distribution are not dissimilar to those reported in industrialised countries. The only other community-based age-stratified data are for Thailand (Suwanjutha et al., 2002), though unfortunately that paper only reported the percentage RSV by age, showing 15% of cases in under 7-month olds, 25% 7–12 months, 32% in 13—24-month olds, and 29% older than 24 months.

Two studies only report age-specific RSV-LRTI incidence, both arise from Moslem societies (Indonesia and Nigeria, Table 2, Fig. 1a) with socio-behavioural characteristics that may have affected the age-incidence pattern. In particular, both report the practice of sheltering infants for the neonatal period. This may have contributed to the lower (observed or real) incidence of RSV in this key age group, although the authors reported this not to have been so. Studies from non-Moslem societies would provide needy comparison. The only two studies reporting age-incidence of RSV-sLRTI (Mozambique and South Africa, Table 2, Fig. 1b) are both hospital-based. Passive surveillance may bias the age-distribution of cases unless the likelihood of presentation to hospital or clinic is independent of age. It seems plausible that parents would be more inclined to take younger children, especially an infant, to hospital in comparison to older children experiencing disease of the same severity, thus inflating estimates of incidence in the younger age groups.

In summary, there remains a dearth of finely age-stratified RSV incidence data from both community and hospital-based studies. However, that which exists suggests that a vaccine delivered to infants older than 2 months, even 6-months olds, would not lead to significant loss of effectiveness.

Do we know enough?

A search for papers from the 75 poorest nations as defined by GAVI (GAVI, 2006) produced 326 references of which 111 papers were of direct relevance to RSV, and 75 of which arose from only 6 countries (China, Kenya, Nigeria, Cuba, India, and Gambia). Out of the 75 GAVI countries, 68% (51) had no references relating directly to RSV. Of the 24 countries with data, 20 reported on the proportion of hospital ARI admissions with a RSV diagnosis, and only 5 with denominator-based RSV incidence estimates. Fig. 3 depicts the regional distribution of the proportion of GAVI countries with at least one article on RSV-LRTI admissions and with RSV denominator-based disease-incidence data.

From this review, it is clear that for those countries eligible for GAVI funding the database on RSV disease burden is poor and grossly deficient in incidence data with none outside of sub-Saharan Africa and East Asia. Even in countries with some data this is in general confined to 1 or only a few papers from hospital surveillance. More generally, there are no studies reporting on the burden of RSV disease in terms of quality-adjusted life years (QALY) or few reporting economic costs. Very few studies have been undertaken in communities for which detailed HIV information is available (Madhi et al., 2000). Finally, given that the argument for vaccine development and implementation may rest upon the burden of RSV-associated deaths, an important question to ask is how good is the data on RSV-associated mortality?

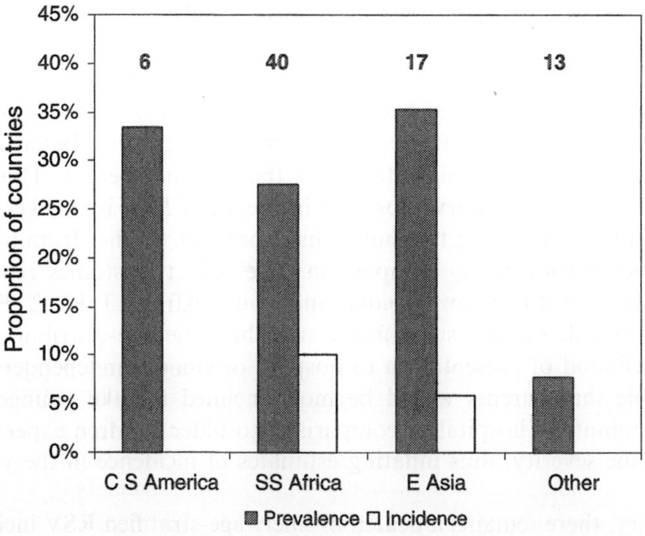

Fig. 3 Proportion of GAVI countries, by region, with one or more papers published on RSV-associated LRTI prevalence in hospital admissions (grey bars) or RSV incidence (open bars). Numbers represent number of GAVI countries in region (total 75), where C S America is Central and South America, SS Africa is sub-Saharan Africa and E Asia is East Asia.

Associated mortality

Two reviews collectively covering 30 studies up to 1995 (Weber et al., 1998b) and 2002 (Stensballe et al., 2003) reported case fatality rates in tropical and developing countries between 0 and 9%; most frequently 0%. The 16 studies summarised in Table 4 are the more recent (onwards from the early 1990s), and were either not included in the above reviews or have comparative data on case fatality rates (CFRs) for RSV-negative cases and/or CFRs for total ARI cases (irrespective of RSV testing). The general picture presented is unaltered from the previous reviews. Five of the studies reported no deaths, and only one exceeded 5%: a small study in South Africa of children admitted to an emergency room with life-threatening illness with a CFR of 14% (Delport and Brisley, 2002). In a comparison of studies, Stensballe et al. (2003) found RSV-associated mortality to be statistically higher in the developing than the developed countries.

Under- or over-estimated?

How reliable are RSV mortality estimates for developing countries? There is in fact considerable uncertainty, arising from two methodological issues. First, there is evidence of a bias in the studies towards sampling less severely ill children for RSV testing. Exhaustive sampling of ARI admissions was not undertaken in four studies in Table 4 and for others this fact is not clear. While CFRs in RSV-negative children are similar to those in RSV-positive children, the rates for total LRTI cases are considerably higher. In Manhica, Mozambique, 27% of eligible ARI patients were not RSV tested, and in Lombok, Indonesia, 84% of paediatric ARI deaths occurred before an RSV test could be undertaken. The CFRs for all ARI admissions in these two studies were 9% and 12%, respectively. In order to assess true mortality, RSV testing of ARI admissions should not be biased towards the less-severely ill. Given that the highest risk of death of very severe ARI patients is soon after admission, early specimen collection is very important.

Second, the extent to which these studies can be described as representative of low resource-settings is debatable. Six studies were set in paediatric intensive-care units or used ventilation (2 reported both), and most offered oxygen therapy. The degree to which even a reliable supply of oxygen for supportive therapy might alter the picture of RSV-associated mortality is potentially considerable. A more general point is that any approved study undertaken to investigate disease aetiology is likely to be accompanied by a minimum of resources that might well exceed the norm for the setting, and as a result lead to an under-estimate of true mortality, and problems in generalising results. This could be gauged by undertaking surveys of oxygen availability in health facilities in the same location in which research was not being conducted, but were otherwise comparable.

Even where RSV can be identified in a child who dies, it is pertinent to ask whether or not the virus was the cause (in main or part). Where authors have given details on the cause or most likely cause of death in RSV cases, this has been

Table 4

Estimates of RSV case fatality rates (CFR)

Location (dates)	Reference	Subjects	CFR% RSV+ (*n*)[a]	CFR% RSV− (*n*)	CFR% ALRTI (*n*)	Comments
Tlaxcala, Mexico (Oct., 1994–Jun., 1995)	Miranda-Novales et al. (*1999*)	IP LRTI <5y	0 (24)	0 (77)		
Sao Paulo, Brazil (Mar., 1995–Aug., 1996)	Vieira et al. (2001))	IP LRTI <15y	0 (100)	0 (139)	2.4 (826)	
Porto Alegre, Brazil (Jun.,–Dec., 1996)	Straliotto et al. (2004)	PICU LRTI <7y	2.8 (71)	2.6 (190)		• Ventilation, oxygen therapy and corticosteroids used
Santiago, Chile (Jan., 1989–Dec., 2000)	Avendano et al., (2003)	IP LRTI <2y	0.1 (1,337)	0.1 (4,607)		• Inclusion: previously healthy children. • Exclusions: chronic lung, heart neurological disease, prematurity, recurrent wheezing or asthma
4 cities, Argentina (Apr., 1993–Dec., 1994)	Carballal et al. (2001)	IP LRTI <5y	1.3 (312)	0.5 (922)		• Exclusions: HIV infected, asthma, cystic fibrosis • 3 of 4 deaths with RFs: CHD + malnutrition (1), preterm (1), previously respiratory disease (1)
Buenos Aires, Argentina (May, 1991–Dec., 1992)	Videla et al., (1998)	IP LRTI <2y	0 (61)	3.7 (107)		
Western Region, The Gambia Oct., 1993–Dec., 1996	Weber et al. (1998a)	IP LRTI <2y	2.5 (511)			• 10/13 deaths probably related to RSV • congenital heart disease (1), neonatal sepsis (1) • Few RF in study population • Oxygen available
Manhica, Mozambique Oct., 1998–May, 2000	Loscertales et al. (2002)	IP, 78% LRTI/ 15% URTI/7% non-ARI <5y	3.4 (116)		9%	• 4 deaths: septicaemia (1), TB and malaria (1), malaria (1), measles (1) • 27% of LRTI cases not tested. No reasons given

Pretoria, South Africa Nov., 1994–Oct., 1995	Delport and Brisley (2002)	Emergency room, PICU sLRTI <6y	14 (7)	37 (16)		• All ventilated • 1 RSV death: premature
Soweto, South Africa Mar., 1997–Mar., 1999	Madhi et al. (2001)	IP sLRTI <5y	2.6 (268)			• 14.6% of RSV cases HIV infected • HIV infected 7.6% (3/39) CFR: pneumococcus (1), no other RFs (2) • HIV uninfected 1.7% (4/229) CFR: premature + CRS (1), premature + CLD (1), CHD (1), nosocomial sepsis (1) • Ventilation available
Cape Town, South Africa Jun., 1995–Aug., 1996	Hussey et al. (2000)	IP LRTI <2y	2.1 (204)	1.9 (1,044)		• Oxygen available
Throughout country, Israel Nov., 2000–Mar., 2001	Prais et al. (2003)	PICU bronchiolitis	4.8 (105)			• Oxygen and ventilation in use • 5 deaths: CHD (2), pre-term (3, with sepsis(1))
Takhli District, Thailand Nov., 1998–Feb., 2001	(Suwanjutha et al., 2002)	LRTI in community <5y	0 (122)	0 (345)		
Lombok, Indonesia Jan., 2000–Dec., 2001	Djelantik et al. (2003a)	IP sLRTI <2y	1.9 (625)	2.9 (2,052)	12%[b]	• 29% admissions not tested, 33% because death before sample could be taken. 60% of children <2m not tested. • 84% of deaths occurred before testing • Oxygen not always available
Hong Kong, China Jan., 1993–Dec., 1997	Chan et al. (1999)	ARI paediatric IP	0.4 (1,340)			• 5 deaths (3 from other underlying causes, 2 attributed to RSV)
Manila, Philippines Mar., 1991–Mar., 1993	Gatchalian et al. (1999)	Severe infection <90d	0 (101)		8 (198)	

[a](n) Denominator (i.e. number of cases).
[b]Djelantik et al., 2003.

included in Table 4. Many studies do not provide details on the probable cause of death in RSV cases and this is an area where future studies could be improved. However, assigning cause may not be easy (particularly in the absence of temporal information) if, for example, one infection is predisposing to severe disease by a subsequent infection. Co-bacterial infection appears to be present in a small fraction of RSV-associated deaths. The review by Weber identified 18 deaths of which there were 3 co-bacterial infections (*Staphylococcus aureus* (2) and *Streptococcus viridans* (1)). Other concurrent infections include HIV and measles.

Finally, other contributory factors to mortality in some studies in Table 4 include CHD, CLD and prematurity; classical RFs for severe disease in developed countries. To what degree these RFs are important co-factors for mortality in developing countries in general cannot easily be gauged from the published literature at present for the reasons of bias in study sites given above.

Alternative lines of enquiry

Post-mortem investigations can be used to identify the proportion of children whose deaths due to pneumonia or bronchiolitis can be ascribed to RSV. A study of 98 children <2 years of age from Mexico City 1989–1997(Bustamante-Calvillo et al., 2001), who died of pneumonia, found using molecular tests on post-mortem lung tissue, 28 (30%) RSV positive. Based on histopathological diagnosis, RSV was identified in 8 of 13 (62%) with viral pneumonia and 21 of 85 (25%) with bacterial pneumonia. In 10 non-pneumonia deaths no evidence of RSV infection was found. Earlier studies (1960s–1980s) in developed countries (Bustamante-Calvillo et al., 2001) have attributed similar proportions of pneumonia and bronchiolitis deaths in young children to RSV. This study suggests that in young children RSV may be the predominant cause of fatality in infants admitted with viral pneumonia, and a common co-infection in deaths due to bacterial infection. However, the marked contrast to mortality estimates reported in Table 4 argues for caution in interpreting these data, for example, there were only 10 controls and there was no association between prevalence of RSV positives and age or season as might be expected. The possibility of persistent virus unrelated to cause of death cannot be discounted (see Schwarze et al., 2004 and references therein).

Puzzling data on the role of RSV in mortality of ARI admissions come from a study in Lombok, Indonesia (Djelantik et al., 2003b). Data over 3 years showed seasonal variation in the case fatality proportion in severe pneumonia (WHO criteria) cases and the proportion of cases tested for RSV found to be RSV positive, with peak admissions during the RSV season. Peaks in case fatalities occurred 2–4 months after peaks in RSV prevalence. Low case fatality proportion occurred in the 2–3 months preceeding the RSV seasonal onset continuing up to the peak in the porportion RSV positive. Low RSV CFR might partially explain the low mortality proportion in severe pneumonia cases occurring during the RSV season, but cannot explain the low mortality in the months immediately preceeding the RSV season. It is plausible that in RSV cases an increased risk of subsequent pneumonia due to highly pathogenic bacteria or exacerbated bacterial infection (Beadling and Slifka, 2004) might explain the rise in pneumonia case fatality proportion shortly after RSV epidemics (a relationship between influenza epidemics an subsequent increase in hospitalisation of severe bacterial infection is well known). These observations deserve further investigations to establish if similar patterns arise elsewhere. Further work is required on secondary bacterial infection post-discharge leading to readmission and further data on the nature of increased pneumonia risk as for The Gambia and whether this leads to increased mortality.

Disease-causing agent or benign co-infection

An important question to ask is how much of the disease of children in whom RSV is identified can be attributed to the virus? Typically, the presence of RSV in nasal specimens from children is associated with symptoms of respiratory disease (Wright and Cutts, 2000) and RSV infection is almost never asymptomatic (Collins et al., 2001). Early studies involving sampling from children without ARI (comparison group) suggested that rarely was RSV isolated from healthy individuals without clinical signs (Chanock et al., 1961).

RSV infection is rarely benign

Table 5 reviews 9 studies from developing countries which investigated the presence of RSV in children attending hospital out-patients or who were admitted with symptoms of ARI (cases) or without ARI symptoms (controls). RSV prevalence in controls is low, ranging from 0 to 6%, usually considerably lower than that in cases. It is difficult to exclude the possibility that the diagnosis of RSV in controls results, at least in part, from false positivity of the laboratory assays, e.g. for most reported studies even an assay of 98% specificity the majority of positives could arise from false laboratory results. Rapid ELISA methods reportedly have lower specificity relative to culture (e.g. 94–97%) (Wright and Cutts, 2000). Culture, the gold standard for specificity, is unlikely to give rise to false positives. However, culture is frequently run together with other assays and papers rarely indicate which of the methods identified the positive samples. The prevalence of RSV in controls is independent of the prevalence in cases, contrary to expectation if both reflected RSV prevalence in the community. At the extreme is the study of Adegbola in Gambia (Adegbola et al., 1994) in which control prevalence was the same as in cases (~6%) for a malnourished study group. This observation adds weight to the assertion of false positivity rather than benign infection in controls.

Nosocomial studies provide a further source of data on the prevalence of benign RSV infection, since sampling is undertaken independent of symptoms. For example, in one study (Madhi et al., 2004), 130 children RSV negative at admission, and repeatedly sampled during their in-stay, 15 were infected with RSV of whom 14 (93%) were clinically symtomatic.

Table 5

Controlled studies of RSV prevalence hospital out-patients or admissions and estimated attributable risk %

Location	Dates of study	Study details	% controls (p/N)[a]	% cases (p/N)[b]	AR%[c]	comments	Reference
Sao Paulo, Brazil	Mar., 1995–Aug., 1996	• Site: IP • Age: < 15y • Controls: no LRTI • Cases: LRTI • Specimen: NPA or NPS • Assay: IFAT & culture	1.7% (3/175)	42.2% (100/237)	98%	Assay which identified control positives not indicated	Vieira et al. (2001)
Coastal Region, Gambia	Nov., 1990–Oct., 1992	• Site: OP clinic • Age: 3–59 ml • Controls: without pneumonia and (a) malnourished or (b) healthy • Cases: pneumonia and (c) malnourished or (d) healthy • Specimen: NPA, LA • Assay: IFAT, culture	(a) 5.9% (7/119) (b) 3.8% (2/52)	(c) 5.7% (9/158) (d) 12.6% (15/119)	M3 %[d] nM 72%	• 4 RSV positives from LA, none in control children • Assay which identified control positives not indicated	Adegbola et al. (1994)

Coastal Region, Gambia	Sep., 1990–Dec., 1992	• Site: OP & IP • Age: <91d • Controls: attending immunization clinic, matched on age, date and location • Cases: Any sign of infection • Specimen: NPA • Assay: IFAT, culture	4.5% (15/333)	11.6% (51/438)	64%	• Assay which identified control positives not indicated	Mulholland et al. (1999a)
Coastal Region, Gambia	Jun., 1987–May, 1988	• Site: IP • Age: <1y • Controls: age and location matched without LRTI • Cases: LRTI • Specimen: NPA • Assay: Culture/ IgG ELISA	4.8% (2/42)	37.2% (32/86)	92%	• Some controls had evidence of URTI • Twofold rise in serum EIA antibody titre as evidence of infection.	(Forgie et al. (1991)
Manhica, Mozambique	Oct., 1998 – May, 2000	• Site: IP • Age <60m • Controls: IP without ARI • Cases: LRTI • Specimen: NWs • Assay: Ag ELISA	2.1% (2/94)	10.7% (107/1,001)	82%	• Commercial Ag ELISA (Testpack, Abbott Labs)	Loscertales et al., (2002)

Table 5 (*continued*)

Location	Dates of study	Study details	% controls (p/N)[a]	% cases (p/N)[b]	AR%[c]	comments	Reference
Kampala & Entebe, Uganda	Apr., 1972–Oct., 1973	• Site: IP/OP • Age: 0–3y • Controls: kwashiorkor • Cases: ARI • Specimen: TS and NS • Assay: culture and CFT	1.7% (1/58)	17% (405)	91%	• CFT results only • One positive control by CFT • Little seasonal variation in prevalence	Sobeslavsky et al. (1977)
Basra, Iraq	Nov., 1992–Apr., 1993	• Site: OP • Age: < 5y • Controls: no ARI in prior month • Cases: ARI • Specimen: NPA • Assay: Ag ELISA	0% (0/57)	37.6% (188/500)	~100%	• Commercial Ag ELISA (Abbott Labs)	Albargish and Hasony, (1999)
Negev Region, Israel	Jan.–Apr. 1986	• Site: IP • Age < 2y • Controls: no ARI • Cases: bronchiolitis • Specimen: NW • Assay: Ag ELISA and Culture/IgG and IgM ELISA	2.5% (1/40)	62.8% (76/121)	98%	• Positive sample identified by culture • Commercial Ag ELISA (Ortho-RSV, Ortho Diag)	Dagan et al. (1993)

Garoka, Papua New Guinea	Jan., 1983–Jun., 1985	• Site: IP & OP • Age: 98% < 59m • Controls: OP non-ARI • Cases: OP LRTI; IP s/vs LRTI[e] • Specimen: NPA • Assay: IFAT and culture	OP 1.2% (5/404)	IP 18.2% (123/675) OP 8.8% (14/160)	IP 94% OP 87%	• AR% for IP calculated using OP controls	Phillips et al., (1990)

[a]% controls (p/N), percent RSV in controls (number RSV positive/number of controls).
[b]% cases (p/N), percent RSV in cases (number RSV positive/number of cases).
[c]AR%, = (OR−1)/OR.100, where OR is odds ratio.
[d]M malnourished, nm not malnourished.
[e]Considered moderate and severe respectively in the report.

The attributable risk percent (AR%) is the proportion of disease in the exposed (RSV positives) which results from that exposure and has been estimated for each of the studies in Table 5 (Hennekens and Buring, 1987). It can be seen that, except for the one study in Gambia (Adegbola et al., 1994) the AR% is always in excess of 60% and in general is over 90%. Thus removal of RSV (the risk factor) from the community through vaccine intervention would be expected to prevent the vast majority of RSV-associated disease of children presenting to hospitals that is presently observed.

Nevertheless, it does not necessarily follow that detection of RSV in a nasal specimen indicates that the virus is the sole infectious agent responsible for the illness. The disease might in part be due to bacterial co-infection or dual viral infection.

Co-infections by bacteria

The prevalence of bacterial co-infection in cases of RSV-associated LRTI (reviewed in Weber et al., 1998b) was found, in general, to be low. However, some studies reported markedly higher rates, e.g. 21% in Bangladesh (Rahman et al., 1990), 31% in Pakistan (Ghafoor et al., 1990), and 50% in Papua New Guinea (Shann et al., 1984). More recently four studies (Weber et al., 1998a; Madhi et al., 2001; Vieira et al., 2001; Loscertales et al., 2002) have shown a low prevalence of bacterial co-infection (<5%) with the exception of one study involving HIV-positive children. The dominant co-infecting bacteria were *Streptococcus pneumoniae* and *S. aureus*. In the Gambia, 9/255 (3.5%) RSV-positive children admitted with LRTI had positive blood cultures (Weber et al., 1998a), including *S. pneumoniae* (4), *Haemophilus influenza* type B (2), *S. aureus* (2), and *Enterobacter agglomeran* (1). Of 107 RSV-positive children with LRTI admitted to hospital in Manhica, Mozambique, 5(4.6%) were co-infected (*S. aureus* (3), Gram-negative bacillus (1), *Pseudomonas aeruginosa* (1)). This was significantly lower than the prevalence of bacteraemia in RSV-negative children (11.2%). 4/100 (4%) of RSV-positive LRTI paediatric hospital admissions in Sao Paulo, Brazil were co-infected with bacteria (*S. pneumoniae* (2), *Neisseria meningitidis* (1), Gram-positive coccus (1)). Finally, a study in Soweto, South Africa of RSV-positive LRTI childhood admissions, identified concurrent bacteraemia in 2.6% (6/227) of those HIV negative (*S. pneumoniae* (3), *S. aureus* (2), *N. meningitidis* (1)) compared with 15.4% (6/39) of those HIV positive (*S. pneumoniae* (5), *S. aureus* (1)). Studies are required to establish which children admitted with RSV are most at risk of bacterial co-infection or secondary infection, whether dually infected children have higher mortality, and, given the generally low prevalence of bacterial isolation, for whom antibiotics might be safely withheld. Persuing this line of enquiry, given the burden of RSV on hospital beds during epidemics, there may be merit in developing an algorithm to determine which children presenting with LRTI are at low risk of bacterial co-infection and disease progression, who might reasonably be sent home, perhaps with oral antibiotics.

Vaccine interventions

It is likely that the contribution of co-bacterial infection to RSV-associated disease is considerably greater than can be determined through classical bacteriological methods which are highly insensitive. Some evidence in support of an extensive role for co- infection with bacteria in RSV disease comes from the results of a double-blind placebo-controlled trial of a 9-valent pneumococcal conjugate vaccine (PncCV) in children of Soweto, South Africa (Madhi and Klugman, 2004). Here it was shown that the PncCV prevented 31% (95% CI 15–43) of pneumonias associated with any of the severe respiratory viruses, and had a specific vaccine efficacy (VE) against RSV-associated pneumonia of 22% although this result was not statistically significant (i.e. 95% CI-3–41, H_0:VE = 0, $P = 0.08$).

It is possible that in fact all disease in which RSV is identified has an alternative aetiology. This circumstance would require that a disease-causing agent predisposes the infected individual to RSV. Reconsidering the PncCV study above, if a specific association betweeen *S. pneumoniae* and RSV (or other viral infections) existed, then it would be hypothesised that the VE of PncCV against non-viral pneumonia would be significantly less than the VE against viral-associated pneumonia. In fact, the VE against pneumonia with any diagnosed virus was higher than for pneumonia without virus, but the association was not statistically significant (VE pneumonia with virus 31% 95% CI 15–43 vs. VE pneumonia without virus 14% 95% CI 2–24).

The prevention of a large proportion of viral pneumonia from an intervention of just one bacterial pathogen (*S. pneumoniae*) is of great interest. This comes from a single study and re-evaluation of other bacterial vaccine interventions (*S. pneumoniae* or *H. influenza* type B), would be worthwhile to confirm the observation and to see if there is a larger proportion of viral infection whose disease is the result of co-infection. What is unclear from the data is whether there is an interaction due to an association between *S. pneumoniae* and viral-associated pneumonia. The alternative is that virus is present in bacterial pneumonia purely by chance, but that does not seem consistent with the results of controlled studies detailed in Table 5.

Co-infections by viruses

Viral pneumonia aetiology studies frequently report the presence of more than one virus in a small proportion of cases. Dual viral infections have been associated with increased disease severity (Aberle et al., 2005). Evidence that RSV disease is modified by viral super-infection is limited to studies of HIV (see section below), the recently identified human metapneumovirus (hMPV) and rhinovirus. In the UK, children under 2 years of age with dual RSV and hMPV were found to have 11-fold higher risk of severe bronchiolitis than children with RSV infection alone (Semple et al., 2005). Co-infection with rhinovirus was associated with a 5-fold increased risk of severe bronchiolitis over single RSV infections in Greek infants (Papadopoulos et al., 2002). There have now been numerous reports of hMPV diagnosed in children with LRTI in developing countries (Cuevas et al., 2003; Madhi et al., 2003; Peiris et al., 2003; Zhu et al., 2003; Chen et al., 2004; Galiano et al., 2004; Ijpma et al., 2004; Serafino et al., 2004; Al-Sonboli et al., 2005), with co-occurrence with RSV observed in some studies, e.g. 4% in Yemen (Al-Sonboli et al., 2005), and 7% in Brazil (Cuevas et al., 2003). Studies reporting on RSV and rhinoviruses in developing countries are few (Doraisingham and Ling, 1981; Ong et al., 1982; Hazlett et al., 1988; Phillips et al., 1990; Nascimento et al., 1991; Gatchalian et al., 1999; Azevedo et al., 2003; Souza et al., 2003). Doraisingham and Ling (1981) reported a strong clinical association of bronchiolitis with RSV and rhinoviruses. In a study of children with ARI in daycare centres in Brazil, 4% of RSV cases had co-infecting rhinoviruses (Souza et al., 2003). Interestingly, a study in Papua New Guinea showed similarly high prevalence of rhinoviruses in children with LRTI admitted or with mild pneumonia (8%), and also in controls, without ARI (9%) (Phillips et al., 1990). Studies are indicated in developing countries to investigate the prevalence of dual RSV and other viral infections and its role in determining the severity of RSV disease.

Risk factors for RSV infection

No attempt will be made to systematically review data on the classical risk factors for RSV disease in developing countries, namely CLD, CHD, immunosuppression and prematurity, although there is an issue as to whether such factors are as prominent in developing as in the developed countries. However, three other factors are of interest given their high or increasing prevalence in much of the developing world.

Malnutrition

Poor nutritional status is identified as a risk factor for increased incidence (Selwyn et al., 1990; Tupasi et al., 1990; Vathanophas et al., 1990; Ballard and Neumann, 1995) and severity (Berman et al., 1991; Singh, 2005) of ARI and LRTI, and mortality due to LRTI (Lehmann et al., 1988; Tupasi et al., 1990) in less-developed countries. However, this risk is not commmon to all pathogens associated with ARI, e.g., Ruutu et al. (1990) found that the presence of viral infection correlated with better nutritional status in <5-year-old children admitted with LRTI in the Philippines. No association between malnutrition status at admission and RSV status was identified in childhood LRTI admissions in Argentina (Videla et al., 1998) and in Papua New Guinea (Phillips et al., 1990). In the Gambia (Adegbola et al., 1994), in general, no difference was identified in the prevalence of viruses in malnourished and well-nourished children with pneumonia, and in the specific case of RSV the virus was more common in well nourished than malnourished children. A similar negative association between RSV infection and malnutrition in children admitted with LRTI was observed in Nigeria (Nwankwo et al., 1994), Mozambique (Loscertales et al., 2002), Indonesia (Djelantik et al., 2003a), and

Mexico (Miranda-Novales et al., 1999). In The Gambia, a case–control study of risk factors for admission with RSV-sLRTI found an interesting protective effect of eating vegetables (although this could have been attributed to a selection bias in controls due to seasonality in availability of vegetables) (Weber et al., 1999b). A study in Chile reported an association between obesity in childhood admissions and more severe RSV-LRTI (Rivera Claros et al., 1999). Only in the case of two studies in South Africa are there reports of increased risk of RSV-LRTI in admissions with malnutrition (Vardas et al., 1999).

Malaria

In endemic locations malaria has the potential for two effects on RSV infection. First, as an influence on estimates of RSV prevalence among LRTI cases or incidence estimation of RSV-associated LRTI. This is because the symptoms of LRTI can be consistent with malaria diagnosis (Redd et al., 1992; Robertson et al., 2004) and, even where microscopy is available, many children who are malaria parasitaemic remain symptomless (Mwangi et al., 2005). In a study of coastal Kenyan infants (Nokes et al., 2004), with seasonal malaria transmission, 5% of children with LRTI (335) had malaria parasitaemia, and in 133 RSV infections only 3 (2.3%) had concurrent malaria. Hence, in this study the effect of misdiagnosis was not great. Second, as a potential risk factor for RSV infection. Possible mechanisms exist for both positive and negative associations between malaria and RSV. In Gambia, placental malaria was associated with reduced transplacental transfer of RSV-specific antibodies (Okoko et al., 2001), which could predispose infants to earlier and more severe RSV. Suppression of malaria infection in children infected with influenza or measles has previously been observed (Rooth and Bjorkman, 1992). Evidence in the RSV literature is meagre, but suggestive of an absence of any association between malaria and RSV. In Mozambique (Loscertales et al., 2002), a study of paediatric IP found a significant negative association between RSV-associated LRTI and falciparum malaria. However, the prevalence of parasitaemia in RSV cases (~30%) was no different from that observed in community cross-sectional bleeds, suggesting the association to be artefact. In an intervention trial in Gambia no difference was observed in the occurrence of sLRTI or ARI mortality in two groups of young children (750 in each) one of which received preventive malaria treatment (Greenwood et al., 1989).

HIV

There is surprisingly little data available on the relationship between HIV status and RSV infection and disease. None of the disease burden studies were conducted in communities in which HIV denominator data was well characterised. Within-hospital studies are confined to South Africa. Data from a large hospital (Chris Hani-Baragwanath) serving the urban black African population of Soweto with high HIV incidence, show that in RSV-positive sLRTI paediatric admissions, mortality is higher (7.6% vs. 1.7%), the median age at admission raised (7 months vs. 4 months), and the prevalence of bacteraemia increased (15% vs. 3%), in HIV-infected (HIV+) relative to HIV-uninfected (HIV–) individuals (Madhi et al., 2001). In other ways the disease spectrum did not differ by HIV status. Furthermore, it was shown that HIV+cases are not restricted to the usual RSV season, and that while the prevalence of RSV (and other viral respiratory pathogens) was lower in HIV+ compared to HIV– cases (in contrast to the relationship with bacterial pathogens), the burden of RSV in the HIV+ population is significantly greater than HIV– population (14 cases sLRTI/1000 vs. 3/1000) (Madhi et al., 2000). In a contrasting study of children under 2 years admitted with LRTI in Cape Town, South Africa (Hussey et al., 2000), no association between HIV and RSV disease severity was identified. However, the prevalence of HIV risk factor was low (3.2% of LRTI admissions) and disease severity of admissions was predominantly (87%) non-severe LRTI, which is in marked difference to the previous studies.

Prolonged shedding of RSV in HIV-positive children, as indeed in immunosuppressed children more generally, has implications epidemiologically in relation to persistence of the virus within communities, and seasonal dynamics of infection (Stensballe et al., 2003). In addition, there are implications of prolonged shedding for within-hospital spread.

Additional burdens of disease

Nosocomial RSV infection is considered in this review as a specific form of health burden which has received little attention to date in the developing world. Furthermore, estimates of disease burden should take into account the sequelae of severe RSV infection in the form of risk of subsequent respiratory disease.

Importance of within-hospital transmission

Past studies in developed countries clearly demonstrate RSV to be highly efficient at transmission within the hospital environment, presumably due to its propensity for transmission on fomites, in particular by health care staff (Hall et al., 1975, 1980, 1983; Collins et al., 2001). In the typical resource-poor setting the recommended treatment regime for a child admitted with suspected LRTI would not alter as a result of diagnosis of RSV or other viral ARI. Consequently, viral diagnosis of ARI admisssions is not a priority. Nevertheless, it would be beneficial to gauge the importance of nosocomial spread, particularly if resources permitted segregation of cases from those most vulnerable such as neonates. A limiting factor remains i.e. the cost of laboratory diagnosis, particularly for rapid tests that would allow quick action to avoid within-hospital spread.

Where resources do permit laboratory diagnosis of viral respiratory infection and space may be available for isolation and cohorting, the importance of nosocomial RSV spread may be of relevance. The literature search identified nine papers in which RSV nosocomial infection was investigated (Almarza et al., 1990;

Avendano et al., 1991; Okuonghae et al., 1992; Nwankwo et al., 1994; Souza et al., 2003; Vieira et al., 2003; Fodha et al., 2004; Madhi et al., 2004; Diniz et al., 2005). The data cannot be generalised to the developing country setting due to a clear resource bias, for example, availability of a neonatal intensive-care unit (NICU) and ventilation, or specific patient profile such a high prevalence of HIV and other risk factors (CHD, CLD, prematurity).

Estimates of risk of nosocomial infection vary in the literature from 6% to 21% (median 11.5%) and appear independent of the type of hospital, on the characteristics of children enrolled (age, severity), on the methods for diagnosis of infections and on the methods used for surveillance, or the prevalence of RSV on admission. Within hospital risk factors identified included long duration of stay, underlying susceptibility (CHD, CLD, prematurity), health care staff, younger age, and HIV– status (in one study because of high associated prevalence of predisposing risk factors in children without HIV). While HIV+ may be less susceptible to RSV infection/disease, increased duration of shedding once infected coupled to long in-patient stay would make them effective as transmitters. Hence identification of RSV status in HIV patients might be of particular importance to control within-hospital spread. In terms of the burden of disease due to nosocomial RSV infection, data are very limited (Table 6). Pinning down the key risk factors for and the burden of disease due to within-hospital transmission requires further investigation.

Respiratory illness subsequent to severe RSV diesease

A single study reported on the frequency of respiratory disease following severe RSV infection. A cohort study of the incidence of pneumonia and wheezing in infants who were previously admitted with RSV-sLRTI (cases) or were not admitted with ARI (comparison group 1) or who were born after the RSV season (comparison group 2), was undertaken in The Gambia (Weber et al., 1999a). Relative to the comparison groups there was an increased incidence of pneumonia, wheezing, and hospital re-admission with pneumonia or wheezing, in the case group (IRR, 95%CI: 3.80 [2.73, 6.10], 7.33 [3.10, 17.54], 3.40 [1.87, 6.15], respectively). Significantly, this increased risk declined with increasing age (time since RSV-sLRTI exposure), and incidence of respiratory disease had declined to low levels in all groups by 3 years of age. It is of interest that the effects of RSV disease were relatively short compared with some studies from developed coutries (e.g. 7–8 years). Any assessment of the the impact of a vaccine intervention needs to take into account this delayed burden of RSV disease. Similar studies of this nature should be undertaken in other developing countries to establish the general nature of these observations.

Temporal dynamics of RSV: Where and how does it persist

There have been two recent reviews of seasonal RSV patterns in tropical and developing countries (Weber et al., 1998b) and worldwide (Stensballe et al., 2003).

Table 6

Studies reporting nosocomial transmission of RSV

Setting (dates)	Ref	Subjects	Nosocomial risk	Admission prevalence	Comments
Newborn Nursery, Benin City, Nigeria (Jul.–Sep., 1988)	Okuonghae et al. (1992)	Babies	19.6% (11/56)	5% (3/56)	• Ag ELISA on NPAs every 4d after admission • Hand-washing between patient contacts • Pre-term and term babies • RFs: long stay, medical personnel • One RSV+ infant died. Preterm
Paediatric ward, Santiago, Chile (May–Aug., 1988)	Almarza et al. (1990)	ARI <2y	16% (5/31)		• Ag IFAT/Ab test on paired sera on NPAs collected 4–5d post admission • Other nosocomial infections: Adenovirus 25%, CMV 16%
Paediatric ARI ward, Santiago, Chile (Jun., 1988–Oct., 1989)	Avendano et al. (1991)	ARI<2y	15% (43/288)	39% (614)	• Ag IFAT and culture on NPAs collected every 2d after admission
NICU, Sao Paulo, Brazil (Nov., 2000–Sep., 2002)	Diniz et al. (2005)	Preterm with respiratory distress	14% (11/78)		• Culture/Ag IFAT on tracheal specimens every 7d after ventilation • All subjects ventilated

					• Cohorting of children with respiratory virus infection (RSV, influenza) • Hand washing enforced • Other nosocomial infections: influenza A 10.2%, mixed viral (RSV/Flu A/Para1) 5.2%
Paediatric IP ward, Soweto, South Africa (Mar–Jun., 2001)	Madhi et al. (2004)	All aged <2y	11.5% (15/130)	11.8% (36/305)	• Ag IFAT on NPA every 2–3d $\geqslant$3d after admission • Medlian age of infected (2.8m) < age uninfected (5.8m) ($P = 0.07$) • Risk of RSV higher in children with under-lying RF (22%) than in those without RF (8%) ($P = 0.036$) (RF: prematurity, CLD, CHD) • Risk higher in HIV-1 uninfected children (because much higher proportion with RFs than HIV infected) • Associated with 54% of clinically diagnosed neonatal sepsis • 2 deaths but with underlying disease

Table 6 (*Continued*)

Setting (dates)	Ref	Subjects	Nosocomial risk	Admission prevalence	Comments
Paediatric IP Ward, Sao Paulo, Brazil (Apr.–Jul., 1996)	Vieira et al. (2003)	All aged 0–15y	8% (4/52)		• Culture/Ag IFAT on NPAs every 5d after admission • Medlian age of infected (6.5m) < age uninfected (24m) ($P<0.05$) • 2/4 cases produced LRTI
Salvador, NE Brazil (urban poor) (May, 1996–Apr., 1997)	Souza et al. (2003)	Day-care centre, <2y, thrice weekly visits		3.6% (5/138)	• Cohort study, incidence of 120/1000cy
Paediatric ward. Benin City, Nigeria (May–Oct.) (year not cited)	(Nwankwo et al. (1994)	Malnourished ARI children ⩽36m	8% (4/51)	8% (4/51)	• Ag ELISA on NPAs every 4d after admission • Admission prevalence in well nourished 55% • All had URTI (No LRTI) • 1 died, with Kwashiorkor/ Septicaemia
Paediatric ward, Sousse, Tunisia (Jun., 2000–Aug., 2002)	Fodha et al. (2004)	LRTI <35d	6.3% (17/268)	10.8% (29/268)	• Ag IFAT on NPAs

Other recent papers of interest include a report on WHO disease burden studies (Robertson et al., 2004), long-term surveillance data from The Gambia (Weber et al., 2002; van der Sande et al., 2004), temporal–spatial data from communities of native Alaskans (Karron et al., 1999), a study of RSV in HIV patients (Madhi et al., 2000), and OP data from Taiwan (Lin et al., 2004). A number of points emerge, (1) the timing of seasonal epidemics varies considerably, and these can only be crudely associated with meteorological patterns at the macro-scale, but almost invariably begin in coastal (low altitude) locations or areas surrounded by water then moving inland (Stensballe et al., 2003); (2) on the micro-scale, locations sharing the same weather patterns and separated by small distances (e.g. Manhica in Mozambique and Agincourt in South Africa separated by 200 km (Robertson et al., 2004)) can experience epidemics completely out of phase; (3) temporal trends in appearance of epidemcs across continents do not appear to result from continuous country to country spread, rather epidemics arise simultaneously over wide geographical space (Stensballe et al., 2003); (4) patterns of transmission and persistence vary markedly, from almost complete absence (Lin et al., 2004), to short discrete and out-of-phase epidemics (around 1 month each) within larger communities (Karron et al., 1999), to typical annual epidemics of 4–5 months duration followed by fade out, to year round occurrence; (5) epidemic behaviour can apparently be altered by interaction with other viruses (Weber et al., 2002) and perturbations to a regular epidemic cycle can result in long-term instability in virus occurrence (van der Sande et al., 2004), (6) prolonged shedding may modify a discrete seasonal pattern towards year-round persistence (Madhi et al., 2000); and finally (7) most data sets are of very short duration, such that trend analysis is practically impossible.

What is clear is that temporal patterns of RSV are complex, and debate will continue as to the mechanisms which drive the epidemic behaviour of RSV and concerning viral persistence within and the re-introduction into communities (e.g. see Stensballe et al., 2003). Improved understanding is more than of academic interest; a better comprehension of the factors-determining RSV transmission dynamics will be of use in predicting the merits of differing control options. Mathematical models which capture, in a quantitative way, what we know about the host–pathogen interaction, have been applied to the interpretation of RSV temporal data (Weber et al., 2001; White et al., 2005). However, models assuming very different assumptions of factors determining population susceptibility to infection can fit time series data equally well, and therefore provide little insight as to the truth. Advances in this area and, eventual use of models to predict the impact of vaccine programmes, will be slow until key factors such rate of loss of immunity, and the magnitude of homologous vs. heterologous immunity, have been quantified.

Conclusions and future research needs

In the course of conducting this literature review it became clear that a large proportion of the papers arise from very few countries. Taking one example, out of

40 GAVI countries in sub-Saharan Africa there were 51 papers identified as relating to RSV, 45 of which were from only 6 countries. Furthermore, the majority (and in 3 of the 6 countries all) emanated from a single centre with long-term international funding. In the typical under-resourced local or even referral hospital setting there is a low priority for viral LRTI dignosis for the reasons that laboratory diagnosis is expensive, the presence of a virus would be unlikely to alter case management (even if co-bacterial infection could be excluded) and space for separate care (isolation) is likely to be limited. It is therefore important to bear in mind that studies of RSV disease burden are unlikely to be representative of the prevailing circumstances, and that estimates of incidence of severe disease and of death may well underestimate the level of burden in truely resource-poor settings. Disease is a function of economics. In the case of RSV, mortality is very likely to be linked to wealth—due for example to its impact on health care-seeking behaviour, and more directly due to health service resources, with issues of affordability and maintenance of supplies of oxygen for supportive therapy.

In many other ways methodology has an impact on what is observed. Disease burden estimates are partly a function of 'the harder you look the more you see'. It is clear from the differential in RSV incidence between active and passive surveillance methods that there is considerable LRTI and probably severe LRTI, due to RSV, occurring in the community that does not come to light from hospital-based studies. Issues of distance, time, and cost, have an important part to play in care-seeking behaviour, and need to be accounted for in burden estimates. In a similar way, uncertainty exists in RSV mortality estimates because of a failure to test a proportion (large in some instances) of fatal ARI admissions. Given the likely importance placed upon mortality as a hard measure of disease burden by health authorities trying to prioritise resources, then mortality incidence estimates of improved accuracy are warranted.

As reviewed here and although quite variable, the available data suggest the burden of RSV morbidity in developing countries is at least as much as in developed countries. Furthermore, mortality appears to be low, although higher than in the developed world, and possibly substantially so. More data are sorely needed from a wider range of countries, particularly from the poorest nations for whom GAVI funding would be available. RSV-LRTI data finely stratified by age are very limited, particularly in the first year of life, where there is a key need to quantify the potential effectiveness of vaccines delivered at different ages: if delivery of RSV vaccine with neonatal tetanus is not possible, due to unacceptable virulence, how effective would be doses delivered at 3–6 months. Presently, age-stratified incidence data are potentially biased by cultural factors (e.g. isolation of neonates in moslem societies) or by the method of surveillance (hospital-based). Unlike in developed countries there has been little emphasis on determining the economic burden of RSV disease; reported studies are not representative of low resource-settings (Chan et al., 1999; Farina et al., 2002; Chan and Abdel-Latif, 2003). Comparison with other infectious disease morbidity would be assisted by use of comparable units such as Quality Adjusted Life Years.

The burden of illness months to years following severe disease is known to be significant for RSV, and may be a crucial consideration in assessing the merits of vaccine intervention (Mulholland et al., 1999b). However, there has been only one study undertaken in a developing country to investigate the longer-term burden of respiratory disease following severe RSV (Weber et al., 1999a). The data from Indonesia suggestive of a delayed impact of RSV epidemics on all-cause pneumonia mortality are perplexing, and require further investigation.

RSV is rarely identified in a child in the absence of symptoms, and it follows that a vaccine-preventing RSV infection will prevent the vast majority of RSV-associated disease. What is less certain is what proportion of RSV disease is the result of concurrent bacterial and viral infection. The situation is uncertain, in the case of bacteria because culture is so insensitive, and in the case of viruses because there are so few studies on important co-morbidities such as HIV, or little emphasis on a pathogenic role of co-infecting respiratory viruses such as hMPV and rhinoviruses. The database is also very sketchy in relation to any association with malaria, and the lack of association (or even negative) association with malnutrition warrants further investigation.

Disease association with certain bacteria, especially *S. pneumoniae* and *H. influenza* type B, is of special interest since vaccines against these pathogens are either in use or available for use through the Expanded Programme on Immunization or are likely to be so within the next few years (Cutts et al., 2005; Madhi et al., 2005). What proportion of RSV disease might be prevented by the use of vaccines against bacterial pneumonia? The pneumococcal vaccine study in South Africa provides a tantalising insight as to what might be the case (Madhi and Klugman, 2004).

As a disease burden issue, the magnitude of the problem of nosocomial infection is yet to be adequately quantified. Studies so far do suggest a significant size to the problem, and further work should be undertaken to identify methods to reduce the risk which are appropriate to implement in resource-poor settings.

The question of where RSV goes in the off season, and what are the key factors that affect persistence and epidemic patterns, remain largely unresolved. There is much fundamental work to do on the determinants of immunity and re-infection that must be undertaken before this can be fully tackled. However, long-term disease surveillance, perhaps in multiple locations within a country, by which to characterise the temporal–spatial spread of the virus, in relation to parasite genotypic structure, will be of great benefit to our understanding. A better understanding of RSV transmission dynamics will assist in developing and refining of future immunization programmes.

Throughout this chapter, areas remaining data-deficient have been highlighted and suggestions for future research given. There remains a considerable amount of work to be undertaken to characterise RSV in developing countries, in particular to support urgently required vaccine trials and interventions (Table 7).

Table 7

Future research needs

Area of concern	Problem	Studies required
Acute morbidity	(i) Poor representation in GAVI countries	Denominator-based studies in GAVI countries
	(ii) Paucity of finely age-stratified data. Insufficient information on incidence in first year of life	More finely age-stratified incidence from cross-sectional cohort designs
	(iii) Effectiveness of surveillance systems at detecting all cases is uncertain	Assessment of detection capability, especially for passive surveillance, e.g. audit referral efficiency, relate incidence to distance/time/cost hospital attendance
	(iv) Lack of economic costs and data suitable to allow comparison with other health priorities	Estimation of burden in QALYs. Direct and opportunity costs of RSV disease. Cost-effectiveness of vaccine intervention
Delayed morbidity	(i) One study to date, which demonstrated significant morbidity following severe RSV. Very important to vaccine assessment	Investigation of respiratory illness after RSV in various locations. Is the duration of effects location specific
Mortality	(i) Possible under-estimation of the true RSV related mortality in under-resourced settings	Comprehensive testing of patients, and especially most severely ill. Or, better information on final diagnosis for case fatalities to identify most likely cause, e.g. malaria rather than LRTI
	(ii) Post-mortem studies using PCR suggest very high prevalence of RSV in ARI deaths	Validation of PCR methods
	(iii) Circumstantial evidence for wave of increased mortality following RSV epidemics	Repeat of study from Indonesia (Djelantik et al., 2003b)—similar phenomenon elsewhere? Investigations of relationship between RSV and subsequent increased risk of mortality
Risk factors for severe disease	(i) Significant proportion of RSV severe disease is due to co-infections with bacteria and viruses. Morbidity and mortality	Evaluation of other bacterial vaccine trials to substantiate data. New trials should explore specific interaction

Table 7 (*continued*)

Area of concern	Problem	Studies required
	due to RSV may be over-estimated? Pneumococcal vaccine trials suggest large proportion of RSV pneumonia might be preventable	with viral pneumonia. True level of RSV disease requires phase 3 trials of RSV vaccines
	(ii) hMPV and rhinoviruses: evidence of exacerbation of disease due to RSV	Hospital- and community-based investigations of association
	(iii) HIV and RSV	Incidence of morbidity and mortality required in a variety of settings of HIV prevalence. Monitor effect of prolonged shedding on RSV epidemiology and control
	(iv) Reasons for absence of positive association between RSV-severe LRTI and malnutrition are unknown	Investigation of mechanism would be worthwhile
	(v) Paucity of data on RSV and malaria	Further descriptive studies required
Nosocomial spread	(i) May be of major importance to burden of disease. Few studies	More studies of within-health facility burden of RSV are needed. IP and OP (latter difficult to assess)
Seasonality	(i) Relationship with seasonal factors, introductions into communities, low season persistence?	Modelling studies which integrate intrinsic transmission dynamics with seasonal forcing
	(ii) Insufficient time-series data to interpret seasonal and longer-term patterns	Longer-term datasets from a variety of countries
Modelling disease dynamics	(i) Few studies, many specific parameters not yet known	More data on effect of infection on individual susceptibility and infectivity. Develop understanding of mechanisms under-lying RSV dynamics and predict impact of vaccination regimes

Abbreviations

Ag/Ab antigen/antibody
ARI acute respiratory infection

AR%	attributable risk percent
CFR	case fatality risk
CFT	complement fixation test
CHD	congential heart disease
CI	confidence interval
CLD	chronic lung disease
com	community
cy	child years
ELISA	enzyme-linked immunosorbent assay
HCW	healthcare worker
HIV	human immunodeficiency virus
hMPV	human metapneumovirus
IFAT	immunofluorescent antibody test
IP	in-patient
LA	lung aspirate
LRTI	lower respiratory tract infection
NPA	nasopharyngeal aspirate
NW	nasopharyngeal wash with or without aspiration
NPS/NS	nasopharyngeal swab/nasal swab
OP	out-patient
OR	odds ratio
PCR	polymerase chain reaction
RF	risk factor
RSV	respiratory syncytial virus
sLRTI	severe LRTI
URTI	upper respiratory tract infection
WHO	World Health Organisation

References

Aberle JH, Aberle SW, Pracher E, Hutter HP, Kundi M, Popow-Kraupp T. Single versus dual respiratory virus infections in hospitalized infants: impact on clinical course of disease and interferon-gamma response. Pediatr Infect Dis J 2005; 24: 605–610.

Adegbola RA, Falade AG, Sam BE, Aidoo M, Baldeh I, Hazlett D, Whittle H, Greenwood BM, Mulholland EK. The etiology of pneumonia in malnourished and well-nourished Gambian children. Pediatr Infect Dis J 1994; 13: 975–982.

Albargish KA, Hasony HJ. Respiratory syncytial virus infection among young children with acute respiratory tract infection in Iraq. East Mediterr Health J 1999; 5: 941–948.

Almarza MI, Wu E, Vicente M, Torres G, Garay B, Alvarez AM. Hospital acute respiratory infections. Rev Chil Pediatr 1990; 61: 185–188.

Al-Sonboli N, Hart CA, Al-Aeryani A, Banajeh SM, Al-Aghbari N, Dove W, Cuevas LE. Respiratory syncytial virus and human metapneumovirus in children with acute respiratory infections in Yemen. Pediatr Infect Dis J 2005; 24: 734–736.

Avendano LF, Larranaga C, Palomino MA, Gaggero A, Montaldo G, Suarez M, Diaz A. Community- and hospital-acquired respiratory syncytial virus infections in Chile. Pediatr Infect Dis J 1991; 10: 564–568.

Avendano LF, Palomino MA, Larranaga C. Surveillance for respiratory syncytial virus in infants hospitalized for acute lower respiratory infection in Chile (1989 to 2000). J Clin Microbiol 2003; 41: 4879–4882.

Azevedo AM, Durigon EL, Okasima V, Queiroz DA, de Moraes-Vasconcelos D, Duarte AJ, Grumach AS. Detection of influenza, parainfluenza, adenovirus and respiratory syncytial virus during asthma attacks in children older than 2 years old. Allergol Immunopathol (Madr) 2003; 31: 311–317.

Ballard T, Neumann MD. The effects of malnutrition, parental literacy and household crowding on acute lower respiratory infections in young Kenyan children. J Trop Pediatr 1995; 41: 8–13.

Beadling C, Slifka MK. How do viral infections predispose patients to bacterial infections? Curr Opin Infect Dis 2004; 17: 185–191.

Belshe RB, Newman FK, Anderson EL, Wright PF, Karron RA, Tollefson S, Henderson FW, Meissner HC, Madhi S, Roberton D, Marshall H, Loh R, Sly P, Murphy B, Tatem JM, Randolph V, Hackell J, Gruber W, Tsai TF. Evaluation of combined live, attenuated respiratory syncytial virus and parainfluenza 3 virus vaccines in infants and young children. J Infect Dis 2004; 190: 2096–2103.

Berman S, Duenas A, Bedoya A, Constain V, Leon S, Borrero I, Murphy J. Acute lower respiratory tract illnesses in Cali, Columbia: a two year ambulatory study. Pediatrics 1983; 71: 210–218.

Berman S. Epidemiology of acute respiratory infections in children of developing countries. Rev Infect Dis 1991; 13 Suppl 6: S454–62.

Bockova J, O'Brien KL, Oski J, Croll J, Reid R, Weatherholtz RC, Santosham M, Karron RA. Respiratory syncytial virus infection in Navajo and White Mountain Apache children. Pediatrics 2002; 110: e20.

Borrero I, Fajardo L, Bedoya A, Zea A, Carmona F, de Borrero MF. Acute respiratory tract infections among a birth cohort of children from Cali, Colombia, who were studied through 17 months of age. Rev Infect Dis 1990; 12(Suppl 8): S950–S956.

Bustamante-Calvillo ME, Velazquez FR, Cabrera-Munoz L, Torres J, Gomez-Delgado A, Moreno JA, Munoz-Hernandez O. Molecular detection of respiratory syncytial virus in postmortem lung tissue samples from Mexican children deceased with pneumonia. Pediatr Infect Dis J 2001; 20: 495–501.

Carballal G, Videla CM, Espinosa MA, Savy V, Uez O, Sequeira MD, Knez V, Requeijo PV, Posse CR, Miceli I. Multicentered study of viral acute lower respiratory infections in children from four cities of Argentina, 1993–1994. J Med Virol 2001; 64: 167–174.

Chan PK, Sung RY, Fung KS, Hui M, Chik KW, Adeyemi-Doro FA, Cheng AF. Epidemiology of respiratory syncytial virus infection among paediatric patients in Hong Kong: seasonality and disease impact. Epidemiol Infect 1999; 123: 257–262.

Chan PW, Abdel-Latif ME. Cost of hospitalization for respiratory syncytial virus chest infection and implications for passive immunization strategies in a developing nation. Acta Paediatr 2003; 92: 481–485.

Chanock R, Kim H, Vargosko A, Deleva A, Johnson K, Cumming C, Parrott R. Respiratory syncytial virus. 1. Virus recovery and other observations during 1960 outbreak of bronchiolitis, pneumonia, and minor respiratory diseases in children. J Am Med Assoc 1961; 176: 647–653.

Chen HZ, Qian Y, Wang TY, Cao L, Yuan Y, Zhu RN, Deng J, Wang F, Hu AZ. Clinical characteristics of bronchiolitis caused by human metapneumovirus in infants. Zhonghua Er Ke Za Zhi 2004; 42: 383–386.

Collins PL, Chanock RM, Murphy BR. Respiratory syncytial virus. Fields Virology 2001; 1(45): 1443–1485.

Cuevas LE, Nasser AM, Dove W, Gurgel RQ, Greensill J, Hart CA. Human metapneumovirus and respiratory syncytial virus, Brazil. Emerg Infect Dis 2003; 9: 1626–1628.

Cutts FT, Zaman SM, Enwere G, Jaffar S, Levine OS, Okoko JB, Oluwalana C, Vaughan A, Obaro SK, Leach A, McAdam KP, Biney E, Saaka M, Onwuchekwa U, Yallop F, Pierce NF, Greenwood BM, Adegbola RA. Efficacy of nine-valent pneumococcal conjugate vaccine against pneumonia and invasive pneumococcal disease in The Gambia: randomised, double-blind, placebo-controlled trial. Lancet 2005; 365: 1139–1146.

Dagan R, Landau D, Haikin H, Tal A. Hospitalization of Jewish and Bedouin infants in southern Israel for bronchiolitis caused by respiratory syncytial virus. Pediatr Infect Dis J 1993; 12: 381–386.

Delport SD, Brisley T. Aetiology and outcome of severe community-acquired pneumonia in children admitted to a paediatric intensive care unit. S Afr Med J 2002; 92: 907–911.

Diniz EM, Vieira RA, Ceccon ME, Ishida MA, Vaz FA. Incidence of respiratory viruses in preterm infants submitted to mechanical ventilation. Rev Inst Med Trop Sao Paulo 2005; 47: 37–44.

Djelantik IGG, Gessner BD, Soewignjo S, Steinhoff M, Sutanto A, Widjaya A, Linehan M, Moniaga V. Incidence and clinical features of hospitalization because of respiratory syncytial virus lower respiratory illness among children less than two years of age in a rural Asian setting. Pediatr Infect Dis J 2003a; 22: 150–156.

Djelantik IGG, Gessner BD, Sutanto A, Steinhoff M, Linehan M, Moulton LH, Arjoso S. Case fatality proportions and predictive factors for mortality among children hospitalized with severe pneumonia in a rural developing country setting. J Trop Pediatr 2003b; 49: 327–332.

Doraisingham S, Ling AE. Acute non-bacterial infections of the respiratory tract in Singapore children: an analysis of three years' laboratory findings. Ann Acad Med Singapore 1981; 10: 69–78.

Farina D, Rodriguez SP, Bauer G, Novali L, Bouzas L, Gonzalez H, Gilli C, Laffaire E. Respiratory syncytial virus prophylaxis: cost-effective analysis in Argentina. Pediatr Infect Dis J 2002; 21: 287–291.

Fisher RG, Gruber WC, Edwards KM, Reed GW, Tollefson SJ, Thompson JM, Wright PF. Twenty years of outpatient respiratory syncytial virus infection: a framework for vaccine efficacy trials. Pediatrics 1997; 99: E7.

Fodha I, Landolsi N, Vabret A, Sboui H, Trabelsi A, Freymuth F. Epidemiology and clinical presentation of respiratory syncytial virus infection in a Tunisian neonatal unit from 2000 to 2002. Ann Trop Paediatr 2004; 24: 219–225.

Forgie IM, O'Neill KP, Lloyd-Evans N, Leinonen M, Campbell H, Whittle HC, Greenwood BM. Etiology of acute lower respiratory tract infections in Gambian children: I. Acute lower respiratory tract infections in infants presenting at the hospital. Pediatr Infect Dis J 1991; 10: 33–41.

Galiano M, Videla C, Puch SS, Martinez A, Echavarria M, Carballal G. Evidence of human metapneumovirus in children in Argentina. J Med Virol 2004; 72: 299–303.

Gatchalian SR, Quiambao BP, Morelos AM, Abraham L, Gepanayao CP, Sombrero LT, Paladin JF, Soriano VC, Obach M, Sunico ES. Bacterial and viral etiology of serious infections in very young Filipino infants. Pediatr Infect Dis J 1999; 18: S50–S55.

GAVI. 2006. Eligible countries. http://www.vaccinealliance.org/.

Ghafoor A, Nomani NK, Ishaq Z, Zaidi SZ, Anwar F, Burney MI, Qureshi AW, Ahmad SA. Diagnoses of acute lower respiratory tract infections in children in Rawalpindi and Islamabad, Pakistan. Rev Infect Dis 1990; 12(Suppl 8): S907–S914.

Glezen W, Paredes A, Allison J, Taber L, Frank A. Risk of respiratory syncytial virus infection for infants from low-income families in relationhsip to age, sex, ethnic group, and maternal antibody level. J Pediatri 1981; 98: 708–715.

Glezen W, Taber L, Frank A, Kasel J. Risk of primary infection and reinfection with respiratory syncytial virus. Am J Dis Children 1986; 140: 543–546.

Greenwood BM, Byass P, Greenwood AM, Hayes RJ, Menon A, Shenton FC, Stephens J, Snow RW. Lack of an association between acute gastroenteritis, acute respiratory infections and malaria in young Gambian children. Trans R Soc Trop Med Hyg 1989; 83: 595–598.

Hall CB. The nosocomial spread of respiratory syncytial viral infections. Annu Rev Med 1983; 34: 311–319.

Hall CB, Douglas Jr. RG, Geiman JM. Possible transmission by fomites of respiratory syncytial virus. J Infect Dis 1980; 141: 98–102.

Hall CB, Douglas Jr. RG, Geiman JM, Messner MK. Nosocomial respiratory syncytial virus infections. N Engl J Med 1975; 293: 1343–1346.

Hazlett DT, Bell TM, Tukei PM, Ademba GR, Ochieng WO, Magana JM, Gathara GW, Wafula EM, Pamba A, Ndinya-Achola JO, et al. Viral etiology and epidemiology of acute respiratory infections in children in Nairobi, Kenya. Am J Trop Med Hyg 1988; 39: 632–640.

Hennekens CH, Buring JE. Epidemiology in Medicine. Boston: Little, Brown & Co; 1987.

Hussey GD, Apolles P, Arendse Z, Yeates J, Robertson A, Swingler G, Zar HJ. Respiratory syncytial virus infection in children hospitalised with acute lower respiratory tract infection. S Afr Med J 2000; 90: 509–512.

Ijpma F, Beekhuis D, Cotton MF, Pieper CH, Kimpen JL, van den Hoogen BG, van Doornum GJ, Osterhaus DM. Human metapneumovirus infection in hospital referred South African children. J Med Virol 2004; 73: 486–493.

Karron RA, Singleton RJ, Bulkow L, Parkinson A, Kruse D, DeSmet I, Indorf C, Petersen KM, Leombruno D, Hurlburt D, Santosham M, Harrison LH. Severe respiratory syncytial virus disease in Alaska native children. RSV Alaska Study Group. J Infect Dis 1999; 180: 41–49.

Karron RA, Wright PF, Belshe RB, Thumar B, Casey R, Newman F, Polack FP, Randolph VB, Deatly A, Hackell J, Gruber W, Murphy BR, Collins PL. Identification of a recombinant live attenuated respiratory syncytial virus vaccine candidate that is highly attenuated in infants. J Infect Dis 2005; 191: 1093–1104.

Lehmann D, Howard P, Heywood P. Nutrition and morbidity: acute lower respiratory tract infections, diarrhoea and malaria. Papua New Guinea Med J 1988; 31: 109.

Lin TY, Huang YC, Ning HC, Tsao KC. Surveillance of respiratory viral infections among pediatric outpatients in northern Taiwan. J Clin Virol 2004; 30: 81–85.

Loscertales MP, Roca A, Ventura PJ, Abacassamo F, Dos Santos F, Sitaube M, Men ndez C, Greenwood BM, Saiz JC, Alonso PL. Epidemiology and clinical presentation of respiratory syncytial virus infection in a rural area of southern Mozambique. Pediatr Infect Dis J 2002; 21: 148–155.

Madhi SA, Ismail K, O'Reilly C, Cutland C. Importance of nosocomial respiratory syncytial virus infections in an African setting. Trop Med Int Health 2004; 9: 491–498.

Madhi SA, Klugman KP. A role for *Streptococcus pneumoniae* in virus-associated pneumonia. Nat Med 2004; 10: 811–813.

Madhi SA, Kuwanda L, Cutland C, Klugman KP. The impact of a 9-valent pneumococcal conjugate vaccine on the public health burden of pneumonia in HIV-infected and -uninfected children. Clin Infect Dis 2005; 40: 1511–1518.

Madhi SA, Ludewick H, Abed Y, Klugman KP, Boivin G. Human metapneumovirus-associated lower respiratory tract infections among hospitalized human immunodeficiency virus type 1 (HIV-1)-infected and HIV-1-uninfected African infants. Clin Infect Dis 2003; 37: 1705–1710.

Madhi SA, Schoub B, Simmank K, Blackburn N, Klugman KP. Increased burden of respiratory viral associated severe lower respiratory tract infections in children infected with human immunodeficiency virus type-1. J Pediatr 2000; 137: 78–84.

Madhi SA, Venter M, Madhi A, Petersen K, Klugman KP. Differing manifestations of respiratory syncytial virus- associated severe lower respiratory tract infections in human immunodeficiency virus type 1-infected and uninfected children. Pediatr Infect Dis J 2001; 20: 164–170.

Miranda-Novales G, Solorzano-Santos F, Leanos-Miranda B, Vazquez-Rosales G, Palafox-Torres M, Guiscafre-Gallardo H. Blood culture and respiratory syncytial virus identification in acute lower respiratory tract infection. Indian J Pediatr 1999; 66: 831–836.

Mulholland EK, Ogunlesi OO, Adegbola RA, Weber M, Sam BE, Palmer A, Manary MJ, Secka O, Aidoo M, Hazlett D, Whittle H, Greenwood BM. Etiology of serious infections in young Gambian infants. Pediatr Infect Dis J 1999a; 18: S35–S41.

Mulholland K, Levine O, Nohynek H, Greenwood BM. Evaluation of vaccines for the prevention of pneumonia in children in developing countries. Epidemiol Rev 1999b; 21: 43–55.

Mwangi TW, Ross A, Snow RW, Marsh K. Case definitions of clinical malaria under different transmission conditions in Kilifi District, Kenya. J Infect Dis 2005; 191: 1932–1939.

Nascimento JP, Siqueira MM, Sutmoller F, Krawczuk MM, de Farias V, Ferreira V, Rodrigues MJ. Longitudinal study of acute respiratory diseases in Rio de Janeiro: occurrence of respiratory viruses during four consecutive years. Rev Inst Med Trop Sao Paulo 1991; 33: 287–296.

Nokes DJ, Okiro EA, Ngama M, White LJ, Ochola R, Scott PD, Cane PA, Medley GF. Respiratory syncytial virus epidemiology in a birth cohort from Kilifi district, Kenya: infection during the first year of life. J Infect Dis 2004; 190: 1828–1832.

Nwankwo MU, Okuonghae HO, Currier G, Schuit KE. Respiratory syncytial virus infections in malnourished children. Ann Trop Paediatr 1994; 14: 125–130.

Okoko BJ, Wesumperuma LH, Ota MOC, Pinder M, Banya W, Gomez SF, McAdam KPJ, Hart AC. The influence of placental malaria infection and maternal hypergammaglobulinemia on transplacental transfer of antibodies and IgG subclasses in a rural West African population. J Infect Dis 2001; 184: 627–632.

Okuonghae HO, Nwankwo MU, Okolo AA, Schuit KE. Nosocomial respiratory syncytial virus infection in a newborn nursery. Ann Trop Paediatr 1992; 12: 185–193.

Ong SB, Lam KL, Lam SK. Viral agents of acute respiratory infections in young children in Kuala Lumpur. Bull World Health Organ 1982; 60: 137–140.

Papadopoulos NG, Moustaki M, Tsolia M, Bossios A, Astra E, Prezerakou A, Gourgiotis D, Kafetzis D. Association of rhinovirus infection with increased disease severity in acute bronchiolitis. Am J Respir Crit Care Med 2002; 165: 1285–1289.

Peiris JS, Tang WH, Chan KH, Khong PL, Guan Y, Lau YL, Chiu SS. Children with respiratory disease associated with metapneumovirus in Hong Kong. Emerg Infect Dis 2003; 9: 628–633.

Phillips PA, Lehmann D, Spooner V, Barker J, Tulloch S, Sungu M, Canil KA, Pratt RD, Lupiwa T, Alpers MP. Viruses associated with acute lower respiratory tract infections in children from the eastern highlands of Papua New Guinea (1983–1985). Southeast Asian J Trop Med Public Health 1990; 21: 373–382.

Prais D, Schonfeld T, Amir J. Admission to the intensive care unit for respiratory syncytial virus bronchiolitis: a national survey before palivizumab use. Pediatrics 2003; 112: 548–552.

Rahman M, Huq F, Sack DA, Butler T, Azad AK, Alam A, Nahar N, Islam M. Acute lower respiratory tract infections in hospitalized patients with diarrhea in Dhaka, Bangladesh. Rev Infect Dis 1990; 12(Suppl 8): S899–S906.

Redd SC, Bloland PB, Kazembe PN, Patrick E, Tembenu R, Campbell CC. Usefulness of clinical case-definitions in guiding therapy for African children with malaria or pneumonia. Lancet 1992; 340: 1140–1143.

Rivera Claros R, Marin V, Castillo-Duran C, Jara L, Guardia S, Diaz N. Nutritional status and clinical evolution of hospitalized Chilean infants with infection by respiratory syncytial virus (RSV). Arch Latinoam Nutr 1999; 49: 326–332.

Robertson SE, Roca A, Alonso P, Simoes EA, Kartasasmita CB, Olaleye DO, Odaibo GN, Collinson M, Venter M, Zhu Y, Wright PF. Respiratory syncytial virus infection: denominator-based studies in Indonesia, Mozambique, Nigeria and South Africa. Bull World Health Organ 2004; 82: 914–922.

Rooth I, Bjorkman A. Suppression of *Plasmodium falciparum* infections during concomitant measles or influenza but not during pertussis. Am J Trop Med Hyg 1992; 47: 675–681.

Rudan I, Tomaskovic L, Boschi-Pinto C, Campbell H. Global estimate of the incidence of clinical pneumonia among children under five years of age. Bull World Health Organ 2004; 82: 895–903.

Ruutu P, Halonen P, Meurman O, Torres C, Paladin F, Yamaoka K, Tupasi TE. Viral lower respiratory tract infections in Filipino children. J Infect Dis 1990; 161: 175–179.

Schwarze J, O'Donnell DR, Rohwedder A, Openshaw PJ. Latency and persistence of respiratory syncytial virus despite T cell immunity. Am J Respir Crit Care Med 2004; 169: 801–805.

Selwyn B, C. D. G. o. B Researchers. The epidemiology of acute respiratory tract infection in young children: comparison of findings from several developing countries. Rev Infecti Dis 1990; 12(Suppl 8): S870–S888.

Semple MG, Cowell A, Dove W, Greensill J, McNamara PS, Halfhide C, Shears P, Smyth RL, Hart CA. Dual infection of infants by human metapneumovirus and human respiratory syncytial virus is strongly associated with severe bronchiolitis. J Infect Dis 2005; 191: 382–386.

Serafino RL, Gurgel RQ, Dove W, Hart CA, Cuevas LE. Respiratory syncytial virus and metapneumovirus in children over two seasons with a high incidence of respiratory infections in Brazil. Ann Trop Paediatr 2004; 24: 213–217.

Shann F, Gratten M, Germer S, Linnemann V, Hazlett D, Payne R. Aetiology of pneumonia in children in Goroka Hospital, Papua New Guinea. Lancet 1984; 2: 537–541.

Singh V. The burden of pneumonia in children: an Asian perspective. Paediatr Respir Rev 2005; 6: 88–93.

Sobeslavsky O, Sebikari SR, Harland PS, Skrtic N, Fayinka OA, Soneji AD. The viral etiology of acute respiratory infections in children in Uganda. Bull World Health Organ 1977; 55: 625–631.

Souza LS, Ramos EA, Carvalho FM, Guedes VM, Rocha CM, Soares AB, Velloso Lde F, Macedo IS, Moura FE, Siqueira M, Fortes S, de Jesus CC, Santiago CM, Carvalho AM, Arruda E. Viral respiratory infections in young children attending day care in urban Northeast Brazil. Pediatr Pulmonol 2003; 35: 184–191.

Stensballe LG, Devasundaram JK, Simoes EA. Respiratory syncytial virus epidemics: the ups and downs of a seasonal virus. Pediatr Infect Dis J 2003; 22: S21–S32.

Straliotto SM, Siqueira MM, Machado V, Maia TM. Respiratory viruses in the pediatric intensive care unit: prevalence and clinical aspects. Mem Inst Oswaldo Cruz 2004; 99: 883–887.

Sutmoller F, Ferro ZP, Asensi MD, Ferreira V, Mazzei IS, Cunha BL. Etiology of acute respiratory tract infections among children in a combined community and hospital study in Rio de Janeiro. Clin Infect Dis 1995; 20: 854–860.

Suwanjutha S, Sunakorn P, Chantarojanasiri T, Siritantikorn S, Nawanoparatkul S, Rattanadilok Na Bhuket T, Teeyapaiboonsilpa P, Preutthipan A, Sareebutr W, Puthavathana P. Respiratory syncytial virus-associated lower respiratory tract infection in under-5-year-old children in a rural community of central Thailand, a population-based study. J Med Assoc Thai 2002; 85(Suppl 4): S1111–S1119.

Tupasi TE, de Leon LE, Lupisan S, Torres CU, Leonor ZA, Sunico ES, Mangubat NV, Miguel CA, Medalla F, Tan ST, et al. Patterns of acute respiratory tract infection in children: a longitudinal study in a depressed community in Metro Manila. Rev Infect Dis 1990; 12(Suppl 8): S940–S949.

van der Sande MAB, Goetghebuer T, Sanneh M, Whittle HC, Weber MW. Seasonal variation in respiratory syncytial virus epidemics in The Gambia, West Africa. Pediatr Infect Dis J 2004; 23: 73–74.

Vardas E, Blaauw D, McAnerney J. The epidemiology of respiratory syncytial virus (RSV) infections in South African children. S Afr Med J 1999; 89: 1079–1084.

Vathanophas K, Sangchai R, Raktham S, Pariyanonda A, Thangsuvan J, Bunyaratabhandu P, Athipanyakom S, Suwanjutha S, Jayanetra P, Wasi C, et al. A community-based study of acute respiratory tract infection in Thai children. Rev Infect Dis 1990; 12(Suppl 8): S957–S965.

Videla C, Carballal G, Misirlian A, Aguilar M. Acute lower respiratory infections due to respiratory syncytial virus and adenovirus among hospitalized children from Argentina. Clin Diagn Virol 1998; 10: 17–23.

Vieira SE, Gilio AE, Miyao CR, Pahl MM, Lotufo JP, Hein N, Betta SL, Durigon EL, Botosso V, Ejzenberg B, Okay Y. Nosocomial respiratory syncytial virus infection in a pediatric ward. Infect Control Hosp Epidemiol 2003; 24: 468–469.

Vieira SE, Stewien KE, Queiroz DA, Durigon EL, Torok TJ, Anderson LJ, Miyao CR, Hein N, Botosso VF, Pahl MM, Gilio AE, Ejzenberg B, Okay Y. Clinical patterns and seasonal trends in respiratory syncytial virus hospitalizations in Sao Paulo, Brazil. Rev Inst Med Trop Sao Paulo 2001; 43: 125–131.

Weber A, Weber M, Milligan P. Modeling epidemics caused by respiratory syncytial virus (RSV). Math Biosci 2001; 172: 95–113.

Weber M, Dackour R, Usen S, Schneider G, Adergbola R, Cane P, Jaffar S, Milligan P, Greenwood B, Whittle H, Mulholland E. The clinical spectrum of respiratory syncytial virus disease in The Gambia. Pediatr Infect Dis J 1998a; 17: 224–230.

Weber M, Mulholland E, Greenwood B. Respiratory syncytial virus infection in tropical and developing countries. Trop Med Int Health 1998b; 3: 268–280.

Weber MW, Milligan P, Giadom B, Pate MA, Kwara A, Sadiq AD, Chanayireh M, Whittle H, Greenwood BM, Mulholland K. Respiratory illness after severe respiratory syncytial virus disease in infancy in The Gambia. J Pediatr 1999a; 135: 683–688.

Weber MW, Milligan P, Hilton S, Lahai G, Whittle H, Mulholland EK, Greenwood BM. Risk factors for severe respiratory syncytial virus infection leading to hospital admission in children in the Western Region of The Gambia. Int J Epidemiol 1999b; 28: 157–162.

Weber MW, Milligan P, Sanneh M, Awemoyi A, Dakour R, Schneider G, Palmer A, Jallow M, Oparaogu A, Whittle H, Mulholland EK, Greenwood BM. An epidemiological study of RSV infection in the Gambia. Bull World Health Organ 2002; 80: 562–568.

White LJ, Waris M, Cane PA, Nokes DJ, Medley GF. The transmission dynamics of groups A and B human respiratory syncytial virus (hRSV) in England & Wales and Finland: seasonality and cross-protection. Epidemiol Infect 2005; 133: 279–289.

Wright P, Cutts F. Generic Protocol to Examine the Incidence of Lower Respiratory Infection (LRI) Due Respiratory Syncytial Virus (RSV) in Children Less than Five Years of Age. Geneva: World Health Organization; 2000.

Zhu RN, Qian Y, Deng J, Wang F, Hu AZ, Lu J, Cao L, Yuan Y, Cheng HZ. Human metapneumovirus may associate with acute respiratory infections in hospitalized pediatric patients in Beijing, China. Zhonghua Er Ke Za Zhi 2003; 41: 441–444.

Respiratory Syncytial Virus
Patricia Cane (Editor)

DOI 10.1016/S0168-7069(06)14008-2

Vaccines against Human Respiratory Syncytial Virus

Peter L. Collins, Brian R. Murphy
Laboratory of Infectious Diseases, National Institute of Allergy and Infectious Diseases, Bethesda, MD 20892-8007, USA

Introduction: the burden of disease and the need for a vaccine

Human respiratory syncytial virus (RSV) is the leading viral agent of serious respiratory disease in infants and young children worldwide, infecting nearly all children one or more times by age 2 (Henderson et al., 1979; Collins et al., 2001; World Health Organization, 2005). RSV can infect very early in life, and the peak of hospitalization for RSV disease occurs at 2–4 months of age. In one prospective study in the United States spanning three decades, RSV was associated with 24% of pediatric hospitalizations for respiratory disease (Murphy et al., 1988). In the United States alone, RSV was estimated to be responsible for 70,000–126,000 pediatric hospitalizations yearly due to bronchiolitis or pneumonia, with an estimated 90–1900 deaths yearly (Shay et al., 1999; World Health Organization, 2005). Mortality due to RSV disease is substantially higher in developing countries due to the limited availability of supportive care. Infants who are premature or have chronic pulmonary disease or congenital heart disease are at increased risk for serious RSV disease, but 60% of serious RSV disease occurs in infants who are without known risk factors. In addition to the morbidity and mortality associated with the acute infection, serious RSV disease frequently is followed by pulmonary abnormality such as a propensity for wheezing that can persist to adolescence. Whether RSV contributes to the development of asthma remains controversial, but it certainly can exacerbate it (Martinez, 2005). Otitis media is another common complication of infection by RSV and other respiratory viruses. Thus, an effective vaccine against RSV would have a major beneficial impact on disease burden in the pediatric population.

RSV is also an important cause of morbidity and mortality in the elderly, where it was estimated to be associated with 14,000–62,000 hospitalizations per year in the

United States with an impact approaching that of non-pandemic influenza (Falsey et al., 2005). RSV also can readily infect and cause serious disease with high mortality in severely immunosuppressed hematopoietic cell transplant recipients (Fouillard et al., 1992).

Although natural infection with RSV does not confer solid long-term protection against re-infection, it does reduce the severity of disease upon re-infection (Henderson et al., 1979). Since it is unlikely that RSV infection can be prevented altogether, the goal of immunization is to provide sufficient protection to prevent serious lower respiratory tract disease leading to hospitalization and to decrease the frequency of complications such as otitis media. In the pediatric population, this can be achieved by immunizing within the first 2 months of life and providing one or more boosts shortly thereafter such as at intervals of 2 months, consistent with the schedule for a number of pediatric vaccines (Centers for Disease Control, 2006). In RSV-experienced individuals at risk for serious disease, such as the elderly, immunization also should provide increased protection against severe disease.

Presently, there is no licensed vaccine against RSV. High-risk infants can be substantially protected by monthly intramuscular injections of a commercially available RSV-neutralizing antibody (palivizumab, Synagis®) administered during the RSV epidemic season (American Academy of Pediatrics, 2003). However, this treatment is too expensive and inconvenient for broader use at the present time. There is also no clinically effective antiviral therapy against RSV. The nucleoside analog ribavirin is effective in cell culture and in experimental animals, but has been disappointing clinically (American Academy of Pediatrics, 1996). Control of RSV by an antiviral agent is challenging because it is a rapid acute infection and by the time the infection is recognized it may be too late to control the disease by antiviral therapy alone. An alternative therapy involving topical administration of RSV-neutralizing antibodies has not been effective therapeutically, probably for the same reason (Rodriguez et al., 1997). In the future, it may be possible to control infection and disease by a combination of antiviral and anti-inflammatory agents (Blanco et al., 2005), but this remains experimental.

Thus, there is a worldwide need for an RSV vaccine, and probably for two different vaccines. The primary need is for a pediatric vaccine, preferably to be administered beginning in the first weeks of life. There also is a need for a vaccine—which likely will be different from the pediatric one—for RSV-experienced individuals at increased risk for serious RSV disease, including the elderly as well as individuals with chronic pulmonary or cardiac disease.

Considerations for vaccine development are described below, and obstacles are summarized in Table 1. Pre-clinical and clinical vaccine studies also are described, and those vaccines that have been evaluated in humans are summarized in Table 2. The vaccines that seem the most feasible are summarized in the final section Perspective.

Table 1

Obstacles to developing an RSV vaccine

1. Factors associated with the need to immunize in the first weeks of life
- Immunosuppression by maternal antibodies
- Reduced immune responses due to immunologic immaturity
- Heightened safety concerns for the very young
- Interference with other pediatric vaccines

2. Factors inherent in RSV
- Highly infectious nature
- Ability to infect very early in life despite the presence of low-to-moderate titers of maternal antibodies
- Inefficient growth *in vitro* and physical instability of the virus
- Lack of convenient permissive animal models
- Presence of two antigenic subgroups

3. Factors inherent in the host response to RSV
- Even natural infection does not confer solid immunity
- Enhanced disease associated with a formalin-inactivated vaccine
- Association with hyper-reactive airway disease

Considerations in developing an RSV vaccine

Correlates of immunity

The G and F proteins are the only RSV neutralization antigens and are major protective antigens (Walsh et al., 1987; Collins et al., 2001). RSV-neutralizing mucosal antibodies, RSV-neutralizing serum antibodies, cytotoxic CD8 + T lymphocytes (CTL), and CD4 + T lymphocytes induced by infection or immunization have been shown to contribute to resistance to challenge virus replication (Mills et al., 1971; Watt et al.,1990; Kulkarni et al., 1995; Plotnicky-Gilquin et al., 2000, 2002). Mucosal antibodies are particularly effective but those induced by a primary infection typically decrease in titer over a period of weeks to several months (Watt et al., 1990). Mucosal antibodies following re-infections can be more long-lived, as suggested by the observation that approximately 50% of adults are highly resistant to RSV challenge (Mills et al., 1971; Watt et al., 1990). Studies in rodents indicated that protection conferred by RSV-specific CTL wanes over a time frame of several weeks (Kulkarni et al., 1995; Murphy, 2005). The protection conferred by serum antibodies is more durable but is less efficient than that of mucosal antibodies because they gain access to the lumen of the respiratory tract by the inefficient process of transudation (Murphy, 2005). Transudation is necessary because RSV replicates in the epithelial lining of the respiratory tract and antibodies must reach

Table 2

RSV vaccine candidates that have been evaluated in humans

Vaccine	Composition	Source and comments (references)
Inactivated or subunit		
FI-RSV	Formalin-inactivated, concentrated whole RSV	NIAID; evaluated in infants and young children in the 1960s; not protective; primed for enhanced disease in RSV-naïve recipients; discontinued (Kapikian et al., 1969, Kim et al., 1969)
PFP-1, -2, and -3	Purified F protein from RSV-infected Vero cells	Wyeth; evaluated in adults, elderly adults, and normal and high-risk RSV-experienced children; safe and immunogenic and may be protective (Belshe et al., 1993; Tristram et al., 1993; Paradiso et al., 1994; Tristram et al., 1994; Falsey and Walsh, 1996; Piedra et al., 1996; Falsey and Walsh, 1997; Groothuis et al., 1998; Piedra et al., 1998; Munoz et al., 2003; Piedra et al., 2003)
FG	Recombinant; fusion of the ectodomains of F and G; expressed in mammalian cells	Glaxo SmithKline; results of clinical studies not reported (Prince et al., 2000)
F, G, and M proteins	Co-formulated purified F, G, and M proteins from RSV-infected cells	Aventis-Pasteur; safe and immunogenic in adults (Ison et al., 2002)
BBG2Na	Recombinant; amino acids 130–230 of G protein fused to a carrier protein; expressed in bacteria	Pierre-Fabre; evaluated in young adults and elderly adults; insufficiently immunogenic; discontinued (Power et al., 2001)
Live, live attenuated or vectored		
Various *cp*, *ts*, and *cpts* mutants	Biologically derived RSV mutants; intranasal	NIAID and Wyeth; safe in adults but usually over or under attenuated in young children, sometimes with genetic instability; one candidate, *cpts*248/404, was safe and immunogenic in young children but insufficiently attenuated in young infants (Friedewald et al., 1968; Kim et al., 1971; Karron et al., 1997b; Wright et al., 2000)
Ts mutants 1B and 1C	Biologically derived RSV mutants; intranasal	University of Warwick; ts1C was safe in adults and immunogenic in some individuals (Watt et al., 1990; Pringle et al., 1993)

Table 2 (*continued*)

Vaccine	Composition	Source and comments (references)
Various r*cpts* and deletion mutants	Recombinant RSV mutants prepared by reverse genetics; intranasal	NIAID and Wyeth; rA2cp248/404/1030ΔSH was safe and immunogenic in young infants; additional candidates are being developed (Karron et al., 2005; Wright et al., 2006)
B/HPIV3-F	Recombinant bovine–human HPIV3 expressing the RSV F protein; bivalent HPIV3/RSV vaccine; intranasal	MedImmune; in progress (Schmidt et al., 2002; Tang et al., 2004)

that surface in order to neutralize virus. Transudation is more effective into the lower versus the upper respiratory tract and thus the level of protection conferred is greater in the lower versus the upper respiratory tract (Prince et al., 1985). In summary, CTL likely contribute to short-term protection, such as against re-infection during the same RSV epidemic; mucosal antibodies appear to play a major role in short-term protection and, in many cases, in long-term protection; and the protection mediated by serum antibodies is more durable but often is not complete, particularly in the upper respiratory tract.

Obstacles to an RSV vaccine

The need to immunize in the first weeks of life for a pediatric RSV vaccine poses a number of obstacles due to the presence of maternal antibodies, immunologic immaturity, and heightened safety concerns. Certain characteristics of the virus and the host response pose additional challenges (Table 1).

Maternal antibodies

Infants are born with transplacentally derived maternal serum IgG antibodies against RSV and other common pathogens. However, the epidemiology of RSV—namely, the ability to infect and cause disease in young infants—indicates that it is less sensitive than other respiratory viruses to control by maternal antibodies, for reasons that are not fully understood. Studies in experimental animals and the clinical experience with palivizumab confirm that a relatively high titer of serum antibodies is necessary to confer substantial protection, reflecting the inefficiency of serum antibody transudation to the respiratory surface as already noted (Prince et al., 1985, 1987). Thus, as the titer of maternal antibodies declines in the RSV-naïve infant, susceptibility to lower respiratory tract disease quickly increases.

While maternal antibodies have limited effectiveness in preventing RSV infection, they partly suppress the immune response to infection. The mechanism of this immunosuppressive effect is not known, but it primarily affects humoral rather than cell-mediated immunity (Siegrist et al., 1998; Crowe et al., 2001). Maternal antibodies also have the potential to neutralize a live vaccine. This prevents efficient vaccination with live RSV by the parenteral route (Belshe et al., 1982; Prince et al., 1982), whereas the replication of a live-attenuated RSV vaccine candidate administered intranasally was not significantly inhibited, at least in the upper respiratory tract (Wright et al., 2000).

Immunologic immaturity

Immune responses in the young infant are reduced in magnitude and effectiveness due to immunologic immaturity (Crowe and Williams, 2003). This effect is particularly evident during the first 6 months of life. For example, in a clinical trial of a live intranasal RSV vaccine candidate, 100% of seronegative vaccinees aged 6 months or greater achieved a 4-fold or greater rise in antibody titer, compared to only 44% of seronegative vaccines aged 2–4 months, even after two doses of vaccine (Karron et al., 2005). Studies with a live intranasal human parainfluenza virus type 3 (HPIV3) vaccine confirmed the reduced immune response in the young infant and in addition showed that protective immunity induced during the first months of life decreased significantly in magnitude over a 3-month interval (Karron et al., 2003). However, these weak responses can be augmented by booster immunizations, as is done for a number of other pediatric vaccines (Centers for Disease Control, 2006). The correlates of immune protection against RSV in the young infant have not been defined, although antibody responses to both F and G have been documented in clinical vaccine trials (Wright et al., 2000; Karron et al., 2005).

Safety

A pediatric RSV vaccine has heightened safety concerns due to the very young age of the recipients. In the interests of safety, live pediatric RSV vaccine candidates in phase I studies are evaluated successively in adults, seropositive older children (~15–60 months of age), seronegative younger children (~6–24 months), and finally young infants (~1–2 months) who are RSV naïve but typically have RSV-specific maternal serum antibodies (Wright et al., 2000; Karron et al., 2005). Studies take place in the off-season for RSV (between March and October in the Northern Hemisphere) to avoid the confounding effects of natural infection on the interpretation of the results of the clinical trial. Because of the multi-step, seasonal requirements, phase I evaluation of a single live vaccine candidate requires approximately 2 years at the present time (although more than one can be evaluated at one time).

The use of a live intranasal RSV vaccine in the early months of life will take place against an existing background incidence of apnea occurring in young infants and will coincide with the existing peak incidence of sudden infant death syndrome at 2–3 months of life. It will be necessary to demonstrate the absence of any association between intranasal RSV vaccination and apnea/sudden infant death syndrome. This will be done during phase 3 and 4 clinical trials as well as by careful monitoring of their incidence in the population before and after the introduction of an RSV vaccine.

Interference with other vaccines

The potential for interference with other immunizations during the crowded pediatric vaccination schedule is another consideration. The topical route of administration of a live RSV vaccine will probably avoid interference with most pediatric vaccines, namely those that are non-replicating and administered parenterally. Compatibility with the newly approved rotavirus vaccine, a live-attenuated vaccine that is administered orally, will have to be addressed experimentally.

A live intransal RSV vaccine probably will be formulated in combination with a live intranasal vaccine under development for HPIV3, the second leading viral agent of pediatric respiratory tract disease, and might also be combined with live intranasal vaccines under development against HPIV1, HPIV2, and human metapneumovirus (HMPV) (Karron et al., 2003; Biacchesi et al., 2005; Nolan et al., 2005). Thus, the possibility of interference among this set of live respiratory vaccines will need to be evaluated during development. Fortunately, when the potential for interference between live intranasal RSV and HPIV3 vaccine candidates was evaluated, it was found to be minimal (Belshe et al., 2004).

Viral factors

RSV does not grow to high titer in cell culture and, depending on conditions, can rapidly lose infectivity during handling (Gupta et al., 1996; Oomens and Wertz, 2004). These properties complicate research and development and pose significant challenges to the formulation, manufacture, and delivery of a live vaccine. There also is a lack of convenient permissive experimental animals for evaluating vaccine safety and efficacy (Collins et al., 2001). For example, RSV is highly restricted for replication in rodents, and thus protection is easily achieved in these animals, giving an overly optimistic conclusions on vaccine efficacy. Chimpanzees are the only experimental animals that approach the human in permissiveness to RSV replication and disease, but are essentially unavailable at the present time. Other non-human primates are much less permissive to wild-type RSV replication and disease and are less informative. Therefore, realistic evaluation of RSV vaccine candidates depends on clinical trials, a requirement that restricts and slows the development of RSV vaccines.

RSV exists as two subgroups, called A and B, that exhibit an approximately 4-fold difference in the efficiency of heterologous versus homologous neutralization with post-infection sera (Coates et al., 1966). The F and G glycoproteins of the two subgroups share approximately 91% and 53% amino acid sequence identity and approximately 5% and 50% antigenic relatedness, respectively (Johnson et al., 1987a, b; Hendry et al., 1988; Collins et al., 2001). This difference is of sufficient magnitude that both subgroups should be reflected in an RSV vaccine, especially for the G protein. This can readily be accommodated in either a live or subunit vaccine, although it does increase the complexity of development.

Vaccine-associated disease enhancement

The development of RSV vaccines also has been complicated by the phenomenon of enhanced RSV disease that was associated with a formalin-inactivated RSV vaccine (Kapikian et al., 1969; Kim et al., 1969), as described next.

Formalin-inactivated RSV (FI-RSV)

FI-RSV consisted of RSV that was grown *in vitro*, inactivated with formalin, and concentrated 100-fold by centrifugation and precipitation with aluminum hydroxide adjuvant (Prince et al., 1986, 2001a). FI-RSV was administered intramuscularly to infants and young children in multi-center trials in the 1960s (Table 2) (Kapikian et al., 1969; Kim et al., 1969). The vaccine did not prevent infection and, in RSV-naïve recipients, had the paradoxical effect of increasing the severity of RSV disease during natural infection. In one center, 80% of the recipients of the FI-RSV vaccine who subsequently became infected with wild-type RSV required hospitalization, compared to 5% of infected control subjects (Kim et al., 1969). The disease observed in the infected vaccinees appeared to resemble that of natural infection, but was of increased frequency and magnitude. This phenomenon of potentiation, in which immunization primes for enhanced disease upon subsequent RSV infection, can be reproduced to some extent in cotton rats and mice (Prince et al., 2001a; Polack et al., 2002; Johnson et al., 2004), as well as in the more authentic model of infant cynomolgus macques (De Swart et al., 2002). The potentiated disease is due to an altered and exaggerated host immune response at the site of RSV replication and does not appear to involve an increase in virus replication.

Our understanding of potentiation is incomplete, but key factors have been identified (for reviews, see (Prince et al., 2001a; Durbin and Karron, 2003; Delgado and Polack, 2004; Openshaw and Tregoning, 2005)). The poor protective efficacy of FI-RSV was important, since enhanced disease is triggered by the expression of RSV antigens during subsequent wild-type RSV replication. Retrospective analysis of post-vaccination sera showed that FI-RSV-induced antibodies that bound efficiently to RSV antigen but did not efficiently neutralize infectivity, in contrast to the efficient neutralization mediated by antibodies induced by RSV infection (Murphy et al., 1986; Murphy and Walsh, 1988). The induction of poorly neutralizing antibodies was confirmed in experimental animals and might reflect either the loss of neutralization epitopes by denaturation of the antigen during preparation or deficient affinity maturation of the RSV-specific antibodies (Delgado and

Polack, 2004). In addition, FI-RSV did not induce a significant CTL response in experimental animals (Nicholas et al., 1990), as often is the case for non-infectious and non-replicating protein vaccines. The deficiency of neutralizing antibodies and CTL, combined with the lack of induction of local IgA antibodies due to the parenteral route of immunization, explains the poor efficacy of FI-RSV.

Analysis of post-vaccination peripheral blood lymphocytes from vaccinees provided evidence of an exaggerated *in vitro* proliferative response to RSV antigens compared to controls (Kim et al., 1976). This was suggestive of an altered T-helper lymphocyte response to the vaccine compared to natural RSV infection. Subsequent studies in experimental animals confirmed and extended these findings by demonstrating a biased stimulation of the Th2 subset of CD4+ T lymphocytes and an increased expression of Th2 cytokines (Tang and Graham, 1994; Waris et al., 1996; De Swart et al., 2002). Depletion of the CD4+ cells or Th2 cytokines in FI-RSV-immunized animals prior to challenge prevented the enhanced response, confirming their role in enhanced disease (Connors et al., 1992b, 1994; Tang and Graham, 1994). Thus, FI-RSV appears to have primed for a delayed-type hypersensitivity response involving Th2 cells that was triggered by the expression of viral antigen during subsequent natural infection. In addition, immune complex formation and complement fixation also have been shown to contribute to enhanced disease in mice (Polack et al., 2002).

Potentiation also has been observed in experimental animals that have been immunized with protein subunit vaccines and later challenged with RSV (Murphy et al., 1990; Connors et al., 1992a; de Waal et al., 2004a), as noted in the next section. In contrast, potentiation is not observed during RSV infection and reinfection (Waris et al., 1997; Wright et al., 2000). An important part of this difference between inactivated virus and subunit vaccines versus viral infection may lie in differences in antigen presentation. In particular, the intracellular synthesis of viral proteins that occurs with viral infection is a much more efficient mode of stimulating virus-specific CTL compared to administration of extracellular antigen. CTL, and possibly natural killer cells, appear to play an important role in regulating the CD4+ lymphocyte response to RSV through the secretion of interferon γ (Hussell et al., 1997; Srikiatkhachorn and Braciale, 1997). At the risk of oversimplification, these studies suggest that efficient stimulation of RSV-specific CTL is an important marker of vaccine safety. Inactivated RSV is not presently being considered further as a vaccine candidate.

Subunit vaccines

Purified viral proteins

Several subunit vaccines have been evaluated involving the F and G neutralization antigens (all based on subgroup A viruses). Initial pre-clinical studies involved F and G proteins purified by immunoaffinity chromatography from lysates of RSV-infected cultured cells (Walsh et al., 1987). Other studies involved a chimeric FG protein in which the signal and extracellular region of F were fused to the extracellular region of G. This was expressed either in insect cells by a recombinant baculovirus or in a stably transfected mammalian cell line, and in either case was purified as a secreted protein from the cell culture medium (Walsh et al., 1987; Wathen et al., 1989a, b; Connors et al., 1992a; Prince et al., 2000). The F protein was also expressed on its own in a transmembrane or secreted form by recombinant baculovirus. When administered intramuscularly to rodents in one to three successive doses (usually mixed with aluminum hydroxide adjuvant), these various preparations induced titers of serum neutralizing antibodies that approached, and in some cases exceeded, that achieved with intranasal RSV infection. These subunit vaccines were highly protective in the lower respiratory tract against intranasal RSV challenge, but only partially protective in the upper respiratory tract. Incomplete protection in the upper respiratory tract is typical for a parenterally administered, non-replicating RSV protein vaccine.

Characterization of the serum antibodies induced in rodents immunized with purified F and G glycoproteins or the chimeric FG glycoprotein revealed a response similar to that induced by FI-RSV, consisting of antibodies that bound efficiently to antigen in an ELISA assay but were inefficient in neutralizing RSV infectivity (Murphy et al., 1989, 1990; Connors et al., 1992a). In addition, animals that were challenged with RSV 3–6 months post immunization had elevated pulmonary histopathology resembling that associated with FI-RSV (Murphy et al., 1990). In studies by the same researchers, enhanced pulmonary histopathology was not observed when the challenge took place only 1 month post immunization, suggesting that the effect was masked immediately post immunization, but could be triggered as protective immunity waned (Murphy et al., 1989). In some studies in rodents and non-human primates, the magnitude of disease enhancement with subunit vaccines was substantially less than with FI-RSV evaluated in parallel (Kakuk et al., 1993; Prince et al., 2000), but the knowledge that the effect can be temporarily masked makes these results difficult to interpret.

Several strategies have been investigated to increase the efficacy of RSV subunit vaccines and to modulate the immune response for improved safety. Intranasal immunization of mice with the F or FG glycoprotein in combination with cholera toxin B chain as an adjuvant provided increased but still incomplete protection in the upper respiratory tract. However, this immunization did not augment the CTL response (Oien et al., 1994; Walsh, 1994). As a refinement, purified F protein was combined with cholera holotoxin that had been genetically detoxified by a point mutation (Tebbey et al., 2000). When administered to mice in three successive intranasal doses, this vaccine conferred complete protection in the upper and lower respiratory tract even at low antigen dose. As another strategy, intramuscular immunization of mice with purified F protein mixed with fraction 12 of *Quillaja saponaria* (QS-21), a saponin adjuvant, induced a response that more closely resembled that of infectious virus with regard to neutralizing antibody and cell-mediated responses (Hancock et al., 1995). In other studies, solubilized RSV proteins were combined with *Quillaja* saponin and lipid to make immune-stimulating complexes (ISCOMs). ISCOMs are ~40 nm particles that provide for improved local and systemic antibody and CTL responses but which can be reactogenic. In one study, parenteral immunization of neonatal mice with ISCOM-RSV was safe and immunogenic, inducing both antibodies and CTL, and was associated with only a small weight loss upon RSV challenge suggestive of minimal disease enhancement (Regner et al., 2004). However, other workers found that ISCOM-RSV administered parenterally or intranasally was protective but did not stimulate a significant CTL response and was associated with enhanced disease upon RSV challenge (Chen et al., 2002). Encapsidation of RSV antigen with liposomes in conjunction with intranasal immunization also have been reported to increase protective efficacy and decrease lung histopathology upon challenge (Mader et al., 2000). A number of compounds that target toll-like receptors (TLRs) have been evaluated as adjuvants. For example, the use of monophosphoryl lipid A (MPL), specific to TLR-4, as an adjuvant prevented disease enhancement by FI-RSV or FG glycoprotein administered intramuscularly to cotton rats (Prince et al., 2000, 2001b). The use of CpG oligonucleotides, specific to TLR-9, as an adjuvant for purified F and G glycoproteins was highly immunogenic when administered intramuscularly to mice and was associated with greatly reduced lung inflammation upon RSV challenge (Hancock et al., 2003). An independent study confirmed that CpG oligonucleotides strongly increased the protective efficacy of purified F protein administered intranasally to cotton rats; however, this study provided evidence of potent disease enhancement upon RSV challenge (Prince et al., 2003). In summary, it is clear that the choice of adjuvant can strongly affect efficacy and reduce disease enhancement associated with RSV subunit vaccines in experimental animal models, although effects on disease enhancement in particular have been inconsistent.

A series of clinical studies to evaluate safety, immunogenicity and, in one case, efficacy have been performed with several versions of a purified F protein vaccine (PFP-1, -2 and -3) prepared from RSV-infected Vero cells (Table 2). These versions of PFP have differences (that probably are not important for this discussion) with regard to some details of preparation, purity (PFP-1 is 90–95% F compared to >98% for PFP-2 and -3), and adjuvant (aluminum hydroxide for PFP-1 and -2 compared to aluminum phosphate for PFP-3).

A single dose of 20 μg ($n = 13$) or 50 μg ($n = 10$) of PFP-1 administered intramuscularly to young children 24–48 months old was well tolerated and induced a ⩾4-fold rise in RSV-neutralizing serum antibodies in 42% and 70% of recipients, respectively (Paradiso et al., 1994). This was confirmed in a second study of 18 to 36-month-old children previously hospitalized for RSV lower respiratory tract disease; in this study, a single intramuscular injection of 50 μg ($n = 13$) resulted in a ⩾4-fold increase in RSV-neutralizing serum antibodies in 82% of recipients (Tristram et al., 1993). A second-year follow-up study documented a decline in RSV-neutralizing serum antibody titers, suggesting that yearly vaccination might be necessary (Tristram et al., 1994). Another study in the same age group indicated that a second dose 1 month after the first did not induce a further increase in antibody titer (Belshe et al., 1993). In general, the RSV-neutralizing serum antibody titers achieved following immunization in these various studies were nearly as high against subgroup B strains as against the subgroup A parent, which is consistent with the antigenic conservation of the F protein and suggests that the vaccine will be cross-protective. Although the studies described above were not designed to measure efficacy, the RSV attack rate appeared to be reduced in vaccinees compared to placebo controls during the first winter following vaccination (Tristram et al., 1993).

The PFP vaccine also has been evaluated in children with underlying pulmonary disease. A single intramuscular injection of 50 μg of PFP-2 to children of 1–12 years with bronchopulmonary dysplasia ($n = 10$) or children of 1–8 years with cystic fibrosis ($n = 17$) was immunogenic, inducing $\geqslant$4-fold rises in RSV-neutralizing serum antibodies in at least two-thirds of recipients, with suggestive evidence of protection against RSV infection (Piedra et al., 1996; Groothuis et al., 1998). A second immunization 1 year later in the cystic fibrosis group ($n = 14$) with PFP-2 was well tolerated and restored the serum neutralizing antibody titers to the level achieved following a first immunization, indicating the safety and efficacy of sequential yearly immunization (Piedra et al., 1998). A phase II multi-center study was performed to evaluate the efficacy of a single intramuscular immunization of 30 μg of PFP-3 in 143 children aged 1–12 years with cystic fibrosis: the vaccine induced a $\geqslant$4-fold rise in RSV-neutralizing serum antibodies in 67% of recipients but, disappointingly, there was no significant difference compared with a control group in the rate of subsequent RSV infection (Piedra et al., 2003).

Two trials were performed with PFP-2 in older adults and the elderly. In 33 adults over 60 years of age, a single 50 μg dose induced a $\geqslant$4-fold rise in RSV-neutralizing serum antibodies in 61% of recipients (Falsey and Walsh, 1996). The response was inversely related to the pre-immunizing serum antibody titer. This suggests that there might be a limit to the titer of antibody that can be achieved, but it also indicates that antibody rises usually were achieved for those most in need. In a second study in frail elderly adults $>$ 65 years of age ($n = 36$), a $\geqslant$4-fold increase in serum neutralizing antibody was induced in 47% of recipients (Falsey and Walsh, 1997).

Another potential use of a subunit vaccine is for immunization of pregnant women to increase the titer of maternal RSV-neutralizing antibodies available for transfer to the infant transplacentally and through breast milk (Munoz et al., 2003). A single 20 μg dose of PFP-2 ($n = 20$) was well tolerated and had no adverse effect on the subsequent delivery or health of the infants. The vaccine induced a $\geqslant$4-fold increase in F-specific serum antibodies in 95% of the vaccinees as well as in their infants at birth and at 2 and 6 months of age. However, the increase in RSV-neutralizing serum antibodies induced by the vaccine in the adult vaccinees in this particular study was unusually low (only 10% of vaccine recipients had a $\geqslant$4-fold increase), and the titer of neutralizing antibodies transferred to the infants was correspondingly low. This indicates that this study should be repeated under conditions where a greater initial neutralizing antibody response is achieved (Munoz et al., 2003).

In the late 1990s, SmithKline Beecham, Belgium (now Glaxo SmithKline) reported that phase I and II clinical studies were underway with the FG chimeric glycoprotein using an adjuvant containing MPL, QS-21, and a proprietary oil in water emulsion (Table 2). However, results from these studies have not been reported. In 2001, Aventis Pasteur, Toronto, has reported phase I trials (Table 2) in which adults were immunized intramuscularly with a subunit vaccine composed of co-purified F, G, and M proteins formulated with either aluminum hydroxide (40 adults) or a poly(di[carboxylatophenoxy]phosphazene) (PCPP) adjuvant (30 adults). The vaccines were well tolerated and were comparable in immunogenicity, inducing a 4-fold or greater rise in RSV-neutralizing serum antibodies in > 80% of recipients (Ison et al., 2002).

Taken together, these studies showed that subunit RSV vaccines were well tolerated and were not associated with enhanced disease upon subsequent RSV infection in the test populations. This was not unexpected since almost all of the recipients had prior natural exposure to RSV. In the FI-RSV trials in the 1960s, disease enhancement was limited to the youngest, RSV-naive infants. In mice, prior exposure to live RSV prevents priming for disease enhancement by subsequent FI-RSV immunization (Waris et al., 1997). Thus, disease enhancement seems to be a risk only for the first immunization in life. Because of this, subunit vaccines are considered to be inappropriate for use in early infancy, at least in their present form. However, they seem to be safe for RSV-experienced individuals, and thus can be used for those at risk for severe RSV disease, such as the elderly as well as older children and adults with chronic pulmonary or cardiac disease.

Pierre Fabre Research Institute (St. Julien en Genevois, France) developed a novel subunit vaccine called BBG2Na in which the central conserved region of the RSV G protein (subgroup A, amino acids 130–230) was fused with the albumin-binding domain of the streptococcal protein G as a carrier (Power et al., 1997). The recombinant protein was produced in bacteria, purified by chromatography, and administered intramuscularly with aluminum hydroxide adjuvant. The prokaryotic source of the protein is noteworthy because the G fragment would lack its usual glycosylation, which might alter and possibly improve its immunogenicity. Also, viral surface proteins expressed in bacteria typically are not folded into an antigenically authentic structure, but this probably is less of a concern for the G protein because it is thought to have a structure that is mostly extended and unfolded (Garcia-Barreno et al., 1989; Collins et al., 2001). In mice and cotton rats, BBG2Na induced low-to-moderate titers of RSV-neutralizing serum antibodies, which was protective against RSV challenge, and did not appear to prime for enhanced disease (Plotnicky-Gilquin et al., 1999). Somewhat unusually, CD4 + lymphocytes appeared to play an important role in the protective response (Plotnicky-Gilquin et al., 2000). Immunization of infant cynomolgus monkeys with two doses of BBG2Na at 4-week intervals did not induce a detectable RSV-neutralizing serum antibody response and, upon RSV challenge 4 months later, was poorly protective (de Waal et al., 2004a). Furthermore, two of the four BBG2Na-immunized RSV-challenged animals had evidence of a Th2-biased response that, although much less than that observed with FI-RSV controls, was suggestive of disease enhancement.

The vaccine was well tolerated in a dose-ranging study in 81 healthy young adults (Table 2) (Power et al., 2001). A single intramuscular injection of the two higher doses, 100 and 300 μg, induced a ≥2-fold increase in RSV-neutralizing serum antibodies in 67% and 72% of recipients, respectively, with a second or third dose providing no significant boosts. The vaccine also was well tolerated in a phase II study in adults aged > 60 years, although these data have not yet been published. However, in a phase III efficacy study in 1330 elderly adults, which also has not been published, the RSV-specific serum antibody response was found to decrease rapidly by 4 weeks post immunization. This will necessitate revision of this strategy for developing a vaccine for the elderly (N. T. Nguyen, personal communication). There also are unconfirmed reports of a few cases of unexpected side effects (purpura) (World Health Organization, 2005).

RSV antigens have also been expressed in plants for the purpose of a subunit vaccine. The complete F protein was expressed in transgenic tomato plants (Sandhu et al., 2000). Mice that were fed the ripe fruit developed both serum and mucosal antibody responses to F, although the virus-neutralizing activity and protective efficacy were not evaluated. Antigenic fragments of the G protein were engineered as fusions with the coat protein of Alfalfa mosaic virus and expressed in tobacco plants, resulting in the formation of antigen-bearing virus particles (Belanger et al., 2000; Yusibov et al., 2005). When administered to mice by three successive intraperitoneal injections, these particles were highly protective against intranasal RSV challenge.

Synthetic peptides have been evaluated as potential RSV vaccines. The most notable was a peptide representing amino acids 174–187 of the G protein (Trudel et al., 1991a; Bastien et al., 1999), which includes most of its central conserved cystine noose (Teng and Collins, 2002). When administered parenterally to mice, this peptide induced RSV-specific antibodies; however, these did not efficiently neutralize RSV infectivity (Trudel et al., 1991a; Bastien et al., 1999). Nonetheless, even after the CTL response was lost, the mice remained protected against RSV challenge. This peptide has some similarities to the BBG2Na antigen described above, which represents a larger fragment of G containing this same cystine noose domain. Immunization of calves with the corresponding 174/187 peptide from bovine RSV also did not induce detectable neutralizing antibody titers but did provide partial protection against BRSV challenge (Bastien et al., 1997). Synthetic peptides against the F protein have been less successful (Trudel et al., 1991b), probably because its major epitopes are dependent on folded structure that cannot be easily recapitulated by a short peptide (Beeler and van Wyke Coelingh, 1989; Garcia-Barreno et al., 1989).

Live-attenuated RSV strains

Advantages and disadvantages

An intranasal live-attenuated RSV vaccine mimics natural infection and presumably induces the same broad array of local and systemic immunity, including innate and cell-mediated immunity as well as mucosal and serum antibodies. Studies in experimental animals confirm that intranasal infection with attenuated strains of RSV is highly immunogenic and protective (Crowe et al., 1993; Whitehead et al., 1998b, 1999a, b; Teng et al., 2000). In addition, the intranasal route of administration partially abrogates the immunosuppressive effects of serum antibodies (Crowe et al., 1995). A live-attenuated RSV vaccine is particularly suitable for pediatric use because there is no association with enhanced disease, as confirmed in the phase I clinical trials performed to date (Wright et al., 2000; Karron et al., 2005). Also, experience with influenza virus vaccines indicates that, for immunologically naïve recipients, live intranasal vaccines induce responses with a greater magnitude and breadth of protection than killed or subunit vaccines.

An intranasal live-attenuated vaccine also might be appropriate for use in RSV-experienced individuals such as the elderly. However, the clinical studies to date indicate that vaccine candidates that approach an acceptable level of attenuation for seronegative infants and children are over attenuated and poorly immunogenic in adults and seropositive children (Gonzalez et al., 2000; Wright et al., 2000, 2006; Karron et al., 2005). Thus, it probably would be necessary to develop a separate, somewhat less-attenuated strain for use in RSV-experienced individuals. In that case, it would be important to establish that such a strain is sufficiently attenuated that it does not readily transmit to susceptible infants and young children. At present, live attenuated RSV strains are being developed primarily for pediatric use.

Disadvantages of the live-attenuated strategy include the poor growth and physical instability of RSV and the need to attenuate the virus without compromising immunogenicity. In addition, attenuation must not substantially decrease the efficiency of growth in cell culture at the risk of making vaccine manufacture unfeasible.

Biologically derived candidates

The development of live-attenuated RSV vaccines began in the 1960s in the National Institute of Allergy and Infectious Diseases (NIAID) in the United States using classical biological methods such as extensive passage at suboptimal temperature to select cold-adapted mutants, or growth in the presence of mutagens and subsequent identification of temperature-sensitive (*ts*) mutants (Table 2). The rationale for cold passage was that adaptation to a sub-optimal temperature might render the virus less fit for natural conditions. The *ts* phenotype provided a marker for identifying progeny that had sustained a mutation. In addition, *ts* viruses often are attenuated *in vivo* and are more highly restricted in the lower respiratory tract because of its higher temperature compared to the upper respiratory tract, a property that enhances the safety of the vaccine. With either strategy, efficient growth *in vitro* can be achieved under the permissive condition of reduced temperature.

Attenuating RSV proved to be an imprecise, laborious task due to its poor growth, its physical instability, the undirected nature of the attenuation methods, and the lack of convenient predictive experimental animals. For example, in early studies, a number of *ts* mutants of strain A2, including ones designated ts-1, ts-1-NG1, and ts-4, were identified and studied in experimental animals and in some cases human volunteers (Table 2) (Wright et al., 1976; Crowe et al., 1993). These proved to be either over or under attenuated and in some cases exhibited genetic instability. A cold-passaged mutant, *cp*RSV, was derived from strain A2 by 52 serial passages *in vitro* at increasingly low temperature, with a final temperature of 26 °C (Friedewald et al., 1968). *Cp*RSV was neither cold adapted (i.e. exhibiting greater growth at low temperature compared to wild type) nor *ts*. It was attenuated in seropositive adults and children but caused upper respiratory tract illness in seronegative young children and thus was insufficiently attenuated (Friedewald et al., 1968; Kim et al., 1971).

In the 1990s, *cp*RSV was used as the starting point for developing the most promising of the biologically derived live vaccine candidates. *Cp*RSV was mutagenized by growth in the presence of 5-flurouracil and derivatives were identified that were *ts* and attenuated, including viruses called *cpts*248 and *cpts*530 (named after plaque numbers) (Crowe et al., 1994b). These *cpts* viruses were subjected to another round of mutagenesis, and derivatives were identified that were both more *ts* and more attenuated, including mutants designated *cpts*248/955, *cpts*530/1030, *cpts*530/1009, and *cpts*248/404 (Crowe et al., 1994a). Pre-clinical evaluation of these viruses in seronegative chimpanzees indicated that they were at least 1000-fold attenuated for replication compared to wild-type RSV. In the clinic, *cpts*248/955 was attenuated in seropositive adults and children, but caused mild upper respiratory tract disease in young seronegative children and could be transmitted from vaccinees to susceptible contacts and thus was insufficiently attenuated (Karron et al., 1997b). A second mutant, *cpts*530/1009, appeared to be satisfactorily attenuated but also was transmitted to susceptible contacts (Karron et al., 1997b). A third virus, *cpts*530/1030, did not appear to be more attenuated in pre-clinical studies and was not studied in humans.

In contrast, *cpts*248/404 seemed to be satisfactorily attenuated in seronegative young children and was not transmitted to susceptible contacts. Therefore, it was chosen to be the first RSV vaccine since FI-RSV to be evaluated in RSV-naïve 1 to 2-month-old infants (Wright et al., 2000). More than 80% of the recipients were infected by the vaccine virus (administered at a dose of 10^4 or 10^5 PFU) and shed 10^3–10^5 PFU of vaccine virus per ml of nasal wash, which is approximately 100–1000-fold less than that observed during natural infection with wild-type RSV. Experience with RSV, HPIV3, and influenza virus live intranasal vaccines has shown that a low-to-moderate level of vaccine virus replication is necessary for satisfactory immunogenicity. The *cpts*248/404 virus was relatively stable genetically: nasal washes from a single vaccinee out of a total of nearly 100 contained a sub-population of virus with a partial loss of the *ts* and attenuation phenotypes. This partial revertant remained significantly attenuated, did not become the predominant viral species in vaccinee nasal wash specimens, and was not associated with increased disease in the vaccinee.

More than 80% of the vaccinees had a ⩾4-fold rise in RSV-specific IgA and a majority was resistant to infection with a second vaccine dose given 1 month later.

However, after receiving the first vaccination, more than 70% of the 1 to 2-month-old infant vaccinees experienced nasal congestion coincident with the peak of vaccine virus shedding (Wright et al., 2000). Thus, *cpts*248/404 was deemed insufficiently attenuated for RSV-naïve young infants, although it did appear to be satisfactorily attenuated for seronegative vaccinees greater than 6 months of age. These studies provided several key observations. This was the first evidence that an attenuated intranasal vaccine can be immunogenic and protective in the young infant, albeit against a second vaccine dose rather than wild-type virus. The magnitude of replication of *cpts*248/404 did not appear to be significantly affected by the titer of maternal RSV-neutralizing antibodies, indicating that they do not significantly interfere with vaccine infectivity and the level of virus replication in the upper respiratory tract. Post-vaccination surveillance in this and other studies provided further support for the absence of enhanced disease.

A second set of biologically derived mutants was developed at the University of Warwick based on the subgroup A strain RSS-2 (Watt et al., 1990; Pringle et al., 1993; Tolley et al., 1996,). RSS-2 was subjected to three rounds of mutagenesis and selection for *ts* mutants. The first round yielded mutant ts1A, which contained five amino acid changes. Ts1A was subjected to a second round of mutagenesis, yielding mutant ts1B, which contained one additional substitution. The third round yielded mutant ts1C that contained seven additional substitutions, for a total of 37 nucleotide changes, 13 of which result in amino acid substitutions. Mutations in the F and L proteins were thought to be particularly important in attenuation. When ts1C was administered intransally to 22 adults at a dose of 10^3 PFU, virus shedding was sporadic and detected in 30% of the recipients, and none of those shedding virus experienced respiratory disease (Pringle et al., 1993). Fifteen (68%) recipients exhibited a $\geqslant$2-fold increase in RSV-neutralizing serum antibodies, with the highest responses occurring in those with the lowest pre-inoculation antibody titers. This suggests that ts1C might be effective as a live-attenuated RSV vaccine in adults, at least for those with a low titer of RSV-specific antibodies.

With the availability of reverse genetics—namely, the capability of producing infectious virus entirely from cloned cDNA (Collins et al., 1995)—all subsequent attenuated strains have been produced by this method.

Vaccine design by reverse genetics

One of the first uses of reverse genetics was to identify a panel of attenuating mutations that could be used to design vaccine candidates. The *cp*RSV, *cpts*248, *cpts*530, *cpts*248/955, *cpts*248/404, *cpts*530/1009, and *cpts*530/1030 viruses described above were sequenced completely to identify putative attenuating mutations, which were characterized by introduction into recombinant wild-type virus. The *cp*RSV mutant was found to contain five amino acid point mutations distributed among the N, F, and L proteins (Whitehead et al., 1998b). The individual contributions of these to the attenuation phenotype could not be readily evaluated because the attenuation phenotype of *cp*RSV is specific to chimpanzees and humans, and the cost of the experimentation that would be required to dissect the phenotype was prohibitive. Therefore, the five mutations are used as a set. The mechanism for attenuation of *cp*RSV remains unknown. The other six viruses yielded a total of six independent attenuating mutations, each of which confers temperature sensitivity. Five of these involve single amino acid substitutions in the L protein (mutations 248, 530, 955, 1009, and 1030, named according to the *cpts* mutant from which they were derived) (Whitehead et al., 1998a, b; Juhasz et al., 1999b). A sixth mutation (designated 404) involves a single nucleotide point mutation in the gene-start motif of the M2 gene, a 10-nucleotide signal that directs transcriptional initiation (Whitehead et al., 1998a). The five *ts* mutations in L presumably exert their attenuating effect at non-permissive temperature by destabilizing the polymerase and reducing viral RNA synthesis. Direct investigation of the 530 and 1009 mutations confirmed that each inhibited RNA replication and transcription and that the 1009 mutation was associated with an increase in readthrough transcription (Juhasz et al., 1999a). The point mutation in the M2 gene-start signal presumably also interferes with RNA synthesis at non-permissive temperatures, although this has not been investigated.

A second source of attenuating mutations has been the deletion of non-essential (accessory) viral genes. An advantage of attenuation by gene deletion is that reversion should not occur. To date, five viral genes have been deleted individually and in various combinations without ablating growth *in vitro*: namely, the major glycoprotein G gene, the non-structural protein NS1 and NS2 genes, the small hydrophobic SH protein gene, and the second open-reading frame of the M2 gene that encodes the M2-2 protein (Bermingham and Collins, 1999; Whitehead et al., 1999a; Jin et al., 2000b; Teng et al., 2000, 2001). Since the G glycoprotein is a major protective antigen, deletion of its gene is not presently being considered for vaccine development. In addition, deletion of G was over-attenuating in rodents and humans and thus probably is too attenuating for a vaccine virus (Karron et al., 1997a; Teng et al., 2001).

Deletion of the SH gene resulted in an approximately 10-fold reduction in virus replication in chimpanzees (Whitehead et al., 1999a). The function of this protein remains unknown. This magnitude of attenuation would not be sufficient on its own in a vaccine strain, but the SH deletion could be used in combination with other attenuating mutations.

The NS1 and NS2 proteins have been shown to inhibit the induction of and response to interferon α/β by the host. Inhibition of interferon induction is achieved by blocking the activation of interferon-regulatory factor 3 (IRF3); NS1 plays the primary role in blocking induction, although the greatest effect is achieved by NS1 and NS2 together (Spann et al., 2004, 2005). RSV inhibits the response to interferon by blocking signal through the JAK/STAT pathway, thus blocking the induction of interferon-regulated genes and development of the antiviral state (Ramaswamy et al., 2004; Lo et al., 2005). This appears to be achieved by destabilization of the transcription factor STAT2. NS2 plays the primary role in blocking JAK/STAT signaling, although the greatest effect is achieved by NS1 and

NS2 together. Recombinant RSV from which NS1 and NS2 have been deleted individually or in combination are attenuated for replication in interferon-competent cells *in vitro* but replicate almost as efficiently as wild type in Vero cells, which lack the interferon structural genes. In chimpanzees, the ΔNS1 and ΔNS2 viruses are reduced in replication by approximately 2000-fold and 500-fold, respectively, compared with a 1000-fold reduction observed for *cpts*248/404 (Whitehead et al., 1999a; Teng et al., 2000). Thus, ΔNS1 virus might be suitable as is for evaluation as a vaccine virus, since it is slightly more attenuated than *cpts*248/404, which as noted above was somewhat too reactogenic in seronegative young infants. The ΔNS2 virus probably would not be sufficiently attenuated as is, but could be further attenuated by the inclusion of one or more additional mutations.

Deletion of NS1 and/or NS2 has the potential to increase the immunogenicity of RSV because it results in an increase in the expression of type I interferon, a cytokine that stimulates innate and adaptive immune responses. Consistent with this idea, infection of calves with ΔNS2 BRSV resulted in an increase in CD4 + cells and virus-specific secretory antibodies compared to wild-type BRSV (Valarcher et al., 2003). However, human RSV lacking ΔNS1 or ΔNS2 individually or together were not noticeably more immunogenic or protective in chimpanzees than comparably attenuated RSV mutants involving other mutations (Whitehead et al., 1999a; Teng et al., 2000).

The M2-2 protein is encoded by a second, overlapping ORF in the M2 mRNA (Collins et al., 1990a). Silencing this ORF by deletion or by the introduction of translational stop codons resulted in a virus that replicates more slowly *in vitro* than its wild-type parent, although it eventually reached a similar titer (Bermingham and Collins, 1999; Jin et al., 2000a). The ΔM2-2 virus exhibited increased transcription and decreased RNA replication, implying that the M2-2 protein plays a role in regulating viral RNA synthesis. The increase in mRNA synthesis results in increased synthesis of the viral proteins relative to the amount of virus replication. This has the potential to increase the immunogenicity of the ΔM2-2 virus compared to a comparably attenuated virus in which transcription was not altered. Importantly, like the ΔNS1 virus, the M2-2 virus appeared to be a very promising candidate based on studies in seronegative chimpanzees.

Reverse genetics can be used to devise other means of attenuation, although at the present time these are not actively being used to develop strains for clinical analysis and therefore will not be described in detail. One strategy is to delete only a portion of a protein. For example, although the M2-1 protein of RSV appears to be essential for viable virus, the N-terminal 67 amino acids can be deleted to yield an attenuated virus (Tang et al., 2001). Another strategy is "charge-to-alanine" mutagenesis, in which a selected protein is systematically modified to change charged residues, individually or in clusters, to an uncharged amino acid such as alanine. This was done with the L protein, resulting in a number of viable mutant viruses, some of which were attenuated (Tang et al., 2002).

Another strategy was based on bovine RSV (BRSV), which is highly attenuated in primates due to a natural host range restriction (Buchholz et al., 2000). Although BRSV shares significant antigenic relatedness to human RSV (Beeler and van

Wyke Coelingh, 1989), it does not appear to be directly suitable as an RSV vaccine because it does not replicate sufficiently well in seronegative chimpanzees to be satisfactorily immunogenic. Somewhat unexpectedly, replacing the G and F surface antigens of BRSV with those of human RSV by reverse genetics did not significantly improve its ability to replicate and induce a satisfactory immune response in chimpanzees (Buchholz et al., 2000). This implies that the surface glycoproteins are not the major determinant of the host range restriction, and indicates that further work would be needed to improve replication and immunogenicity. At the present time, studies are in progress to replace additional BRSV genes with their human RSV counterparts with the aim of developing a chimeric virus that combines the G and F major protective antigens of human RSV with one or more BRSV genes that confer a satisfactory balance between attenuation and immunogenicity.

Other means of attenuating RSV, such as by modifying the F protein so that its cleavage would be suboptimal, or modifying the gene order to make gene expression suboptimal, are possible but have not been reported.

The magnitude of expression of the F and G protective antigen genes can be increased by moving them to a promoter-proximal location (Krempl et al., 2002). Expression might also be improved by adding additional copies of these protective antigen genes, as has been done for human metapneumovirus (Biacchesi et al., 2004). Features such as the secreted form of RSV G (Johnson et al., 1998) or the fractalkine-like domain of G (Tripp et al., 2001), either of which might be involved in increasing viral pathogenesis or altering the host immune response, can readily be ablated in infectious vaccine virus (Teng et al., 2001; Teng and Collins, 2002). However, it is not yet clear whether this would necessarily be helpful.

Cross-protection between the two RSV subgroups is incomplete, and ideally both should be included in a live vaccine, at least with regard to the G protein and preferably both the G and F proteins. One strategy to achieve this was to express the RSV-B G protein from an RSV-A virus as an added gene, making the virus bivalent with respect to G (Jin et al., 1998). A second strategy was to replace the G and F genes of recombinant RSV-A virus with their RSV-B counterparts. This resulted in an AB chimeric virus that replicated with wild-type-like efficiency and could be attenuated by inserting known mutations into the RSV-A backbone (Whitehead et al., 1999c). A third strategy would be to develop a complete attenuated recombinant RSV-B virus.

The ability to generate vaccine virus from DNA provides a stable seed. Recovery can be achieved under highly controlled laboratory conditions using Vero cells that have been qualified for human use and using a plasmid expressing T7 RNA polymerase to drive expression of the plasmids encoding the viral components. Vaccine candidates can be modified as necessary in response to clinical data, and vaccine viruses can be modified to accommodate whatever changes might occur in circulating strains.

Recombinant live-attenuated vaccine candidates

Fig. 1A and B show two lineages of recombinant vaccine candidates. The lineage in Fig. 1A is based on the biologically derived *cpts*248/404 virus, which seemed to be under attenuated by a small margin as noted above. In an effort to introduce an incremental increase in attenuation, a recombinant version of *cpts*248/404 was modified by deletion of the SH gene, yielding the virus rA2cp248/404ΔSH (Karron et al., 2005). This virus thus has four attenuating elements: the set of cp mutations, the 248 and 404 mutations, and the SH deletion. However, when evaluated in seronegative children, the rA2cp248/404ΔSH virus was not more attenuated that its biological parent *cpts*248/404 (Karron et al., 2005). This indicates that the attenuating effect of the ΔSH mutation was not additive to that of the *cpts*248/404 background.

The rA2cp248/404ΔSH virus was then further modified by the inclusion of the 1030 amino acid point mutation in the L protein, yielding the rA2cp248/404/1030ΔSH virus that thus contains five attenuating elements (Whitehead et al., 1999b; Karron et al., 2005) (Fig. 1A). The rA2cp248/404/1030ΔSH virus indeed proved to be more attenuated in seronegative children than its *cpts*248/404 and *cpts*248/404ΔSH predecessors (Fig. 2) (Karron et al., 2005). In these studies, the magnitude of reactogenicity appeared to be directly related to the magnitude of vaccine virus shedding, emphasizing the importance of quantitative virology in evaluating vaccine candidates. Thus, rA2cp248/404/1030ΔSH was deemed suitable for further evaluation in 1–2-month-old RSV naïve infants, the target vaccine age group. In this young age group, the vaccine was infectious and well tolerated. A $\geq$4-fold rise in RSV-specific antibodies was observed in 44% of RSV-naïve infants compared to 100% of seronegative children of 6 months age or greater, reflecting the effects of immunological immaturity and antibody-mediated immunosuppression, as already mentioned. Nonetheless, a second vaccine dose administered within two months was highly restricted, indicating that significant protective immunity had been induced in a majority of vaccinees even if the mediators remained unidentified by the available assays.

However, evaluation of vaccine virus shed from vaccinees provided evidence of genetic and phenotypic instability. The rA2cp248/404/1030ΔSH virus is highly temperature sensitive and did not form plaques above 34 °C, whereas wild-type RSV readily forms plaques at temperatures above and including 40 °C. Evaluation of 141 nasal swab specimens showed that 48 (34%) contained virus that had a shift in the maximum temperature at which plaques can form; specifically, 21, 26, and 1 of the specimens contained virus with a maximum temperature of plaque formation of 35°, 36°, and 37 °C, respectively. Sequence analysis of nine specimens showed that six contained virus in which either the 248 or the 1030 mutation had reverted to wild type or changed to another assignment (Karron et al., 2005). Thus, each of these revertant viruses retained four of the five attenuating elements and remained highly attenuated, approximately equivalent to *cpts*248/404. The kinetics of appearance of these revertant viruses appeared to be coincident with peak virus replication. They sometimes became the predominant species but even then they remained at low levels of $\leq 10^3$ PFU per ml and were not associated with disease, consistent with being highly attenuated.

Thus, rA2cp248/404/1030ΔSH is the first live-attenuated vaccine candidate to exhibit a satisfactory level of attenuation in young infants and to be moderately immunogenic. In principle, this virus might be suitable as is for the development as a pediatric vaccine. Although revertants appeared, they did not replicate efficiently and were not associated with disease, and they do not present an unusual risk to vaccinees or to the environment, given the high prevalence of wild-type RSV. One potential concern would be the possibility of transmission of revertant virus to susceptible contacts. This might not be a serious concern, since attenuated virus is transmitted inefficiently and would be restricted in replication in contacts. To obviate these concerns, the rA2cp248/404/1030ΔSH virus is presently being modified by reverse genetics to increase the stability of the 248 and 1030 mutations using a general strategy previously developed for HPIV1 (McAuliffe et al., 2004).

Concurrent with the studies involving rA2cp248/404/1030ΔSH, a second series of mutants was developed based on deletion of the NS2 gene (Fig. 1B) (Wright et al., 2006). Specifically, the NS2 gene was deleted from recombinant versions of three previously tested viruses, namely *cp*RSV, *cpts*248/404, and *cpts*530/1009. This yielded viruses called rA2cpΔNS2, rA2cp248/404ΔNS2, and rA2cp530/1009ΔNS2, respectively (Fig. 1B). The rA2cpΔNS2 mutant was not shed by any of the adults tested, and only 13% had a detectable serological response. However, this virus replicated to a moderate titer ($10^{3.4}$ PFU/ml nasal wash fluid) in three of eight seropositive children and was deemed insufficiently attenuated for evaluation in seronegative children or infants. Thus, the rA2cpΔNS2 virus appeared to be over attenuated for use as an adult vaccine but under attenuated for use as a pediatric vaccine (Wright et al., 2006).

In contrast, the rA2cp248/404ΔNS2 and rA2cp530/1009ΔNS viruses were sufficiently attenuated to be evaluated in seronegative children. In that population, they infected only 50% and 20%, respectively, of recipients, compared to 100% for

---

Fig. 1 Attenuation of RSV for infants and young children. (A) Wild-type RSV (top line) was attenuated by classical biological methods of cold passage and chemical mutagenesis to yield *cpts*248/404 (second line), which exhibited reduced replication and virulence. Sequence analysis in conjunction with reverse genetics showed that *cpts*248/404 has three attenuating elements: the set of five *cp* mutations and the 404 and 248 mutations. A recombinant version of this virus (designated by the letters "rA2" in the virus name) was made and modified by deletion of the SH gene (boxed), yielding the virus rA2cp248/404ΔSH (third line). This virus did not exhibit a further reduction in replication or virulence. It was then modified by the introduction of the 1030 mutation (boxed), yielding rA2cp248/404/1030ΔSH (fourth line), which was well tolerated in young infants. (B) A second lineage of viruses was constructed that each had deletion of the NS2 gene. The top virus combined the NS2 gene deletion with the *cp* mutations; the middle one added the 248 and 404 mutations; and the bottom one added instead the 530 and 1009 mutations. (A and B) The magnitude of virus replication was assayed by virus titer in nasal swabs, and virulence indicates respiratory disease signs: these are scored from 0 to + + + +. Replication of + or more was necessary for immunogenicity. A virulence score of + or greater is an unsatisfactory level. The *cp* mutations are: Val-267-Ile (N), Glu-218-Ala (F), Thr-523-Ile (F), Cys-319-Tyr (L), and His-1690-Tyr (L). The other point mutations shown are: 248, Gln-831-Leu (L); 1030, Tyr-1321-Asn (L); 404, T to C at position 9 in the M2 gene start signal; 530, Phe-521-Leu (L); and 1009, Met-1169-Val (L).

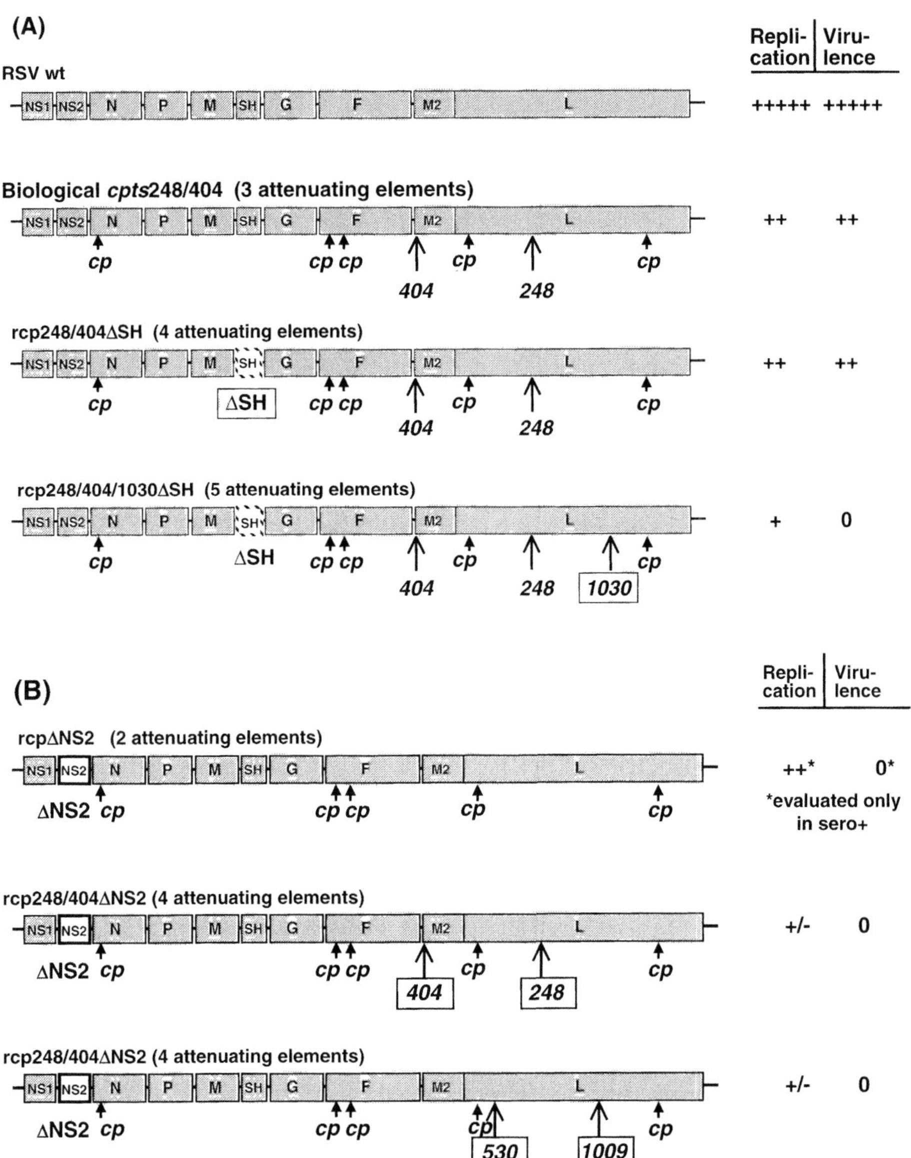
(A)
Repli- cation | Viru- lence
RSV wt
NS1 NS2 N P M SH G F M2 L
+++++ +++++
Biological cpts248/404 (3 attenuating elements)
cp cp cp cp cp
404 248
++ ++
rcp248/404ΔSH (4 attenuating elements)
ΔSH
404 248
++ ++
rcp248/404/1030ΔSH (5 attenuating elements)
ΔSH
404 248 1030
+ 0
(B)
Repli- cation | Viru- lence
rcpΔNS2 (2 attenuating elements)
ΔNS2 cp cp cp cp cp
++* 0*
*evaluated only in sero+
rcp248/404ΔNS2 (4 attenuating elements)
404 248
+/- 0
rcp248/404ΔNS2 (4 attenuating elements)
530 1009
+/- 0

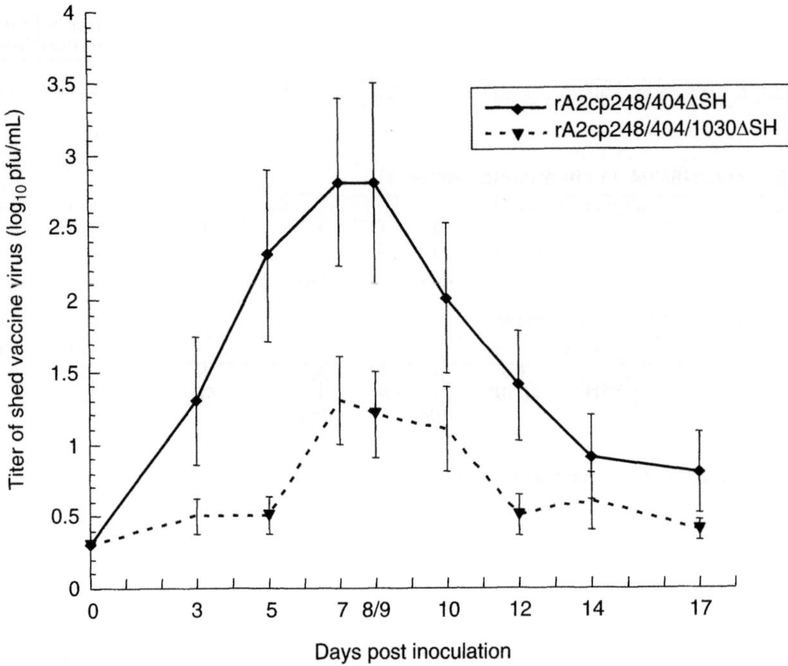

Fig. 2 Replication of the rA2cp248/404ΔSH and rA2cp248/404/1030ΔSH candidate vaccine viruses in RSV-seronegative children ($n = 8$ for each vaccine). Children were inoculated intranasally with $10^{5.0}$ PFU of rA2cp248/404ΔSH or $10^{5.3}$ PFU of rA2cp248/404/1030ΔSH on day 0, and nasopharyngeal washes were taken on the indicated days and assayed for the titer of infectious virus, which is presented as $\log_{10}$ mean titer with standard error indicated. The level of replication of the rA2cp248/404ΔSH virus was essentially indistinguishable from that of its biological *cpts*248/404 predecessor (see Fig. 1A), which differs by the presence of the SH gene and which caused mild upper respiratory tract illness in young infants (Wright et al., 2000). The rA2cp248/404/1030ΔSH virus, which has the addition of the 1030 point mutation in L (see Fig. 1A), did not cause illness in young infants and was immunogenic (Karron et al., 2005). This illustrates that a low level of shedding is to be expected for a satisfactorily immunogenic live RSV vaccine, and that the level of reactogenicity is related to the level of virus replication. Thus, quantitation of vaccine virus shedding plays a key role in clinical evaluation. Adapted from Karron et al. (2005), courtesy of Ruth Karron.

their biological *cpts*248/404 and *cpts*530/1009 parents. Thus, these viruses appear to be over attenuated for use as a pediatric vaccine, especially rA2cp530/1009ΔNS2 (Wright et al., 2006).

While these particular candidates containing the NS2 deletion were not satisfactory for further evaluation, these studies did establish that deletion of NS2 is attenuating for humans and that an attenuation strategy based on deletion of an interferon antagonist is feasible. This strategy is somewhat unusual because attenuation depends on the host interferon system rather than a viral factor. This raises the questions of (i) whether the magnitude of attenuation might be reduced in

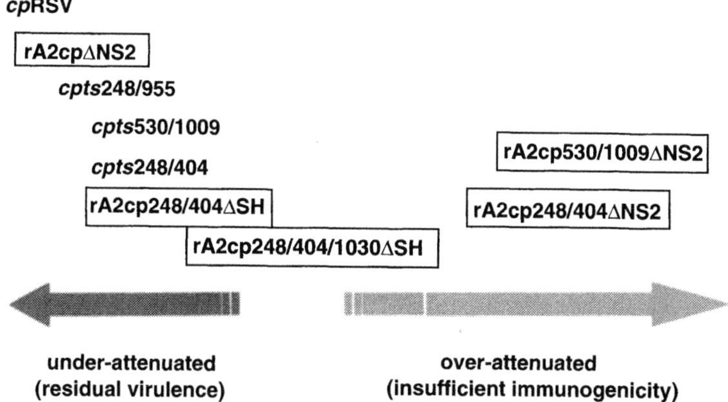

Fig. 3 Listing of most of the biological and recombinant (the latter boxed) RSV vaccine candidates that have been evaluated in humans. These are displayed in the horizontal dimension according to the magnitude of their attenuation phenotype (under attenuated to the left, over attenuated to the right).

infants due to possible immaturity of the type I interferon response, and (ii) whether the magnitude of attenuation might be less in some individuals due to polymorphism in the interferon system.

These studies illustrate the difficulty in identifying a vaccine candidate that has an appropriate level of attenuation. There appears to be a narrow window between being under attenuated and possessing residual virulence versus being over attenuated and insufficiently infectious and immunogenic. This is illustrated in Fig. 3, which shows most of the biological and recombinant vaccine candidates that have been evaluated clinically. In this regard, reverse genetics may be the only feasible avenue for developing an appropriately attenuated strain, since it provides a means for incrementally adding, removing, and substituting mutations to achieve an appropriate level of attenuation, immunogenicity, and genetic stability.

Other promising candidates that are being prepared for clinical trials are viruses whose sole mutation is deletion of the NS1 gene or M2-2 ORF (rA2ΔNS1 and rA2ΔM2-2 viruses). As noted above, each of these was incrementally more attenuated in chimpanzees than the benchmark *cpts*248/404 virus. In addition, the ΔNS2 deletion will be combined with a single *ts* attenuating point mutation.

Parenteral immunization with live wild-type RSV

Another strategy for immunization that was evaluated involved intramuscular administration of live wild-type RSV. Studies in cotton rats indicated that wild-type RSV that is administered intramuscularly undergoes a single cycle of abortive replication, such that infectious virus could not be recovered (Prince et al., 1979). A single immunization of seronegative animals was highly protective against intranasal RSV challenge. However, immunization was very sensitive to RSV-specific serum antibodies, presumably because they neutralized the viral inoculum (Prince et al., 1982). This vaccine was administered to 233 children 6–47 months of age. It was found to be very sensitive to serum antibodies, was poorly immunogenic in most of the recipients, and did not protect against RSV infection or disease (Belshe et al., 1982).

Live-vectored RSV vaccines

Advantages and disadvantages

A number of microbes—mostly viruses—have been evaluated as live vectors for expressing RSV antigens. The use of a heterologous vector in place of RSV itself avoids the problems of poor growth and physical instability characteristic of RSV. This has the potential to greatly simplify vaccine manufacture and delivery. For example, a live RSV vaccine will likely be administered at a dose of 10^5 PFU/ml. Considering that the maximum yields of vaccine virus in cell culture likely will not exceed 10^7–10^8 PFU/ml, and that there will be considerable losses in the infectivity of this labile virus during filtration, lyophilization, packaging, storage, and rehydration, the feasibility of manufacture remains a concern.

Conversely, a potential disadvantage of a vectored RSV vaccine is that typically only one or two of the 11 RSV proteins will be represented, namely the F and G neutralization antigens. This would provide a reduced set of antigens for cellular immunity. Since the correlates of immunity in young infants have not been defined and since cell-mediated responses can provide significant protection at least in the short term, it would be preferable to have as many viral antigens as possible . A second challenge with a vectored vaccine is that the vector must be satisfactorily attenuated in humans yet sufficiently immunogenic for the expressed RSV antigen(s).

Early lessons with DNA viral vectors

Vaccinia virus, a live viral vaccine against smallpox, was the first vector to be evaluated to express RSV antigens in studies beginning in the early 1980s. The vector system available at that time was based on the mouse-adapted WR laboratory strain rather than one specifically approved for immunization of humans. Vaccinia-WR recombinants were constructed that individually expressed each of the RSV proteins except L (Connors et al., 1991). Evaluation of these recombinants in rodents helped to define the roles of the viral proteins in inducing protective immunity and to identify and characterize the correlates of protection, as has already been described. Intradermal immunization of rodents with recombinants expressing the RSV G or F protein was highly immunogenic and induced durable protection (Connors et al., 1991). These recombinants were also safe, immunogenic, and protective in several species of monkeys (Olmsted et al., 1988). However, intradermal immunization of chimpanzees with WR-F and WR-G induced only a moderate titer of serum antibodies, provided inconsistent protection in the lower respiratory tract against intranasal challenge with RSV, and failed to protect the upper respiratory tract (Collins et al., 1990c; Crowe et al., 1993). In comparison, intranasal immunization with an attenuated RSV strain induced a substantially higher level of RSV-neutralizing serum antibodies and a high level of protection against intranasal RSV challenge (Crowe et al., 1993). It was surprising to find that a powerful expression vector such as vaccinia virus was less immunogenic and protective than an attenuated strain of RSV administered intranasally.

Recombinants expressing the RSV F and G glycoproteins were also constructed based on the more highly attenuated MVA strain of vaccinia virus (Wyatt et al., 1999). The MVA strain, which was derived by extensive passage in cell culture, is defective for virus production in most mammalian cells including human cells and has been administered to humans as a smallpox vaccine. This increased attenuation provides increased safety and might make intranasal immunization possible. Like their WR-based counterparts, the MVA-G and MVA-F recombinants were immunogenic and protective in rodents (Wyatt et al., 1999). However, when administered to infant rhesus monkeys simultaneously by the intramuscular and intranasal routes in a two-dose schedule, MVA-G and MVA-F induced low or undetectable titers of RSV-neutralizing serum antibodies and were not significantly protective against RSV challenge (De Waal et al., 2004b).

Adenovirus also was evaluated as an RSV vaccine vector. The adenovirus type 4 and 7 vaccine that has been used in the military consists of a coated tablet of live, replication-competent wild-type virus that is taken orally and initiates an asymptomatic intestinal infection that induces protection against subsequent adenovirus respiratory infection (Gutekunst et al., 1967). The RSV F glycoprotein gene was inserted into the non-essential E3 region of adenovirus types 4, 5, and 7, yielding replication-competent viruses. In initial studies in cotton rats, ferrets and dogs, administration of adenovirus-F recombinants by the enteric, intranasal, or intratracheal route was immunogenic and protective in the upper and lower respiratory tracts against RSV challenge (Collins et al., 1990b; Hsu et al., 1992, 1994). However, sequential oral immunization of a chimpanzee with the adenovirus-4, -5, and -7 recombinants expressing RSV F was poorly immunogenic (Hsu et al., 1992). This was another situation of a powerful expression vector proving to be less immunogenic than anticipated.

Parainfluenza virus vectors

Recombinant parainfluenza viruses (PIVs) such as HPIV3 and Sendai virus (SeV) also have been evaluated as vectors for expressing the protective F and G antigens of RSV, among other foreign antigens. By this strategy, each foreign ORF is placed under the control of PIV transcription signals and inserted into the viral genome as an additional gene (Skiadopoulos et al., 2002b). The foreign gene(s) usually is placed in the first or second position in the gene order in order to have full advantage of the polar gradient of gene transcription. Studies with wild-type HPIV3 showed that three foreign genes totaling 7.5 kb (almost 50% the size of the

HPIV3 genome) could be accommodated with only a minimal reduction in replication in cell culture, although in some cases the attenuating effect of additional genes was more pronounced *in vivo* (Skiadopoulos et al., 2002b). The foreign genes also were surprisingly stable genetically, although point mutations and in some cases biased hypermutation occurred, necessitating careful monitoring of such vaccines during manufacture and use in humans.

To develop an attenuated vectored RSV vaccine, the RSV F and G genes were inserted individually and in combination into positions 1 or 2 of a recombinant virus called B/HPIV3 that is being evaluated on its own as a candidate vaccine against HPIV3 (Schmidt et al., 2001, 2002; Tang et al., 2003). B/HPIV3 is a version of bovine PIV3—which is attenuated in primates due to a natural host range restriction—in which the F and HN genes were replaced by their counterparts from HPIV3. Thus, B/HPIV3 combines the attenuated background of BPIV3 with the major protective antigens of HPIV3. B/HPIV3 expressing RSV F and/or G replicated efficiently *in vitro* and expressed a higher level of RSV G and F protein than did RSV evaluated in parallel. The foreign RSV proteins did not appear to be incorporated into the vector particle based on the lack of sensitivity to neutralization by RSV-specific antibodies in the presence of complement. B/HPIV3 expressing G and/or F exhibited a modest increase in attenuation in rhesus monkeys compared to the B/HPIV3 parent, but were highly immunogenic against both HPIV3 and RSV (Schmidt et al., 2002). B/HPIV3 expressing RSV F was shown to be effective against RSV challenge in African green monkeys (Tang et al., 2004).

The use of B/HPIV3 as a vector to express protective antigens of RSV has a number of advantages. The vector itself is a needed vaccine that is based on an attenuated version of a ubiquitous pediatric pathogen, and hence its use does not expose infants to a new virus. This provides a bivalent vaccine against the two leading viral agents of pediatric respiratory tract disease, RSV and HPIV3. Combining vaccines against RSV and HPIV3 is appropriate because each is a pediatric respiratory pathogen against which immunization should begin within the first few weeks of life. A PIV-vectored RSV vaccine has the additional advantage that PIVs replicate much more efficiently in cell culture than does RSV and do not share its physical lability, thus avoiding these obstacles to manufacture and delivery. The B/HPIV3-F virus is presently being evaluated as a bivalent RSV/HPIV3 vaccine in clinical trials by MedImmune (Table 2).

SeV, a murine PIV that is closely related to HPIV1, also is being evaluated as an intranasal vaccine and vector. SeV is a potential vaccine against HPIV1, based on its antigenic relatedness (Hurwitz et al., 1997). In addition, recombinant SeV has been modified by insertion of the RSV G gene into the fifth gene position, yielding a potential bivalent vaccine against HPIV1 and RSV (Takimoto et al., 2004, 2005). This recombinant was immunogenic and protective against RSV challenge in cotton rats. The use of SeV as a vaccine or vector is based on the presumption that this murine pathogen will be attenuated in primates due to a host range restriction. However, when this possibility was evaluated in non-human primates, SeV replicated as efficiently as wild-type HPIV1 in the respiratory tract of African green monkeys and was only slightly attenuated in chimpanzees (Skiadopoulos et al., 2002a). Therefore, it is not clear whether SeV will be attenuated in humans. SeV did not cause disease when administered intranasally to adults (Slobod et al., 2004), but this would be expected since these individuals had serum antibodies that reacted with SeV that presumably arose from previous natural exposure to HPIV1. Young infants and children, the vaccine target population, will for the most part lack this protection due to prior exposure to HPIV1, and further studies will be needed to determine the safety of SeV in this population. Based on the primate studies described above, studies in HPIV1-seronegative humans should proceed with caution.

Attenuated, recombinant versions of HPIV1 and HPIV2 also have the potential to serve as vectors for RSV antigens (Skiadopoulos et al., 2004). These viruses share the advantage with HPIV3 of being needed pediatric vaccines, and attenuated derivatives of HPIV1 and 2 presently are being developed by reverse genetics (Bartlett et al., 2005; Nolan et al., 2005). HPIV1 and 2 infect and cause disease beginning at approximately 6 months of age, which is somewhat later than for RSV and HPIV3. Thus, it might be possible to use HPIV1 and 2 vectors for expressing RSV G and F protein in order to boost immunity induced by earlier immunization with attenuated RSV or HPIV3-vectored G and F. Studies in hamsters showed that boosting with a PIV vector expressing RSV G and F was substantially more effective compared to successive doses of an attenuated RSV strain (B.R. Murphy et al., unpublished data).

Other vectored vaccines

Recombinant wild-type vesicular stomatitis virus (VSV) was modified so that the RSV F or G ORF was expressed from an added gene (Kahn et al., 1999). In contrast to the results with the PIV vectors, either RSV protein was incorporated into the viral vector particle and the F protein was functional in directing entry (Kahn et al., 1999). When inoculated intranasally into mice, the VSV-G and VSV-F vectors were immunogenic and protective against RSV challenge. For the purpose of attenuation, non-propagating versions were made in which the G glycoprotein gene of the VSV backbone was deleted and replaced by the RSV F or G gene (Kahn et al., 2001). Neither of these viruses produced significant infectious virus in cell culture unless complemented by cDNA encoding the VSV G protein. These non-propagating vectors were substantially less immunogenic in mice than the replication-competent versions, but nonetheless were highly protective. It will be important to evaluate immunogenicity in the presence of passively transferred RSV-specific antibodies. There is little experience with infection of humans with VSV vectors, and the clinical potential of these vectors is unknown. Also, unlike HPIV3 or SeV, the VSV vector does not provide a needed vaccine and thus provides only a monovalent vaccine involving a vector to which infants otherwise would not be exposed.

Other viral vectors have been evaluated in preliminary studies. Non-propagating alphavirus vectors expressing the F and G glycoproteins (whose replication-limited nature resembles that of the non-propagating VSV vectors mentioned above) were highly immunogenic and protective in mice against RSV challenge, particularly when the vectors were administered intranasally (Chen et al., 2002). A recombinant version of the avian paramyxovirus Newcastle disease virus expressing the RSV F protein was partially protective when administered intransally in mice, inducing a 10-fold decrease in RSV challenge virus replication (Martinez-Sobrido et al., 2006). Human rhinovirus type 14 successfully expressed the RSV F protein in cell culture, suggesting as a potential vaccine delivery system (Dollenmaier et al., 2001).

Bacterial vectors have also been considered (Martin-Gallardo et al., 1993; Crowe, 1995; Cano et al., 2000). In one interesting application, three fragments of the G protein were expressed individually fused with part of the cholera B subunit as surface-exposed antigens in non-pathogenic *Staphylococcus carnosus* (Cano et al., 2000). This provides the potential for a live bacterially vectored RSV vaccine that might be administered orally or intranasally. However, when administered to mice in three successive intranasal doses, the vaccine induced only inconsistent, partial protection against RSV challenge virus replication.

In principle, any live vector probably could be engineered to express RSV antigen in a form that is at least somewhat immunogenic and protective in an experimental animal like mice. It is much more difficult to design a strategy that will be safe and effective in the target populations.

DNA vaccines

RSV DNA vaccines usually involve the F and/or G neutralization antigens, although sometimes fragments are used and sometimes other RSV proteins have been expressed from multiple plasmids (Li et al., 1998, 2000; Bembridge et al., 2000a, b; Kumar et al., 2002; Iqbal et al., 2003). Pre-clinical studies to date have involved administration of naked DNA by the intramuscular or intradermal route, or DNA adsorbed onto gold particles and delivered into the skin by a gene gun, or DNA complexed with carbohydrate or abumin to make particles for intranasal delivery. The use of particles for delivery increases the efficiency of immunization and allows for substantially reduced plasmid dose (Iqbal et al., 2003; Harcourt et al., 2004).

A DNA vaccine resembles a live virus or vector in providing for *in situ* intracellular expression of viral antigens. Unlike live virus, attenuation is not an issue. In addition, a DNA vaccine would not be subject to neutralization by maternal antibodies, although immunosuppression by maternal antibodies is a concern as with other RSV vaccines (Siegrist et al., 1998). Another potential advantage is that expression of antigens by parenteral DNA vaccines has been found to persist over several months in animal studies. Conversely, DNA vaccines usually involve only a subset of RSV antigens, which might reduce efficacy. More than one dose is needed frequently, and antibody responses to DNA vaccines often are delayed and reduced compared with virus infection. These are significant drawbacks for a vaccine that should be effective in the first weeks of life. The use of a parenteral route of administration would not directly stimulate local respiratory tract immunity. While DNA vaccines generally are well tolerated, one must be convinced of very low risk before administering an expression plasmid into young infants, a population in which DNA vaccination is without precedent.

Depending on the details of the experiment, RSV DNA vaccines have been found to be weak- to-moderately immunogenic and weak- to-strongly protective in mice, a model that does not provide a rigorous test of efficacy (Li et al., 1998, 2000; Iqbal et al., 2003; Harcourt et al., 2004). In general, DNA vaccines seem to induce a balanced Th1/Th2 response and are not associated with disease enhancement upon RSV challenge. However, the quality of the response seems to be sensitive to variables, such as the route of administration, that are not well defined. Two studies noted increased Th2 stimulation or enhanced disease associated with gene gun delivery (Bembridge et al., 2000b; Bartholdy et al., 2004). Thus, any candidate RSV DNA vaccine for humans will need to be carefully monitored in pre-clinical and clinical trials.

When a DNA vaccine expressing the BRSV F protein was administered intramuscularly or intradermally in two large doses to young calves, it induced a reduced and delayed response of BRSV-specific serum antibodies compared to intranasal BRSV infection and was only moderately protective (Bartholdy et al., 2004). DNA vaccines expressing the BRSV F and N proteins also were administered in two large doses to infant rhesus monkeys (Vaughan et al., 2005). This reduced the level of replication of a human RSV challenge, but only 6-fold. Better efficacy might have been achieved had the DNA vaccine expressed homologous human RSV antigens.

Thus, DNA vaccines have not been very effective so far in the most realistic trials (namely, those in calves and primates). They offer tremendous flexibility with regard to composition and delivery but would require substantial improvement to rapidly induce a protective immune response in young infants.

Perspective

The primary worldwide need is for a pediatric RSV vaccine, one that optimally would be administered during the first weeks of life. The secondary need is for a vaccine for RSV-experienced individuals at high risk of serious RSV disease. It is likely that the two needs will require different vaccines.

The only vaccines under clinical evaluation for pediatric use at the present time are live intranasal vaccines based on (i) attenuated RSV or (ii) attenuated PIV3 expressing the RSV F protein as a bivalent RSV/HPIV3 vaccine. The most important advantages of the live intranasal strategy are the direct stimulation of local respiratory tract immunity and the lack of associated disease enhancement. Identifying a satisfactorily attenuated and immunogenic candidate has proven to be a difficult task. Nonetheless, one such candidate, the rA2cp248/404/1030ΔSH virus, has now been identified. The PIV-vectored bivalent strategy may also hold promise. Whether any other vectors, such as SeV or replication-limited alphaviruses or adenoviruses, prove to be feasible remains to be seen.

Inactivated or subunit vaccines are not presently being considered for pediatric use because of their association with disease potentiation. Improved adjuvants might be able to improve their safety for RSV-naïve recipients, although this remains to be demonstrated. Given the indirect and sometimes speculative association between proposed markers of disease enhancement observed in experimental animals versus the authentic phenomenon in human infants, it will be difficult to devise pre-clinical testing that can confidently determine that a subunit vaccine is sufficiently safe to be evaluated in seronegative infants.

With regard to RSV-experienced individuals, it is not known whether a live-attenuated strain can be developed that will be suitably infectious and immunogenic in that population without risk of transmission to younger, more-susceptible contacts. Vectored vaccines, particularly ones based on vectors such as alphaviruses to which adults would lack immunity, might be an alternative. Subunit vaccines also may be a promising alternative. As already noted, disease enhancement is not associated with their use in RSV-experienced recipients. The subunit vaccines based on PFP or co-formulated F, G and M proteins appear to be immunogenic in RSV-experienced children and adults, but their efficacy remains to be established. A subunit RSV vaccine might be administered yearly in combination with or concurrently with the influenza vaccine.

Acknowledgment

We thank Alexander Schmidt for careful review. The authors were funded as part of the NIAID Intramural Program.

References

American Academy of Pediatrics, C. O. I. D. A. C. O. F. A. N. Reassessment of the indications for ribavirin therapy in respiratory syncytial virus infections. American Academy of Pediatrics Committee on Infectious Diseases. Pediatrics 1996; 97: 137.

American Academy of Pediatrics, C. O. I. D. A. C. O. F. A. N. Revised indications for the use of palivizumab and respiratory syncytial virus immune globulin intravenous for the prevention of respiratory syncytial virus infections. Pediatrics 2003; 112: 1442.

Bartholdy C, Olszewska W, Stryhn A, Thomsen AR, Openshaw PJ. Gene-gun DNA vaccination aggravates respiratory syncytial virus-induced pneumonitis. J Gen Virol 2004; 85: 3017.

Bartlett EJ, Amaro-Carambot E, Surman SR, Newman JT, Collins PL, Murphy BR, Skiadopoulos MH. Human parainfluenza virus type I (HPIV1) vaccine candidates designed by reverse genetics are attenuated and efficacious in African green monkeys. Vaccine 2005; 23: 4631.

Bastien N, Taylor G, Thomas LH, Wyld SG, Simard C, Trudel M. Immunization with a peptide derived from the G glycoprotein of bovine respiratory syncytial virus (BRSV) reduces the incidence of BRSV-associated pneumonia in the natural host. Vaccine 1997; 15: 1385.

Bastien N, Trudel M, Simard C. Complete protection of mice from respiratory syncytial virus infection following mucosal delivery of synthetic peptide vaccines. Vaccine 1999; 17: 832.

Beeler JA, Van Wyke Coelingh K. Neutralization epitopes of the F glycoprotein of respiratory syncytial virus: effect of mutation upon fusion function. J Virol 1989; 63: 2941.

Belanger H, Fleysh N, Cox S, Bartman G, Deka D, Trudel M, Koprowski H, Yusibov V. Human respiratory syncytial virus vaccine antigen produced in plants. FASEB J 2000; 14: 2323.

Belshe RB, Anderson EL, Walsh EE. Immunogenicity of purified F glycoprotein of respiratory syncytial virus: clinical and immune responses to subsequent natural infection in children. J Infect Dis 1993; 168: 1024.

Belshe RB, Newman FK, Anderson EL, Wright PF, Karron RA, Tollefson S, Henderson FW, Meissner HC, Madhi S, Roberton D, Marshall H, Loh R, Sly P, Murphy B, Tatem JM, Randolph V, Hackell J, Gruber W, Tsai TF. Evaluation of combined live, attenuated respiratory syncytial virus and parainfluenza 3 virus vaccines in infants and young children. J Infect Dis 2004; 190: 2096.

Belshe RB, Van Voris LP, Mufson MA. Parenteral administration of live respiratory syncytial virus vaccine: results of a field trial. J Infect Dis 1982; 145: 311.

Bembridge GP, Rodriguez N, Garcia-Beato R, Nicolson C, Melero JA, Taylor G. DNA encoding the attachment (G) or fusion (F) protein of respiratory syncytial virus induces protection in the absence of pulmonary inflammation. J Gen Virol 2000a; 81: 2519.

Bembridge GP, Rodriguez N, Garcia-Beato R, Nicolson C, Melero JA, Taylor G. Respiratory syncytial virus infection of gene gun vaccinated mice induces Th2-driven pulmonary eosinophilia even in the absence of sensitisation to the fusion (F) or attachment (G) protein. Vaccine 2000b; 19: 1038.

Bermingham A, Collins PL. The M2-2 protein of human respiratory syncytial virus is a regulatory factor involved in the balance between RNA replication and transcription. Proc Natl Acad Sci USA 1999; 96: 11259.

Biacchesi S, Pham QN, Skiadopoulos MH, Murphy BR, Collins PL, Buchholz UJ. Infection of non-human primates with recombinant human metapneumovirus lacking the SH, G or M2-2 protein catagorizes each as a nonessential accessory protein and identifies a vaccine candidate. J Virol 2005; 79: 12608.

Biacchesi S, Skiadopoulos MH, Tran KC, Murphy BR, Collins PL, Buchholz UJ. Recovery of human metapneumovirus from cDNA: optimization of growth *in vitro* and expression of additional genes. Virology 2004; 321: 247.

Blanco JC, Boukhvalova MS, Hemming P, Ottolini MG, Prince GA. Prospects of antiviral and anti-inflammatory therapy for respiratory syncytial virus infection. Expert Rev Anti Infect Ther 2005; 3: 945.

Buchholz UJ, Granzow H, Schuldt K, Whitehead SS, Murphy BR, Collins PL. Chimeric bovine respiratory syncytial virus with glycoprotein gene substitutions from human respiratory syncytial virus (HRSV): effects on host range and evaluation as a live-attenuated HRSV vaccine. J Virol 2000; 74: 1187.

Cano F, Plotnicky-Gilquin H, Nguyen TN, Liljeqvist S, Samuelson P, Bonnefoy J, Stahl S, Robert A. Partial protection to respiratory syncytial virus (RSV) elicited in mice by intranasal immunization using live staphylococci with surface- displayed RSV-peptides. Vaccine 2000; 18: 2743.

Centers for Disease Control and Prevention, United States. Recommended childhood and adolescent immunization schedule, 2006. www.immunize.org/cdc/child.

Chen M, Hu KF, Rozell B, Orvell C, Morein B, Liljestrom P. Vaccination with recombinant alphavirus or immune-stimulating complex antigen against respiratory syncytial virus. J Immunol 2002; 169: 3208.

Coates HV, Alling DW, Chanock RM. An antigenic analysis of respiratory syncytial virus isolates by a plaque reduction neutralization test. Am J Epidemiol 1966; 83: 299.

Collins PL, Chanock RM, Murphy BR. Respiratory syncytial virus. In: Fields Virology (Knipe DM, Howley PM, editors). 4th ed. Philadelphia: Lippincott, Williams & Wilkins; 2001.

Collins PL, Hill MG, Camargo E, Grosfeld H, Chanock RM, Murphy BR. Production of infectious human respiratory syncytial virus from cloned cDNA confirms an essential role for the transcription elongation factor from the 5′ proximal open reading frame of the M2 mRNA in gene expression and provides a capability for vaccine development. Proc Natl Acad Sci USA 1995; 92: 11563.

Collins PL, Hill MG, Johnson PR. The two open reading frames of the 22 K mRNA of human respiratory syncytial virus: sequence comparison of antigenic subgroups A and B and expression *in vitro*. J Gen Virol 1990a; 71(Pt 12): 3015.

Collins PL, Prince GA, Camargo E, Purcell RH, Chanock RM, Murphy BR, Davis AR, Lubeck MD, Mizutani S, Hung PP. Evaluation of the protective efficacy of recombinant vaccinia viruses and adenoviruses that express respiratory syncytial virus glycoproteins. In: Vaccines (Brown F, Chanock RM, Ginsberg HS, Lerner RA, editors). 90. New York: Cold Spring Harbor Laboratory Press; 1990b.

Collins PL, Purcell RH, London WT, Lawrence LA, Chanock RM, Murphy BR. Evaluation in chimpanzees of vaccinia virus recombinants that express the surface glycoproteins of human respiratory syncytial virus. Vaccine 1990c; 8: 164.

Connors M, Collins PL, Firestone CY, Murphy BR. Respiratory syncytial virus (RSV) F, G, M2 (22 K), and N proteins each induce resistance to RSV challenge, but resistance induced by M2 and N proteins is relatively short-lived. J Virol 1991; 65: 1634.

Connors M, Collins PL, Firestone CY, Sotnikov AV, Waitze A, Davis AR, Hung PP, Chanock RM, Murphy BR. Cotton rats previously immunized with a chimeric RSV FG glycoprotein develop enhanced pulmonary pathology when infected with RSV, a phenomenon not encountered following immunization with vaccinia–RSV recombinants or RSV. Vaccine 1992a; 10: 475.

Connors M, Giese NA, Kulkarni AB, Firestone CY, Morse HCR, Murphy BR. Enhanced pulmonary histopathology induced by respiratory syncytial virus (RSV) challenge of formalin-inactivated RSV-immunized BALB/c mice is abrogated by depletion of interleukin-4 (IL-4) and IL-10. J Virol 1994; 68: 5321.

Connors M, Kulkarni AB, Firestone CY, Holmes KL, Morse HCD, Sotnikov AV, Murphy BR. Pulmonary histopathology induced by respiratory syncytial virus (RSV) challenge of formalin-inactivated RSV-immunized BALB/c mice is abrogated by depletion of CD4+T cells. J Virol 1992b; 66: 7444.

Crowe Jr. JE. Current approaches to the development of vaccines against disease caused by respiratory syncytial virus (RSV) and parainfluenza virus (PIV). A meeting report of the WHO programme for vaccine development. Vaccine 1995; 13: 415.

Crowe Jr. JE, Bui PT, Davis AR, Chanock RM, Murphy BR. A further attenuated derivative of a cold-passaged temperature-sensitive mutant of human respiratory syncytial virus retains immunogenicity and protective efficacy against wild-type challenge in seronegative chimpanzees. Vaccine 1994a; 12: 783.

Crowe Jr. JE, Bui PT, London WT, Davis AR, Hung PP, Chanock RM, Murphy BR. Satisfactorily attenuated and protective mutants derived from a partially attenuated cold-passaged respiratory syncytial virus mutant by introduction of additional attenuating mutations during chemical mutagenesis. Vaccine 1994b; 12: 691.

Crowe Jr. JE, Bui PT, Siber GR, Elkins WR, Chanock RM, Murphy BR. Cold-passaged, temperature-sensitive mutants of human respiratory syncytial virus (RSV) are highly attenuated, immunogenic, and protective in seronegative chimpanzees, even when RSV antibodies are infused shortly before immunization. Vaccine 1995; 13: 847.

Crowe Jr. JE, Collins PL, London WT, Chanock RM, Murphy BR. A comparison in chimpanzees of the immunogenicity and efficacy of live attenuated respiratory syncytial virus (RSV) temperature-sensitive mutant vaccines and vaccinia virus recombinants that express the surface glycoproteins of RSV. Vaccine 1993; 11: 1395.

Crowe Jr. JE, Firestone CY, Murphy BR. Passively acquired antibodies suppress humoral but not cell-mediated immunity in mice immunized with live attenuated respiratory syncytial virus vaccines. J Immunol 2001; 167: 3910.

Crowe Jr. JE, Williams JV. Immunology of viral respiratory tract infection in infancy. Paediatr Respir Rev 2003; 4: 112.

De Swart RL, Kuiken T, Timmerman HH, Amerongen Gv G, Van Den Hoogen BG, Vos HW, Neijens HJ, Andeweg AC, Osterhaus AD. Immunization of macaques with formalin-inactivated respiratory syncytial virus (RSV) induces interleukin-13-associated hypersensitivity to subsequent RSV infection. J Virol 2002; 76: 11561.

De Waal L, Power UF, Yuksel S, Van Amerongen G, Nguyen TN, Niesters HG, De Swart RL, Osterhaus AD. Evaluation of BBG2Na in infant macaques: specific immune responses after vaccination and RSV challenge. Vaccine 2004a; 22: 915.

De Waal L, Wyatt LS, Yuksel S, Van Amerongen G, Moss B, Niesters HG, Osterhaus AD, De Swart RL. Vaccination of infant macaques with a recombinant modified vaccinia virus Ankara expressing the respiratory syncytial virus F and G genes does not predispose for immunopathology. Vaccine 2004b; 22: 923.

Delgado MF, Polack FP. Involvement of antibody, complement and cellular immunity in the pathogenesis of enhanced respiratory syncytial virus disease. Expert Rev Vaccines 2004; 3: 693.

Dollenmaier G, Mosier SM, Scholle F, Sharma N, Mcknight KL, Lemon SM. Membrane-associated respiratory syncytial virus F protein expressed from a human rhinovirus type 14 vector is immunogenic. Virology 2001; 281: 216.

Durbin AP, Karron RA. Progress in the development of respiratory syncytial virus and parainfluenza virus vaccines. Clin Infect Dis 2003; 37: 1668.

Falsey AR, Hennessey PA, Formica MA, Cox C, Walsh EE. Respiratory syncytial virus infection in elderly and high-risk adults. N Engl J Med 2005; 352: 1749.

Falsey AR, Walsh EE. Safety and immunogenicity of a respiratory syncytial virus subunit vaccine (PFP-2) in ambulatory adults over age 60. Vaccine 1996; 14: 1214.

Falsey AR, Walsh EE. Safety and immunogenicity of a respiratory syncytial virus subunit vaccine (PFP-2) in the institutionalized elderly. Vaccine 1997; 15: 1130.

Fouillard L, Mouthon L, Laporte JP, Isnard F, Stachowiak J, Aoudjhane M, Lucet JC, Wolf M, Bricourt F, Douay L, Lopez M, Marche C, Najman A, Gorin NC. Severe respiratory syncytial virus pneumonia after autologous bone marrow transplantation: a report of three cases and review. Bone Marrow Transplant 1992; 9: 97.

Friedewald WT, Forsyth BR, Smith CB, Gharpure MA, Chanock RM. Low-temperature-grown RS virus in adult volunteers. JAMA 1968; 203: 690.

Garcia-Barreno B, Palomo C, Penas C, Delgado T, Perez-Brena P, Melero JA. Marked differences in the antigenic structure of human respiratory syncytial virus F and G glycoproteins. J Virol 1989; 63: 925.

Gonzalez IM, Karron RA, Eichelberger M, Walsh EE, Delagarza VW, Bennett R, Chanock RM, Murphy BR, Clements-Mann ML, Falsey AR. Evaluation of the live attenuated cpts 248/404 RSV vaccine in combination with a subunit RSV vaccine (PFP-2) in healthy young and older adults. Vaccine 2000; 18: 1763.

Groothuis JR, King SJ, Hogerman DA, Paradiso PR, Simoes EA. Safety and immunogenicity of a purified F protein respiratory syncytial virus (PFP-2) vaccine in seropositive children with bronchopulmonary dysplasia. J Infect Dis 1998; 177: 467.

Gupta CK, Leszczynski J, Gupta RK, Siber GR. Stabilization of respiratory syncytial virus (RSV) against thermal inactivation and freeze–thaw cycles for development and control of RSV vaccines and immune globulin [published erratum appears in Vaccine 1997; 15(2): 247]. Vaccine 1996; 14: 1417.

Gutekunst RR, White RJ, Edmondson WP, Chanock RM. Immunization with live type 4 adenovirus: determination of infectious virus dose and protective effect of enteric infection. Am J Epidemiol 1967; 86: 341.

Hancock GE, Heers KM, Pryharski KS, Smith JD, Tiberio L. Adjuvants recognized by toll-like receptors inhibit the induction of polarized type 2 T cell responses by natural attachment (G) protein of respiratory syncytial virus. Vaccine 2003; 21: 4348.

Hancock GE, Speelman DJ, Frenchick PJ, Mineo-Kuhn MM, Baggs RB, Hahn DJ. Formulation of the purified fusion protein of respiratory syncytial virus with the saponin QS-21 induces protective immune responses in Balb/c mice that are similar to those generated by experimental infection. Vaccine 1995; 13: 391.

Harcourt JL, Anderson LJ, Sullender W, Tripp RA. Pulmonary delivery of respiratory syncytial virus DNA vaccines using macroaggregated albumin particles. Vaccine 2004; 22: 2248.

Henderson FW, Collier AM, Clyde Jr. WA, Denny FW. Respiratory-syncytial-virus infections, reinfections and immunity. A prospective, longitudinal study in young children. N Engl J Med 1979; 300: 530.

Hendry RM, Burns JC, Walsh EE, Graham BS, Wright PF, Hemming VG, Rodriguez WJ, Kim HW, Prince GA, McIntosh K, Chanock RM, Murphy BR. Strain-specific serum antibody responses in infants undergoing primary infection with respiratory syncytial virus. J Infect Dis 1988; 157: 640.

Hsu KH, Lubeck MD, Bhat BM, Bhat RA, Kostek B, Selling BH, Mizutani S, Davis AR, Hung PP. Efficacy of adenovirus-vectored respiratory syncytial virus vaccines in a new ferret model. Vaccine 1994; 12: 607.

Hsu KH, Lubeck MD, Davis AR, Bhat RA, Selling BH, Bhat BM, Mizutani S, Murphy BR, Collins PL, Chanock RM, Hung PP. Immunogenicity of recombinant adenovirus-respiratory syncytial virus vaccines with adenovirus types 4, 5, and 7 vectors in dogs and a chimpanzee. J Infect Dis 1992; 166: 769.

Hurwitz JL, Soike KF, Sangster MY, Portner A, Sealy RE, Dawson DH, Coleclough C. Intranasal Sendai virus vaccine protects African green monkeys from infection with human parainfluenza virus-type one. Vaccine 1997; 15: 533.

Hussell T, Baldwin CJ, O'garra A, Openshaw PJ. CD8+ T cells control Th2-driven pathology during pulmonary respiratory syncytial virus infection. Eur J Immunol 1997; 27: 3341.

Iqbal M, Lin W, Jabbal-Gill I, Davis SS, Steward MW, Illum L. Nasal delivery of chitosan-DNA plasmid expressing epitopes of respiratory syncytial virus (RSV) induces protective CTL responses in BALB/c mice. Vaccine 2003; 21: 1478.

Ison MG, Mills J, Openshaw P, Zambon M, Osterhaus A, Hayden F. Current research on respiratory viral infections: Fourth International Symposium. Antiviral Res 2002; 55: 227.

Jin H, Cheng X, Zhou HZ, Li S, Seddiqui A. Respiratory syncytial virus that lacks open reading frame 2 of the M2 gene (M2-2) has altered growth characteristics and is attenuated in rodents. J Virol 2000a; 74: 74.

Jin H, Clarke D, Zhou HZ, Cheng X, Coelingh K, Bryant M, Li S. Recombinant human respiratory syncytial virus (RSV) from cDNA and construction of subgroup A and B chimeric RSV. Virology 1998; 251: 206.

Jin H, Zhou H, Cheng X, Tang R, Munoz M, Nguyen N. Recombinant respiratory syncytial viruses with deletions in the NS1, NS2, SH, and M2-2 genes are attenuated *in vitro* and *in vivo*. Virology 2000b; 273: 210.

Johnson Jr. PR, Olmsted RA, Prince GA, Murphy BR, Alling DW, Walsh EE, Collins PL. Antigenic relatedness between glycoproteins of human respiratory syncytial virus subgroups A and B: evaluation of the contributions of F and G glycoproteins to immunity. J Virol 1987a; 61: 3163.

Johnson PR, Spriggs MK, Olmsted RA, Collins PL. The G glycoprotein of human respiratory syncytial viruses of subgroups A and B: extensive sequence divergence between antigenically related proteins. Proc Natl Acad Sci USA 1987b; 84: 5625.

Johnson TR, Johnson JE, Roberts SR, Wertz GW, Parker RA, Graham BS. Priming with secreted glycoprotein G of respiratory syncytial virus (RSV) augments interleukin-5 production and tissue eosinophilia after RSV challenge. J Virol 1998; 72: 2871.

Johnson TR, Teng MN, Collins PL, Graham BS. Respiratory syncytial virus (RSV) G glycoprotein is not necessary for vaccine-enhanced disease induced by immunization with formalin-inactivated RSV. J Virol 2004; 78: 6024.

Juhasz K, Murphy BR, Collins PL. The major attenuating mutations of the respiratory syncytial virus vaccine candidate cpts530/1009 specify temperature-sensitive defects in transcription and replication and a non-temperature-sensitive alteration in mRNA termination. J Virol 1999a; 73: 5176.

Juhasz K, Whitehead SS, Boulanger CA, Firestone CY, Collins PL, Murphy BR. The two amino acid substitutions in the L protein of cpts530/1009, a live-attenuated respiratory syncytial virus candidate vaccine, are independent temperature-sensitive and attenuation mutations. Vaccine 1999b; 17: 1416.

Kahn JS, Roberts A, Weibel C, Buonocore L, Rose JK. Replication-competent or attenuated, nonpropagating vesicular stomatitis viruses expressing respiratory syncytial virus (RSV) antigens protect mice against RSV challenge. J Virol 2001; 75: 11079.

Kahn JS, Schnell MJ, Buonocore L, Rose JK. Recombinant vesicular stomatitis virus expressing respiratory syncytial virus (RSV) glycoproteins: RSV fusion protein can mediate infection and cell fusion. Virology 1999; 254: 81.

Kakuk TJ, Soike K, Brideau RJ, Zaya RM, Cole SL, Zhang JY, Roberts ED, Wells PA, Wathen MW. A human respiratory syncytial virus (RSV) primate model of enhanced pulmonary pathology induced with a formalin-inactivated RSV vaccine but not a recombinant FG subunit vaccine. J Infect Dis 1993; 167: 553.

Kapikian AZ, Mitchell RH, Chanock RM, Shvedoff RA, Stewart CE. An epidemiologic study of altered clinical reactivity to respiratory syncytial (RS) virus infection in children previously vaccinated with an inactivated RS virus vaccine. Am J Epidemiol 1969; 89: 405.

Karron RA, Belshe RB, Wright PF, Thumar B, Burns B, Newman F, Cannon JC, Thompson J, Tsai T, Paschalis M, Wu SL, Mitcho Y, Hackell J, Murphy BR, Tatem JM. A live human parainfluenza type 3 virus vaccine is attenuated and immunogenic in young infants. Pediatr Infect Dis J 2003; 22: 394.

Karron RA, Buonagurio DA, Georgiu AF, Whitehead SS, Adamus JE, Clements-Mann ML, Harris DO, Randolph VB, Udem SA, Murphy BR, Sidhu MS. Respiratory syncytial virus (RSV) SH and G proteins are not essential for viral replication *in vitro*: clinical evaluation and molecular characterization of a cold-passaged, attenuated RSV subgroup B mutant. Proc Natl Acad Sci USA 1997a; 94: 13961.

Karron RA, Wright PF, Belshe RB, Thumar B, Casey R, Newman F, Polack FP, Randolph VB, Deatly A, Hackell J, Gruber W, Murphy BR, Collins PL. Identification of a recombinant live attenuated respiratory syncytial virus vaccine candidate that is highly attenuated in infants. J Infect Dis 2005; 191: 1093.

Karron RA, Wright PF, Crowe Jr. JE, Clements ML, Thompson J, Makhene M, Casey R, Murphy BR. Evaluation of two live, cold-passaged, temperature-sensitive respiratory syncytial virus (RSV) vaccines in chimpanzees, adults, infants and children. J Infect Dis 1997b; 176: 1428.

Kim HW, Arrobio JO, Pyles G, Brandt CD, Camargo E, Chanock RM, Parrott RH. Clinical and immunological response of infants and children to administration of low-temperature adapted respiratory syncytial virus. Pediatrics 1971; 48: 745.

Kim HW, Canchola JG, Brandt CD, Pyles G, Chanock RM, Jensen K, Parrott RH. Respiratory syncytial virus disease in infants despite prior administration of antigenic inactivated vaccine. Am J Epidemiol 1969; 89: 422.

Kim HW, Leikin SL, Arrobio J, Brandt CD, Chanock RM, Parrott RH. Cell-mediated immunity to respiratory syncytial virus induced by inactivated vaccine or by infection. Pediatr Res 1976; 10: 75.

Krempl C, Murphy BR, Collins PL. Recombinant respiratory syncytial virus with the G and F genes shifted to the promoter-proximal positions. J Virol 2002; 76: 11931.

Kulkarni AB, Collins PL, Bacik I, Yewdell JW, Bennink JR, Crowe Jr. JE, Murphy BR. Cytotoxic T cells specific for a single peptide on the M2 protein of respiratory syncytial virus are the sole mediators of resistance induced by immunization with M2 encoded by a recombinant vaccinia virus. J Virol 1995; 69: 1261.

Kumar M, Behera AK, Lockey RF, Zhang J, Bhullar G, De La Cruz CP, Chen LC, Leong KW, Huang SK, Mohapatra SS. Intranasal gene transfer by chitosan-DNA nanospheres protects BALB/c mice against acute respiratory syncytial virus infection. Hum Gene Ther 2002; 13: 1415.

Li X, Sambhara S, Li CX, Ettorre L, Switzer I, Cates G, James O, Parrington M, Oomen R, Du RP, Klein M. Plasmid DNA encoding the respiratory syncytial virus G protein is a promising vaccine candidate. Virology 2000; 269: 54.

Li X, Sambhara S, Li CX, Ewasyshyn M, Parrington M, Caterini J, James O, Cates G, Du RP, Klein M. Protection against respiratory syncytial virus infection by DNA immunization. J Exp Med 1998; 188: 681.

Lo MS, Brazas RM, Holtzman MJ. Respiratory syncytial virus nonstructural proteins NS1 and NS2 mediate inhibition of Stat2 expression and alpha/beta interferon responsiveness. J Virol 2005; 79: 9315.

Mader D, Huang Y, Wang C, Fraser R, Issekutz AC, Stadnyk AW, Anderson R. Liposome encapsulation of a soluble recombinant fragment of the respiratory syncytial virus (RSV) G protein enhances immune protection and reduces lung eosinophilia associated with virus challenge. Vaccine 2000; 18: 1110.

Martin-Gallardo A, Fleischer E, Doyle SA, Arumugham R, Collins PL, Hildreth SW, Paradiso PR. Expression of the G glycoprotein gene of human respiratory syncytial virus in *Salmonella typhimurium*. J Gen Virol 1993; 74: 453.

Martinez FD. Heterogeneity of the association between lower respiratory illness in infancy and subsequent asthma. Proc Am Thorac Soc 2005; 2: 157.

Martinez-Sobrido L, Gitiban N, Fernandez-Sesma A, Cros J, Mertz SE, Jewell NA, Hammond S, Flano E, Durbin RK, Garcia-Sastre A, Durbin JE. Protection against respiratory syncytial virus by a recombinant Newcastle disease virus vector. J Virol 2006; 80: 1130.

Mcauliffe JM, Surman SR, Newman JT, Riggs JM, Collins PL, Murphy BR, Skiadopoulos MH. Codon substitution mutations at two positions in the L polymerase protein of human parainfluenza virus type 1 yield viruses with a spectrum of attenuation *in vivo* and increased phenotypic stability *in vitro*. J Virol 2004; 78: 2029.

Mills J, Van Kirk JE, Wright PF, Chanock RM. Experimental respiratory syncytial virus infection of adults. Possible mechanisms of resistance to infection and illness. J Immunol 1971; 107: 123.

Munoz FM, Piedra PA, Glezen WP. Safety and immunogenicity of respiratory syncytial virus purified fusion protein-2 vaccine in pregnant women. Vaccine 2003; 21: 3465.

Murphy B. Mucosal immunity to viruses. In: Mucosal Immunology (Mestecky JEA, editor). Amsterdam: Elsevier Academic Press; 2005.

Murphy BR, Prince GA, Collins PL, Van Wyke Coelingh K, Olmsted RA, Spriggs MK, Parrott RH, Kim HW, Brandt CD, Chanock RM. Current approaches to the development of vaccines effective against parainfluenza and respiratory syncytial viruses. Virus Res 1988; 11: 1.

Murphy BR, Prince GA, Walsh EE, Kim HW, Parrott RH, Hemming VG, Rodriguez WJ, Chanock RM. Dissociation between serum neutralizing and glycoprotein antibody responses of infants and children who received inactivated respiratory syncytial virus vaccine. J Clin Microbiol 1986; 24: 197.

Murphy BR, Sotnikov A, Paradiso PR, Hildreth SW, Jenson AB, Baggs RB, Lawrence L, Zubak JJ, Chanock RM, Beeler JA, Prince GA. Immunization of cotton rats with the fusion (F) and large (G) glycoproteins of respiratory syncytial virus (RSV) protects against RSV challenge without potentiating RSV disease. Vaccine 1989; 7: 533.

Murphy BR, Sotnikov AV, Lawrence LA, Banks SM, Prince GA. Enhanced pulmonary histopathology is observed in cotton rats immunized with formalin-inactivated respiratory syncytial virus (RSV) or purified F glycoprotein and challenged with RSV 3-6 months after immunization. Vaccine 1990; 8: 497.

Murphy BR, Walsh EE. Formalin-inactivated respiratory syncytial virus vaccine induces antibodies to the fusion glycoprotein that are deficient in fusion-inhibiting activity. J Clin Microbiol 1988; 26: 1595.

Nicholas JA, Rubino KL, Levely ME, Adams EG, Collins PL. Cytolytic T-lymphocyte responses to respiratory syncytial virus: effector cell phenotype and target proteins. J Virol 1990; 64: 4232.

Nolan SM, Surman SR, Amaro-Carambot E, Collins PL, Murphy BR, Skiadopoulos MH. Live-attenuated intranasal parainfluenza virus type 2 vaccine candidates developed by reverse genetics containing L polymerase protein mutations imported from heterologous paramyxoviruses. Vaccine 2005; 23: 4765.

Oien NL, Brideau RJ, Walsh EE, Wathen MW. Induction of local and systemic immunity against human respiratory syncytial virus using a chimeric FG glycoprotein and cholera toxin B subunit. Vaccine 1994; 12: 731.

Olmsted RA, Buller RM, Collins PL, London WT, Beeler JA, Prince GA, Chanock RM, Murphy BR. Evaluation in non-human primates of the safety, immunogenicity and efficacy of recombinant vaccinia viruses expressing the F or G glycoprotein of respiratory syncytial virus. Vaccine 1988; 6: 519.

Oomens AG, Wertz GW. The baculovirus GP64 protein mediates highly stable infectivity of a human respiratory syncytial virus lacking its homologous transmembrane glycoproteins. J Virol 2004; 78: 124.

Openshaw PJ, Tregoning JS. Immune responses and disease enhancement during respiratory syncytial virus infection. Clin Microbiol Rev 2005; 18: 541.

Paradiso PR, Hildreth SW, Hogerman DA, Speelman DJ, Lewin EB, Oren J, Smith DH. Safety and immunogenicity of a subunit respiratory syncytial virus vaccine in children 24 to 48 months old. Pediatr Infect Dis J 1994; 13: 792.

Piedra PA, Cron SG, Jewell A, Hamblett N, Mcbride R, Palacio MA, Ginsberg R, Oermann CM, Hiatt PW. Immunogenicity of a new purified fusion protein vaccine to respiratory syncytial virus: a multi-center trial in children with cystic fibrosis. Vaccine 2003; 21: 2448.

Piedra PA, Grace S, Jewell A, Spinelli S, Bunting D, Hogerman DA, Malinoski F, Hiatt PW. Purified fusion protein vaccine protects against lower respiratory tract illness during respiratory syncytial virus season in children with cystic fibrosis. Pediatr Infect Dis J 1996; 15: 23.

Piedra PA, Grace S, Jewell A, Spinelli S, Hogerman DA, Malinoski F, Hiatt PW. Sequential annual administration of purified fusion protein vaccine against respiratory syncytial virus in children with cystic fibrosis. Pediatr Infect Dis J 1998; 17: 217.

Plotnicky-Gilquin H, Cyblat-Chanal D, Aubry JP, Champion T, Beck A, Nguyen T, Bonnefoy JY, Corvaia N. Gamma interferon-dependent protection of the mouse upper respiratory tract following parenteral immunization with a respiratory syncytial virus G protein fragment. J Virol 2002; 76: 10203.

Plotnicky-Gilquin H, Huss T, Aubry JP, Haeuw JF, Beck A, Bonnefoy JY, Nguyen TN, Power UF. Absence of lung immunopathology following respiratory syncytial virus (RSV) challenge in mice immunized with a recombinant RSV G protein fragment. Virology 1999; 258: 128.

Plotnicky-Gilquin H, Robert A, Chevalet L, Haeuw JF, Beck A, Bonnefoy JY, Brandt C, Siegrist CA, Nguyen TN, Power UF. CD4(+) T-cell-mediated antiviral protection of the upper respiratory tract in BALB/c mice following parenteral immunization with a recombinant respiratory syncytial virus G protein fragment. J Virol 2000; 74: 3455.

Polack FP, Teng MN, Collins PL, Prince GA, Exner M, Regele H, Lirman DD, Rabold R, Hoffman SJ, Karp CL, Kleeberger SR, Wills-Karp M, Karron RA. A role for immune complexes in enhanced respiratory syncytial virus disease. J Exp Med 2002; 196: 859.

Power UF, Nguyen TN, Rietveld E, De Swart RL, Groen J, Osterhaus AD, De Groot R, Corvaia N, Beck A, Bouveret-Le-Cam N, Bonnefoy JY. Safety and immunogenicity of a novel recombinant subunit respiratory syncytial virus vaccine (BBG2Na) in healthy young adults. J Infect Dis 2001; 184: 1456.

Power UF, Plotnicky-Gilquin H, Huss T, Robert A, Trudel M, St~Ahl S, Uhlen M, Nguyen TN, Binz H. Induction of protective immunity in rodents by vaccination with a prokaryotically expressed recombinant fusion protein containing a respiratory syncytial virus G protein fragment. Virology 1997; 230: 155.

Prince GA, Capiau C, Deschamps M, Fabry L, Garcon N, Gheysen D, Prieels JP, Thiry G, Van Opstal O, Porter DD. Efficacy and safety studies of a recombinant chimeric respiratory syncytial virus FG glycoprotein vaccine in cotton rats. J Virol 2000; 74: 10287.

Prince GA, Curtis SJ, Yim KC, Porter DD. Vaccine-enhanced respiratory syncytial virus disease in cotton rats following immunization with Lot 100 or a newly prepared reference vaccine. J Gen Virol 2001a; 82: 2881.

Prince GA, Denamur F, Deschamps M, Garcon N, Prieels JP, Slaoui M, Thiriart C, Porter DD. Monophosphoryl lipid A adjuvant reverses a principal histologic parameter of formalin-inactivated respiratory syncytial virus vaccine-induced disease. Vaccine 2001b; 19: 2048.

Prince GA, Hemming VG, Horswood RL, Baron PA, Chanock RM. Effectiveness of topically administered neutralizing antibodies in experimental immunotherapy of respiratory syncytial virus infection in cotton rats. J Virol 1987; 61: 1851.

Prince GA, Horswood RL, Camargo E, Suffin SC, Chanock RM. Parenteral immunization with live respiratory syncytial virus is blocked in seropositive cotton rats. Infect Immun 1982; 37: 1074.

Prince GA, Horswood RL, Chanock RM. Quantitative aspects of passive immunity to respiratory syncytial virus infection in infant cotton rats. J Virol 1985; 55: 517.

Prince GA, Jenson AB, Hemming VG, Murphy BR, Walsh EE, Horswood RL, Chanock RM. Enhancement of respiratory syncytial virus pulmonary pathology in cotton rats by prior intramuscular inoculation of formalin-inactivated virus. J Virol 1986; 57: 721.

Prince GA, Mond JJ, Porter DD, Yim KC, Lan SJ, Klinman DM. Immunoprotective activity and safety of a respiratory syncytial virus vaccine: mucosal delivery of fusion glycoprotein with a CpG oligodeoxynucleotide adjuvant. J Virol 2003; 77: 13156.

Prince GA, Potash L, Horswood RL, Camargo E, Suffin SC, Johnson RA, Chanock RM. Intramuscular inoculation of live respiratory syncytial virus induces immunity in cotton rats. Infect Immun 1979; 23: 723.

Pringle CR, Filipiuk AH, Robinson BS, Watt PJ, Higgins P, Tyrrell DA. Immunogenicity and pathogenicity of a triple temperature-sensitive modified respiratory syncytial virus in adult volunteers. Vaccine 1993; 11: 473.

Ramaswamy M, Shi L, Monick MM, Hunninghake GW, Look DC. Specific inhibition of type I interferon signal transduction by respiratory syncytial virus. Am J Respir Cell Mol Biol 2004; 30: 893.

Regner M, Culley F, Fontannaz P, Hu K, Morein B, Lambert PH, Openshaw P, Siegrist CA. Safety and efficacy of immune-stimulating complex-based antigen delivery systems for neonatal immunisation against respiratory syncytial virus infection. Microbes Infect 2004; 6: 666.

Rodriguez WJ, Gruber WC, Groothuis JR, Simoes EA, Rosas AJ, Lepow M, Kramer A, Hemming V. Respiratory syncytial virus immune globulin treatment of RSV lower respiratory tract infection in previously healthy children. Pediatrics 1997; 100: 937.

Sandhu JS, Krasnyanski SF, Domier LL, Korban SS, Osadjan MD, Buetow DE. Oral immunization of mice with transgenic tomato fruit expressing respiratory syncytial virus-F protein induces a systemic immune response. Transgenic Res 2000; 9: 127.

Schmidt AC, Mcauliffe JM, Murphy BR, Collins PL. Recombinant bovine/human parainfluenza virus type 3 (B/HPIV3) expressing the respiratory syncytial virus (RSV) G and F proteins can be used to achieve simultaneous mucosal immunization against RSV and HPIV3. J Virol 2001; 75: 4594.

Schmidt AC, Wenzke DR, Mcauliffe JM, St. Clair M, Elkins WR, Murphy BR, Collins PL. Mucosal immunization of rhesus monkeys against respiratory syncytial virus subgroups A and B and human parainfluenza virus type 3 using a live cDNA-derived vaccine based on a host range-attenuated bovine parainfluenza virus type 3 vector backbone. J Virol 2002; 76.

Shay DK, Holman RC, Newman RD, Liu LL, Stout JW, Anderson LJ. Bronchiolitis-associated hospitalizations among US children, 1980–1996. J Am Med Assoc 1999; 282: 1440.

Siegrist CA, Barrios C, Martinez X, Brandt C, Berney M, Cordova M, Kovarik J, Lambert PH. Influence of maternal antibodies on vaccine responses: inhibition of antibody but not T cell responses allows successful early prime-boost strategies in mice. Eur J Immunol 1998; 28: 4138.

Skiadopoulos MH, Biacchesi S, Buchholz UJ, Riggs JM, Surman SR, Amaro-Carambot E, Mcauliffe JM, Elkins WR, St Claire M, Collins PL, Murphy BR. The two major human metapneumovirus genetic lineages are highly related antigenically, and the fusion (F) protein is a major contributor to this antigenic relatedness. J Virol 2004; 78: 6927.

Skiadopoulos MH, Surman SR, Riggs JM, Elkins WR, St Claire M, Nishio M, Garcin D, Kolakofsky D, Collins PL, Murphy BR. Sendai virus, a murine parainfluenza virus type 1, replicates to a level similar to human PIV1 in the upper and lower respiratory tract of African green monkeys and chimpanzees. Virology 2002a; 297: 153.

Skiadopoulos MH, Surman SR, Riggs JM, Orvell C, Collins PL, Murphy BR. Evaluation of the replication and immunogenicity of recombinant human parainfluenza virus type 3 vectors expressing up to three foreign glycoproteins. Virology 2002b; 297: 136.

Slobod KS, Shenep JL, Lujan-Zilbermann J, Allison K, Brown B, Scroggs RA, Portner A, Coleclough C, Hurwitz JL. Safety and immunogenicity of intranasal murine parainfluenza virus type 1 (Sendai virus) in healthy human adults. Vaccine 2004; 22: 3182.

Spann KM, Tran KC, Chi B, Rabin RL, Collins PL. Suppression of the induction of alpha, beta, and lambda interferons by the NS1 and NS2 proteins of human respiratory syncytial virus in human epithelial cells and macrophage. J Virol 2004; 78: 4363.

Spann KM, Tran KC, Collins PL. Effects of nonstructural proteins NS1 and NS2 of human respiratory syncytial virus on interferon regulatory factor 3, NF-kappaB, and proinflammatory cytokines. J Virol 2005; 79: 5353.

Srikiatkhachorn A, Braciale TJ. Virus-specific CD8+ T lymphocytes downregulate T helper cell type 2 cytokine secretion and pulmonary eosinophilia during experimental murine respiratory syncytial virus infection. J Exp Med 1997; 186: 421.

Takimoto T, Hurwitz JL, Coleclough C, Prouser C, Krishnamurthy S, Zhan X, Boyd K, Scroggs RA, Brown B, Nagai Y, Portner A, Slobod KS. Recombinant Sendai virus expressing the G glycoprotein of respiratory syncytial virus (RSV) elicits immune protection against RSV. J Virol 2004; 78: 6043.

Takimoto T, Hurwitz JL, Zhan X, Krishnamurthy S, Prouser C, Brown B, Coleclough C, Boyd K, Scroggs RA, Portner A, Slobod KS. Recombinant Sendai virus as a novel vaccine candidate for respiratory syncytial virus. Viral Immunol 2005; 18: 255.

Tang RS, Macphail M, Schickli JH, Kaur J, Robinson CL, Lawlor HA, Guzzetta JM, Spaete RR, Haller AA. Parainfluenza virus type 3 expressing the native or soluble fusion (F) protein of respiratory syncytial virus (RSV) confers protection from RSV infection in African green monkeys. J Virol 2004; 78: 11198.

Tang RS, Nguyen N, Cheng X, Jin H. Requirement of cysteines and length of the human respiratory syncytial virus m2-1 protein for protein function and virus viability. J Virol 2001; 75: 11328.

Tang RS, Nguyen N, Zhou H, Jin H. Clustered charge-to-alanine mutagenesis of human respiratory syncytial virus L polymerase generates temperature-sensitive viruses. Virology 2002; 302: 207.

Tang RS, Schickli JH, Macphail M, Fernandes F, Bicha L, Spaete J, Fouchier RA, Osterhaus AD, Spaete R, Haller AA. Effects of human metapneumovirus and respiratory syncytial virus antigen insertion in two 3′ proximal genome positions of bovine/human parainfluenza virus type 3 on virus replication and immunogenicity. J Virol 2003; 77: 10819.

Tang YW, Graham BS. Anti-IL-4 treatment at immunization modulates cytokine expression, reduces illness, and increases cytotoxic T lymphocyte activity in mice challenged with respiratory syncytial virus. J Clin Invest 1994; 94: 1953.

Tebbey PW, Scheuer CA, Peek JA, Zhu D, Lapierre NA, Green BA, Phillips ED, Ibraghimov AR, Eldridge JH, Hancock GE. Effective mucosal immunization against respiratory syncytial virus using purified F protein and a genetically detoxified cholera holotoxin, CT-E29 H. Vaccine 2000; 18: 2723.

Teng MN, Collins PL. The central conserved cystine noose of the attachment G protein of human respiratory syncytial virus is not required for efficient viral infection *in vitro* or *in vivo*. J Virol 2002; 76: 6164.

Teng MN, Whitehead SS, Bermingham A, Clair MS, Elkins WR, Murphy BR, Collins PL. Recombinant respiratory syncytial virus that does not express the NS1 or M2-2 protein is highly attenuated and immunogenic in chimpanzees. J Virol 2000; 74: 9317.

Teng MN, Whitehead SS, Collins PL. Contribution of the respiratory syncytial virus G glycoprotein and its secreted and membrane-bound forms to virus replication *in vitro* and *in vivo*. Virology 2001; 289: 283.

Tolley KP, Marriott AC, Simpson A, Plows DJ, Matthews DA, Longhurst SJ, Evans JE, Johnson JL, Cane PA, Randolph VB, Easton AJ, Pringle CR. Identification of mutations contributing to the reduced virulence of a modified strain of respiratory syncytial virus. Vaccine 1996; 14: 1637.

Tripp RA, Jones LP, Haynes LM, Zheng H, Murphy PM, Anderson LJ. CX3C chemokine mimicry by respiratory syncytial virus G glycoprotein. Nat Immunol 2001; 2: 732.

Tristram DA, Welliver RC, Hogerman DA, Hildreth SW, Paradiso P. Second-year surveillance of recipients of a respiratory syncytial virus (RSV) F protein subunit vaccine, PFP-1: evaluation of antibody persistence and possible disease enhancement. Vaccine 1994; 12: 551.

Tristram DA, Welliver RC, Mohar CK, Hogerman DA, Hildreth SW, Paradiso P. Immunogenicity and safety of respiratory syncytial virus subunit vaccine in seropositive children 18–36 months old. J Infect Dis 1993; 167: 191.

Trudel M, Nadon F, Seguin C, Binz H. Protection of BALB/c mice from respiratory syncytial virus infection by immunization with a synthetic peptide derived from the G glycoprotein. Virology 1991a; 185: 749.

Trudel M, Stott EJ, Taylor G, Oth D, Mercier G, Nadon F, Seguin C, Simard C, Lacroix M. Synthetic peptides corresponding to the F protein of RSV stimulate murine B and T cells but fail to confer protection. Arch Virol 1991b; 117: 59.

Valarcher JF, Furze J, Wyld S, Cook R, Conzelmann KK, Taylor G. Role of alpha/beta interferons in the attenuation and immunogenicity of recombinant bovine respiratory syncytial viruses lacking NS proteins. J Virol 2003; 77: 8426.

Vaughan K, Rhodes GH, Gershwin LJ. DNA immunization against respiratory syncytial virus (RSV) in infant rhesus monkeys. Vaccine 2005; 23: 2928.

Walsh EE. Humoral, mucosal, and cellular immune response to topical immunization with a subunit respiratory syncytial virus vaccine. J Infect Dis 1994; 170: 345.

Walsh EE, Hall CB, Briselli M, Brandriss MW, Schlesinger JJ. Immunization with glycoprotein subunits of respiratory syncytial virus to protect cotton rats against viral infection. J Infect Dis 1987; 155: 1198.

Waris ME, Tsou C, Erdman DD, Day DB, Anderson LJ. Priming with live respiratory syncytial virus (RSV) prevents the enhanced pulmonary inflammatory response seen after RSV challenge in BALB/c mice immunized with formalin-inactivated RSV. J Virol 1997; 71: 6935.

Waris ME, Tsou C, Erdman DD, Zaki SR, Anderson LJ. Respiratory synctial virus infection in BALB/c mice previously immunized with formalin-inactivated virus induces enhanced pulmonary inflammatory response with a predominant Th2-like cytokine pattern. J Virol 1996; 70: 2852.

Wathen MW, Brideau RJ, Thomsen DR. Immunization of cotton rats with the human respiratory syncytial virus F glycoprotein produced using a baculovirus vector. J Infect Dis 1989a; 159: 255.

Wathen MW, Brideau RJ, Thomsen DR, Murphy BR. Characterization of a novel human respiratory syncytial virus chimeric FG glycoprotein expressed using a baculovirus vector. J Gen Virol 1989b; 70: 2625.

Watt PJ, Robinson BS, Pringle CR, Tyrrell DA. Determinants of susceptibility to challenge and the antibody response of adult volunteers given experimental respiratory syncytial virus vaccines. Vaccine 1990; 8: 231.

Whitehead SS, Bukreyev A, Teng MN, Firestone CY, St Claire M, Elkins WR, Collins PL, Murphy BR. Recombinant respiratory syncytial virus bearing a deletion of either the NS2 or SH gene is attenuated in chimpanzees. J Virol 1999a; 73: 3438.

Whitehead SS, Firestone CY, Collins PL, Murphy BR. A single nucleotide substitution in the transcription start signal of the M2 gene of respiratory syncytial virus vaccine candidate cpts248/404 is the major determinant of the temperature-sensitive and attenuation phenotypes. Virology 1998a; 247: 232.

Whitehead SS, Firestone CY, Karron RA, Crowe Jr. JE, Elkins WR, Collins PL, Murphy BR. Addition of a missense mutation present in the L gene of respiratory syncytial virus (RSV) cpts530/1030 to RSV vaccine candidate cpts248/404 increases its attenuation and temperature sensitivity. J Virol 1999b; 73: 871.

Whitehead SS, Hill MG, Firestone CY, St Claire M, Elkins WR, Murphy BR, Collins PL. Replacement of the F and G proteins of respiratory syncytial virus (RSV) subgroup A with those of subgroup B generates chimeric live attenuated RSV subgroup B vaccine candidates. J Virol 1999c; 73: 9773.

Whitehead SS, Juhasz K, Firestone CY, Collins PL, Murphy BR. Recombinant respiratory syncytial virus (RSV) bearing a set of mutations from cold-passaged RSV is attenuated in chimpanzees. J Virol 1998b; 72: 4467.

World Health Organization Initiaitive for vaccine research: respiratory syncytial virus (RSV), 2005. http://www.who.int/vaccine_research/diseases/ari/en/index3.html.

Wright PF, Karron RA, Belshe RB, Thompson J, Crowe Jr. JE, Boyce TG, Halburnt LL, Reed GW, Whitehead SS, Anderson EL, Wittek AE, Casey R, Eichelberger M, Thumar B, Randolph VB, Udem SA, Chanock RM, Murphy BR. Evaluation of a live, cold-passaged, temperature-sensitive, respiratory syncytial virus vaccine candidate in infancy. J Infect Dis 2000; 182: 1331.

Wright PF, Karron RA, Madhi SA, Treanor JJ, King JC, O'shea A, Ikizler MR, Zhu Y, Collins PL, Cutland C, Randolph VB, Deatly AM, Hackell JG, Gruber WC, Murphy B. The interferon antagonist NS2 protein of respiratory syncytial virus is an important virulence determinant for humans. J Infect Dis 2006; 193.

Wright PF, Shinozaki T, Fleet W, Sell SH, Thompson J, Karzon DT. Evaluation of a live, attenuated respiratory syncytial virus vaccine in infants. J Pediatr 1976; 88: 931.

Wyatt LS, Whitehead SS, Venanzi KA, Murphy BR, Moss B. Priming and boosting immunity to respiratory syncytial virus by recombinant replication-defective vaccinia virus MVA. Vaccine 1999; 18: 392.

Yusibov V, Mett V, Mett V, Davidson C, Musiychuk K, Gilliam S, Farese A, Macvittie T, Mann D. Peptide-based candidate vaccine against respiratory syncytial virus. Vaccine 2005; 23: 2261.

Respiratory Syncytial Virus
Patricia Cane (Editor)

DOI 10.1016/S0168-7069(06)14009-4

Development of Antivirals against Respiratory Syncytial Virus

Kenneth L. Powell, Dagmar Alber
Arrow Therapeutics Ltd., 7 Trinity Street, Borough, London SE1 1DA, UK

Introduction

The previous chapters in this book demonstrate the crucial need for new antiviral drugs to treat the victims of infection by respiratory syncytial virus (RSV). Historically the search for such treatments has been focussed on the most visible patients—small infants, but over the last decade there has been increasing awareness of the importance of this virus in other patient populations, particularly the elderly, those with chronic heart or lung conditions and the immunocompromised. This awareness means that there is no longer any question that the prospects for an RSV drug would justify its research and development costs.

The evolutionary position of RSV as a fairly isolated member of Paramyxoviruses makes it unlikely that a drug developed for this virus would be used to treat other infections (with the possible exception of bovine or ovine RSV in their respective hosts). Even its apparently most similar human pathogen, human metapneumo virus (HMPV, van den Hoogen et al., 2002) has a significantly different RNA sequence. Selectivity for RSV on the other hand would indicate the possibility of safe treatment with a specific molecule.

In this review, we will discuss the reasons behind the paucity of treatment options for RSV infection and the balance between research on vaccines and antiviral approaches. We will then review the history, current state and future of anti-RSV chemotherapy.

Slow progress

Although it is some quarter of a century since the discovery of ribavirin's *in vitro* activity against RSV, there have been no new treatments for the infection which have reached the market. There are many reasons for this lack of success, the major ones being:

1. *Varying enthusiasm*: It took almost 20 years of research before the first truly selective antiviral, acyclovir, reached the clinic. During this period up to the late 1970s there was much scepticism that compounds could be made which would discriminate between a virus and its host cell. As this eased and indeed as ribavirin was discovered to have activity against RSV *in vitro* (Hruska et al., 1980), first the emergence of the AIDS epidemic and then the discovery of Hepatitis C diverted attention from RSV to antivirals that combat these more obvious threats. In the 1990s, the lack of commercial success for the influenza drugs Tamiflu and Relenza dealt a blow to the enthusiasm for the development of drugs to treat respiratory virus infection. This was despite the huge differences in both the window of opportunity for treatment and in the markets for agents to treat infections by these viruses. This pessimism was enhanced by the clinical failure of the antirhinovirus agent, Pleconaril, due to problems of drug–drug interaction (Hayden et al., 2003).
2. The lack of good animal models for human RSV infection is a major hurdle for the field. There is no small animal in which the virus replicates well. Although RSV replicates well in the chimpanzee, it produces few symptoms. These animals are difficult to obtain free of RSV infection (and hence pre-existing antibodies), are expensive and present ethical issues which make their use prohibitive. Large animal models are available for bovine RSV but these are expensive and require large amounts of test drugs and facilities as well as expertise for handling large animals.
3. Clinical trials for RSV infection present some interesting problems. The most obvious patient group (neonates and infants) are a very difficult group in which to do any study and are not suitable for the earliest trials. Adults who are immunocompromised—stem cell transplant patients for example—are an obvious treatment group as their infections are serious and prolonged. Trials in this group are complicated as patients are often being treated with many other drugs.
4. A lack of sensitive 'point of care' diagnostic tests led to an underestimate of the prevalence of RSV infection and the perception that development of new drugs would be difficult.
5. Finally, the perception that RSV is a trivial infection without major morbidity and mortality impact is only gradually being dispelled.

The time is now ripe for the development of new RSV drugs. The need is evident and new tools and techniques make the discovery of new drugs more likely than in the past.

Vaccines versus antivirals

Despite extensive research expenditure over the years since the discovery of RSV, we are still a long way from an effective vaccine (Hall, 1980). This is not surprising given the relatively poor protection provided by prior exposure to the virus in natural infection. RSV vaccine research was dealt a major blow early in its development, when clinical trials of an inactivated viral vaccine led to vaccinated children having more severe disease than those not in receipt of vaccine (Kapikian et al., 1969). These events led to an extremely cautious approach to novel RSV vaccines. The key problems of RSV vaccine research (dealt with in the chapter by Collins & Murphy in this volume) are providing an effective, protective immune response, while ensuring the vaccine is entirely safe. Since immune responses to natural RSV infection are short lived, another major issue is getting vaccine dosage frequency to practically achievable levels of a yearly vaccination.

In the absence of a vaccine, prevention of infection using a passive vaccination with polyclonal or monoclonal antibodies has been shown to be a practical approach. First a polyclonal human antibody—Respigam (Groothius et al., 1993), and then a monoclonal antibody palivizumab (Synagis, The Impact-RSV Study Group, 1998), were shown to offer significant protection from RSV infection in community studies in infants. About 50% of infants could be protected from hospitalisation due to RSV infection during an RSV season by a course of antibody therapy involving monthly injections. Because of the expense of such a prophylactic approach (where many of the patients treated will never catch the virus), its use is limited to prematurely born infants or those with a serious congenital condition. Even with these cost-based restrictions, the use of the antibody is widespread only in a small number of developed countries, including the USA.

Antivirals offer the possibility of treating the infection after it has occurred. This is a major advantage from a cost basis since only infected patients will be treated. Treatment in otherwise healthy adults is challenging, where the virus replication is limited in extent and duration, but less so in infants and the immunocompromised, where the virus replication is enhanced and of much greater duration. There is also the long-term prospect of using therapeutic drugs for prophylaxis in a community outbreak setting.

Many serious infections with RSV occur in countries where the use of expensive drugs or antibodies is totally beyond the means of local healthcare delivery systems. Here the development of a low-cost vaccine requiring a single administration would be ideal but, while this remains impractical, consideration needs to be given to mechanisms to provide novel drugs at reasonable cost in these territories.

Brief history of RSV antiviral development

Prior to the genomics era, the discovery of anti-infective drugs relied on the screening of chemical libraries or natural products using classic virology assays—sometimes modified to provide marginally higher throughput. Consequently, there is a not a huge range of chemotypes in the armoury against viruses. Indeed, most of the early antiviral compounds were based on analogues of nucleic acid precursors or nucleosides. It was by testing such a compound against RSV that the activity of ribavirin was discovered (Hruska et al., 1980). Subsequent to this work many compounds have been identified with interesting activity against RSV. Table 1 lists the most important of these compounds, as far as is possible, by the target with which they interact.

Modern approaches to antiviral discovery

With the advent of viral genome sequencing the possibility of direct analysis of each viral gene product as a target for therapy became possible. Such approaches have largely dominated antiviral discovery for the last 15 years. Although this approach is very successful as part of the discovery process, no antiviral drug has yet been designed entirely *de novo*. Rather it has been the intelligent use of compound testing of small focussed libraries, and the use of biochemical information on enzyme substrates and products combined with good chemistry and biology, which have yielded success. The success against some viruses has been impressive—for HIV—for example we already have some 20 FDA approved therapies available (http://www.niaid.nih.gov/factsheets/hivinf.htm). This success depended on resources and the inherent tractability of the virus/host system in question. Unfortunately, for RSV the funding has been sparse and the virus has been difficult to study. Comparing the polymerase enzymes of the two viruses: for HIV, it was relatively straightforward to express the reverse transcriptase as a heterodimer and to make large quantities of active enzyme in *Escherichia coli*. (Larder et al., 1987). For the Paramyxoviruses, it is difficult to isolate the RNA polymerase complex and establishing an enzyme assay in the laboratory has been anything but straightforward (Mason et al., 2004). In another RNA virus, Hepatitis C, progress has been rapid in the discovery of compounds with activity against at least three well understood viral protein targets; for RSV, it has been slow with only the external fusion protein being widely used as a target.

Fortunately, the commercial success of Synagis has rekindled the interest of the pharmaceutical industry in the possibility of selective antivirals for RSV. Consequently, more resources for academic studies of the virus and for the development of new antiviral molecules inhibiting at least some of the, as yet poorly understood, targets can be expected. Research at Arrow Therapeutics has used traditional screening methods to discover a lead molecule, which has then been refined through medicinal chemistry prior to identifying mechanism, using modern molecular methods. We would expect to see more of such approaches in the future.

Models of RSV disease

Background

The lack of a good animal model has been a major barrier to the development of effective antiviral drugs for RSV disease. In fact, having sub-optimal animal models has probably been worse for the field than having no models at all! Modern developments of antiviral drugs have been mostly achieved without the use of

Table 1

Compounds identified with anti-RSV activity

Target	Compound	Stage of development	Reference
F-fusion protein	RD3-0028	Animal models	Watanabe et al. (1998)
F-fusion protein	VP14637	Phase 1	McKimm-Breschkin (2000)
F-fusion protein	JNJ2408068	Preclinical	Andries et al. (2003)
F-fusion protein	BMS-433771	Preclinical	Cianci et al. (2004a, b)
F-fusion protein	RFI-641	Preclinical	Nikitenko et al. (2001)
F-fusion protein	DATEM	Research	Ohki et al. (2003)
F-fusion protein	Not yet released	Research	Bond et al. (2005)
F-fusion protein	Not identified individually	Research	Lackey et al. (2002) A1 Trimeris Inc.
F-fusion protein	Benzodithiin derivative	Research	Watanabe et al. (1998)
G-glycoprotein	NMSO3	Research	Kimura et al. (2000)
G-glycoprotein?	SP-303, Provir, Virend, Crofelemer—plant flavanoid	Phase III clinical (discontinued?)	Barnard et al. (1993)
Entry	PAMPS	Research	Ikeda et al. (1994)
Entry	Polyoxometalates	Research	Barnard et al. (1997)
Entry	Rho peptides	Research	Budge et al. (2004)
Entry	Dendrimers	Research	Starpharma Web site
Entry	Bis (5-amidino-2-benzimidazolyl) methane (BABIM)	Research	Dubovi et al. (1980)
Entry	Lovastatin	Research	Gower and Graham (2001)
L-Protein	YM-53403	Research	Sudo et al. (2005)
N-Protein	A-60444 (RSV604)	Phase II	Carter et al. (2006)
Unknown	Pyridobenzazoles and pyrimidobenzimadazoles	Research	Chiba et al. (1995)
Unknown	3-cyclopentyl-1-adamantanamines	Research	Fytas et al. (1994)
Unknown	Carbocyclic 3-azaadenosine	Research	Wyde et al. (1990a)
Unknown	LY253963	Research	Wyde et al. (1990b)
Unknown	6-diazo-5-oxo-L-norleucine	Research	Huang et al. (1994)
Unknown	N-(phophonoacetyl)-L-aspartate	Research	Wyde et al. (1995)
Multiple	Ribavirin	Approved	Hruska et al. (1980)
Multiple	Ribavirin analogues	Research	Gabrielsen et al.(1992)
Host cell	VMX-497	Research	Markland et al. (2000)
Host cell	CCL5 and CCL5 mimics	Research	Hancock and Tebbey (2005)

animal models. The models available for HIV and Hepatitis C viruses were so poor that their use has largely been bypassed to go from *in vitro* models, via appropriate preclinical studies of safety and pharmacokinetics, directly to the clinic. With the much-improved quality of measurement of viral replication in humans (through the use of quantitative PCR on the relevant samples), it has been possible to prove in HIV studies that reduction in viral load correlates with clinical benefit. Thus, such clinical Phase II studies can be small, rapid and largely predictive of future Phase III studies. This may indeed be the future of antiviral development, except where predictive rodent models of a human virus infection are available.

Prior to discussing the models of RSV disease, we need to examine what we mean by a good animal model. An example of a good model is the mouse model of human herpes virus infection (Field et al., 1979). In such models the key characteristics are:

- a biologically relevant inoculum size;
- animals which are readily available, preferably rodent in origin and which can be used in sufficient numbers to yield significant data;
- the ability of human clinical isolates of the virus, unadapted in the laboratory, to produce disease;
- development of symptoms similar to the human condition;
- significant replication of the virus *in vivo*;
- a yield of virus in >10-fold excess over the inoculum; and
- the ability to detect sites of replication *in vivo*.

The significance of the majority of these issues is obvious, but we need to emphasise the importance of the first one. It is essential to avoid the use of large inocula of unpurified viruses. Such samples contain a huge mixture of cell debris, including cytokines and their inducers, with a very small amount of virus. Using such inocula will almost inevitably yield misleading results especially when considering symptoms and the host response to infection.

If we consider the best animal models for HIV—such as the SCID/hu mouse or the chimaeric mouse/human liver model for Hepatitis C it can be seen that these do not meet important criteria largely because they involve very small numbers of animals, created at great expense and with variable degrees of virus replication. This had led to the unsatisfactory use of surrogate animal viruses, such as the simian immunodeficiency virus (SIV) for HIV and bovine viral diarrhoea virus (BVDV) for Hepatitis C. Although these viruses produce good replication in their hosts, they are sufficiently divergent from the human viruses to make them poor models for the human disease.

RSV models

The mouse model

The mouse model of human RSV infection does not meet our criteria for a good model. The inoculum is large, viral replication is very restricted and only a very small amount of virus can be recovered from infected animals (Prince et al., 1979; Taylor et al., 1984). Surprisingly, these defects are almost totally ignored in the literature, probably reflecting the convenience of working with a small animal model and its widespread use to examine immunological phenomena. A comparison of pneumonia virus of mice (PVM) and human RSV infection in the mouse is very revealing (Cook et al., 1998). This clearly shows the abundant replication of the PVM virus in its natural host and the very restricted nature of the human virus in the mouse. Quantitative studies of human RSV infection would suggest the virus is highly productive in its natural host (Di Vincenzo et al., 2005; Lee et al., 2004; Perkins et al., 2005).

The cotton rat

The cotton rat is by far the most widely used animal model for RSV infections (Wyde et al., 1987) however the criticisms of the mouse model largely apply to it (Collins et al., 2001). A key question in both these models is the fate of the administered virus. Is replication really being measured or are both models measuring the survival of the virus over time? Does human RSV replicate in rodent cells or is an abortive, non-productive infection being observed? If the latter, what are the mechanisms by which the virus survives in the animals? These questions can and should now be addressed given the availability of modern PCR methods for quantitative virus load determination.

The PVM model

Although PVM is only somewhat related to human RSV it does offer a virus which replicates well in its natural host. Success has been reported in making hybrid N protein between PVM and RSV—at least in the minigenome replication model (this offers the possibility of making PVM viruses containing portions of the RSV genome relevant to the compound under test). Although complex, exploration of such models could well be rewarding and may create an affordable small animal model for exploring therapies.

The bovine RSV model

Bovine RSV is closely related to human RSV. It is also an economically important pathogen in its own host (Taylor et al., 1997; Woolums et al., 1999; Antonis et al., 2003). Bovine RSV offers a model which is much more relevant to human RSV than the rodent models; however, it is not without considerable problems:

- it is a relatively unexplored model which has not been used to develop antiviral compounds;
- as the animals are large (calves weigh about 70 kg at 4 weeks), it requires large amounts of the test compounds;

- as the animals are expensive, group sizes must be small;
- bovine g.i. tract adsorption and metabolism undergoes drastic changes during development and experiments must deal with these issues; and
- stocks of virus for these experiments need to be carefully prepared, be passaged to minimum amounts in tissue culture and be free of adventitious agents.

Alternative model of human RSV in tissue culture

The lack of good animal models frustrates the desire for more detailed understanding of the replication of this virus. Most laboratory studies of the virus are done in simple monolayer cell cultures yielding little information on the cell specificity of infection. To overcome partially this drawback, Zhang et al. (2002) have studied the replication of the virus in differentiated human primary epithelial cell cultures. The experiment is to study the differentiation of biopsy-derived human nasal epithelium in culture, which is brought about by growing the explanted cells at an air–liquid interface. The cultures are then infected and observed. They discovered that the luminal columnar (especially ciliated epithelial) cells of these cultures were targeted by RSV. The virus only infected the apical side of the culture, and the virus produced was released from this side of the culture. The released virus was spread by the beating of the cilia of these columnar epithelial cells.

These differentiated cultures make an interesting laboratory model of infection. Virus can be used to infect the culture from the apical side, while potential inhibitors are given in the medium from the basal side. Inhibition of the virus indicates that the drug can penetrate the potential barriers to infection present in a complete epithelium.

Clinical trials of RSV agents

The development of a new drug for the treatment of RSV infection requires the development of new clinical trial designs. It has been common practice in trials of potential drugs for human respiratory disease to use human challenge studies. In such studies, validated stocks of virus are carefully safety checked and then used to infect human volunteers. Challenge studies like these were used in the development of inhibitors of both influenza virus and human rhinovirus infection (Hayden et al., 1992, 1999; Calfee et al., 1999). Similar studies have been shown to be possible with RSV (Falsey et al., 2003; Lee et al., 2004). Unfortunately, the conduct of these studies requires a preparation of challenge virus to be available and this has been a consistent problem for RSV. Although the US NIH prepared a small quantity of a virus pool for human studies (as used in the Lee et al. (2004) study), this virus stock is no longer available. Preparation of another stock is both technically challenging and very expensive, making these desirable studies impractical in the short term.

While children are the obvious target of RSV therapies they are not suitable for initial clinical trials. This makes it most likely that Phase IIa studies will be done in patients who are immunocompromised and produce high virus loads for prolonged periods.

Early Phase II clinical trials for antivirals now almost exclusively use virus load determinations to provide evidence of efficacy endpoints. Such an approach has been well validated with both HIV and Hepatitis C. Falsey et al. (2003) have used quantitative PCR methods to detect and quantify infection in RSV infected volunteers, and Perkins et al. (2005) have used similar techniques to follow RSV infections in infants. We have examined the possibility of using such a PCR approach with RSV clinical trials. Using a simple nasal swab we have been able to follow virus infection over the course of naturally acquired RSV infection and quantify virus by a quantitative PCR approach (J. Dent et al., personal communication). This method has also worked well in similar trials of bovine RSV infection.

Phase II trials of RSV inhibitors will have to involve studies in children. Given the higher yields of virus and the more consistent levels of replication, this should present fewer technical problems than adult trials. Careful assessment of side effect profiles will be a very important part of studies in such vulnerable populations.

It is likely that clinical trials of treatments for RSV infections will remain complex but the establishment of well-developed methods for viral load detection should simplify the development of the next generation of compounds.

Drugs in development

Fusion inhibitors

In vitro screening in tissue culture for activity against RSV has been used in many attempts to discover small molecule inhibitors of virus function. In almost all such attempts, the result has been the discovery of multiple inhibitors of the viral fusion protein. A screen at Arrow of our 'in-house' compound library also resulted in several hits with similar properties. Recent detailed structural work on the mechanism of action of some well-characterised fusion inhibitors has revealed why they may be relatively easy to discover. Examples of such compounds have been shown to bind to a well conserved and relatively accommodating hydrophobic pocket on the F protein formed by its HR1 and HR2 peptides (Douglas et al., 2005; Cianci et al., 2004c; Cianci et al., 2005), destabilizing the trimer-of-hairpins structure required for fusion. This mechanism seems to apply to multiple structural classes of fusion protein inhibitors.

For convenience, we will divide this discussion into two groups of compounds. The first are all derived from benzimadazoles—ironically the first such compound to show RSV activity was described more than 25 years ago by Dubovi et al. (1980). The compound (BABIM) was shown to inhibit the early stage of infection and to have limited activity in the cotton rat model of infection (Tidwell et al., 1984), but little further information is available on the compound. Modern compounds of this type were described in patents filed by Johnson and Johnson,

Trimeris and Bristol–Myers Squibb (BMS) and additional patents describing similar compounds have recently been published by Biota and Tibotec. These compounds are often extremely potent in antiviral assays, provided they are given before or during the infection process; for example, JNJ2408068 has sub-nanomolar activity against RSV. Both this compound and the BMS compound BMS-433771 need to be present before or during the virus infection process in order to demonstrate their potency; added after infection they are ineffective (Andries et al., 2003; Wyde et al., 2003; Cianci et al., 2004a, b, 2005). This is very consistent with the mode of action of these compounds and may mean they are more suited to prophylactic than therapeutic use. Although little data are available on the Trimeris compounds, our own observations on those from the Biota patent suggest they have similar properties.

Both BMS-433771 and JNJ2408068 have been studied extensively in the various animal models of RSV infection with a confusing array of results. JNJ2408068 was effective in the cotton rat model either given as a prophylactic or on the final day of treatment prior to culling animals (but not on the previous day) (Wyde et al., 2003). The authors attribute this result to carry-over of the drug into the *in vitro* assays at the end of the experiment. Such carry-over is always a problem in animal model experiments and especially so with such potent compounds. BMS-433771 needed to be dosed prior to virus infection in order to demonstrate antiviral activity *in vivo*. The dose of the compound required for activity was huge compared to the potency of the compound observed in laboratory assays and there was a poor dose-response relationship (Cianci et al., 2004a, b). In our view these compounds would require testing in the bovine model or in humans in order to understand their real utility in therapy.

It is relatively easy to isolate mutants resistant to fusion inhibitors (even in the presence of high concentrations of the compounds ($>1000 \times IC_{50}$)). Such mutants have point mutations within the F1 domain of the fusion protein and may arise in a single passage *in vitro* (Cianci et al., 2004c). This ready isolation of mutants raises concerns about how effective the fusion protein inhibitors would be in a clinical situation.

The second group of fusion inhibitors are a diverse array of chemical structures; VP-14637 is the best characterised of these molecules. It is a triphenol compound which, although completely unrelated to the benzimadazole group chemically, has been shown to have a very similar mechanism (Douglas et al., 2005). This compound has similar activity to the benzimadazoles in laboratory studies but differs greatly in its *in vivo* properties (Wyde et al., 2005). Thus it has no prophylactic activity at all, but seems effective when given in divided doses as a small particle aerosol to infected cotton rats. Unfortunately, this compound is highly insoluble and has to be given in a vehicle containing 85% alcohol. It might be interesting to examine the effect of this carrier on the *in vivo* activity of other potential antivirals in the model.

RFI-641 a biphenyl triazine anionic compound was also discovered through modifying a hit from a high-throughput screen (Huntley et al., 2002). The compound has a high molecular weight, but is water soluble. Like the other fusion inhibitors the compound is active given prior to viral infection and inactive given later. In animal models, the compound was seen to have prophylactic activity against RSV in the mouse, cotton rat and African green monkey models and a very moderate therapeutic effect in the monkey but not the other models. The compound is not as selective as the other compounds discussed in this section and had some moderate activity against the herpes viruses. Mutants of RSV lacking the other membrane proteins of the virus were insensitive to the compound. Watanabe et al. (1998) reported a benzodithiin series with activity against RSV. This series has relatively weak antiviral activity—the best compound having an IC_{50} of about 4.5 μM. Nevertheless, the authors report activity in the mouse model of infection. The compound appears to have an entirely different mechanism to other fusion protein inhibitors in that it acts very late in the replication cycle. Mutants resistant to the compound had a mutation at position 276 of the F1 protein (Sudo et al., 2001). More information on this series of compounds would be interesting.

There are numerous other compounds which have been described as inhibitors of RSV entry or cell fusion. Unfortunately there is little information on the mechanism of most of these compounds or their promise for further development. DATEM (diacetyltartaric acid esters of mono and diglycerides) was shown to inhibit RSV induced cell fusion; Bis (5-amidino-2-benzimidazolyl) methane (BABIM), for the reasons discussed above, also probably works through modulation of fusion protein function (Cianci et al., 2004a).

Compounds inhibiting virus adsorbtion and penetration

While there has been much less activity in this area, some compounds have been reported to inhibit virus entry by mechanisms independent of the fusion protein. NMSO3, a sulphated sialyl lipid, has been reported as a potent inhibitor of RSV (Kimura et al., 2000, 2004). This compound inhibited both virus binding to cells and cell penetration. Given prior to and during infection, the compound produced a modest reduction of virus titre in the cotton-rat model. Mutants of RSV resistant to this compound developed mutations in a conserved region of the RSV G protein but not in the fusion protein. Such mutants were cross resistant with heparin (see below).

SP-303 is a natural polyphenolic compound with moderate activity against RSV (Barnard et al., 1993). The compound inhibited virus penetration, but a detailed molecular mechanism has not been determined. Although only moderately active *in vitro,* the compound was active in the cotton-rat model when given by the intra-peritoneal but not the oral route of administration. The compound was quite toxic and the therapeutic index moderate (Wyde et al., 1993). This compound is not selective for RSV and has been widely studied as an antiviral against other virus families.

Many negatively charged polymers inhibit the adsorbtion and penetration of a range of viruses, including RSV; these include heparin, dextran sulphate and a range of polyanionic peptides (Budge et al., 2004). Initially the activity of rhoA-derived peptides suggested inhibition through an F protein mechanism, but subsequent studies have clearly shown that these peptides inhibit entry through interaction with the virus G protein (Pastey et al., 2000; Budge et al., 2004). Similar mechanisms probably account for the antiviral activities observed for the sulphonic acid polymer PAMPS (Ikeda et al., 1994), the polyoxometalates (Barnard et al., 1997) and high concentrations of Lovastatin (Gower and Graham, 2001).

Compounds affecting virus replication

Given the success of enzyme inhibitors as antiviral compounds against other virus families, it is perhaps surprising that there has been so little success with inhibitors of RNA replication for the Paramyxoviruses. The problem here is that there has been relatively little progress in understanding the replication of these viruses at the protein level. The viral polymerase function is composed of at least five components: the viral proteins N (nucleocapsid), L (catalytic subunit), two transcription factors P protein and the M2-1 protein, as well as viral RNA in the form of ribonucleoprotein (Collins et al., 2001; Mason et al., 2004). Although crude extracts of infected cells can be prepared which are capable of making viral RNA (Herman, 1989), the enzyme complex has not been reassembled from recombinant expressed pure subunits. Nevertheless, Mason et al. (2004) have reported a moderate-throughput screen of potential inhibitors against a crude lysate assay in which they found hits from three distinct chemical classes. These authors report that one of their hit compounds—compound A, specifically inhibited the capping of viral RNA molecules; however, its therapeutic index was poor suggesting other mechanisms at work.

Using a traditional antiviral screening approach, Sudo et al. (2005) discovered an inhibitor of the polymerase catalytic subunit (L protein). This compound YM-53403 is a benzazepine with potent RSV activity. Virus mutants resistant to the compound were found to have mutations in the L protein gene. Consistent with this mechanism, the compound was highly specific for RSV and worked relatively late in the virus replication cycle as determined by time of addition studies.

Our own screen for RSV inhibitors largely revealed new structures which inhibited virus fusion; however we also observed a benzodiazepine which worked much later in the virus growth cycle. Optimisation of this compound led to the discovery of A-60444, a chiral benzodiazepine compound currently in Phase II clinical trials. A-60444 has consistent activity of about 700 nM IC_{50} against a large range of clinical isolates of both the RSV A and B sub-types as well as a large therapeutic index (Carter et al., 2006, Henderson et al., 2006 submitted to Journal of Medicinal Chemistry). The activity of the compound is restricted to human and bovine RSV with no activity against PVM or other Paramyxoviruses. *In vitro* mutants of RSV resistant to the compound have been isolated and have been shown to have acquired mutations in the N protein—the nucleocapsid protein of the virus. The compound showed potent activity in the differentiated human epithelium model (Zhang et al., 2002). The compound was found to have a combination of good pharmacokinetic properties and low toxicity, facilitating its evaluation in human trials. A considered decision was made to avoid the use of animal models (given their lack of validation for inhibitors of virus replication), and to gain sufficient pre-clinical data to enable the entry of the compound into human trials.

Phase 1 clinical trials of A-60444 have shown it to be well absorbed in the presence of food. A single daily dose of the compound provides plasma concentrations in excess of the IC_{90} for 24 h. No safety issues were identified in the Phase 1 trials (Dent et al., 2005). Currently, A-60444 is undergoing a Phase II clinical trial in stem cell transplant recipients who have become infected with RSV. Results from this latter trial are expected during 2006.

Miscellaneous (unknown) mechanisms

Given the relative simplicity with which compounds can be tested for activity against RSV and the difficulty of developing biochemical assays for individual virus components, it is not surprising that there is a list of compounds for which no mechanism has been elucidated. These compounds include: (1) pyridobenzazoles (Chiba et al., 1995); (2) cyclopentyl-adamantanamines (Fytas et al., 1994); (3) carbocyclic 3-deazaadenosine (Wyde et al., 1990a); (4) thiadiazol–cyanamide (Wyde et al., 1990b); (5) glutamine analogues (Huang et al., 1994) and (6) phosphonacetyl-N-Aspartate (Wyde et al., 1995). For most of these compounds the only data available is *in vitro* and *in vivo* antiviral efficacy. The lack of attention to these compounds is probably due to their lack of chemical tractability or attractiveness.

Inhibiting host cell functions

There is considerable interest in inhibiting host cell functions, which are obligate for virus replication but which can be inhibited without affecting cell viability. Such compounds may have considerable potential to avoid the development of antiviral resistance. The best-known inhibitor of RSV, ribavirin, may itself work through host cell functions but little is known of the detail even after many years of clinical use. One mechanism proposed for ribavirin was inhibition of IMPDH (IMP dehydrogenase), which caused Vertex to synthesise VX-497, a compound with much improved activity against this enzyme. Unfortunately, although the compound was more potent against RSV, its therapeutic index was not improved.

Our view is that, while host cell functions may indeed be future targets of antiviral drugs, we need to know far more about human cell functions before such compounds can be reliably designed.

Antisense compounds and siRNA

The seductive theoretical selectivity of using nucleic acid sequences to inhibit viral functions has caused a lot of R&D expenditure over the years. It is relatively easy to demonstrate extreme selectivity of these approaches *in vitro* but careful controls often show that the actual mechanisms differ from the theoretical. Antisense approaches have been unsuccessful because of such off-target activity and the extreme technical difficulty of delivery of nucleic acid-based drugs to target organs *in vivo*. Nevertheless Leaman et al. (2002) claimed to produce a positive result in the African green monkey model of RSV infection.

The recent advent of siRNA approaches has rekindled interest in this area. Indeed the first demonstration of the antiviral effects of siRNA was claimed by Bitko and Barik (2001) for RSV in a reverse genetics study. Extension of this work to *in vivo* studies showed an apparent effect of the siRNA in the mouse model of RSV infection (Bitko et al., 2005). In this approach, the authors used siRNAs that had *in vitro* IC_{50}s of 15–20 nM simply delivered to the mouse nasal passages in a transfection reagent. Their experiments seem to demonstrate excellent control of infection in both prophylactic and therapeutic modes. Unfortunately, the usual criticisms of the mouse model apply (see the section on Animal models) and it would be interesting to see if similar siRNAs could control a PVM infection in its natural host or the bovine virus in the calf model. Importantly no controls were done to look at carry-over from the treated mouse to the virology assays *in vitro.*

In another approach, Zhang et al. (2005) used DNA vector-derived siRNAs targeted at the NS1 protein in similar experiments. In this case, nanoparticles were used to deliver the DNA vectors *in vivo*. The potency of the different siRNAs was not determined but a significant reduction in virus yield was seen in interferon-producing A549 cells but not in Vero cells. The authors think these siRNAs work by abrogating the anti-interferon response of NS1. The *in vivo* effects were again assayed in the mouse model. The results were less impressive and less specific than those seen by Bitko et al. (2005). Again, it is frustrating not to see the same approach explored in the PVM model, which is absolutely suitable for such molecules.

These early experiments in the mouse model have led a US biotechnology company Alnylam (http://www.alnylam.com/) to file an IND with the FDA for human studies of such a siRNA. There is limited information on the molecule(s) they intend to study but the general data would suggest this would be a chemically modified short siRNA delivered in a vehicle via the intranasal route. Alnylam have not disclosed their preferred clinical trial plan. It will be interesting to see if clinical success ensues.

There are many general concerns about siRNA, partly because this approach is so new.

- *Safety*. There are many off-target effects of these molecules (Eckstein, 2005). Those on RNA expression can and need to be fully evaluated by array analysis. Unfortunately, siRNAs can also function as miRNAs, which exert their function at the translational level requiring a fuller analysis of protein effects. This may be important for example in controlling tumour growth requiring long-term toxicological analysis.
- *Pharmacodynamics*. Delivery of these molecules in a safe and effective manner is not a trivial task. The most compelling evidence for *in vivo* activity required high-pressure i.v. delivery to the mouse.

- *Resistance*. Because an almost 100% base match is required for siRNA activity, it may be easy for viruses like RSV to escape from the effects of single or even combinations of siRNAs.

It will be interesting to see how these challenges to a novel approach are dealt with.

Future prospects

As recently as last year, Maggon and Barik (2004) presented a rather pessimistic picture of the position of new drug development for RSV. This was more than justified at the time, as there had been a considerable lack of pharmaceutical discovery effort in this area. The last year has seen the emergence of several promising programmes at least one of which has reached clinical trials (Carter et al., 2006). While it remains to be seen how effective these new entities will prove in the only relevant model—man—we can be more optimistic. The success of Synagis has proven the market for new RSV therapies and re-energised the search for novel therapies. The fruits of this activity should be seen flowing through to the clinic over the next few years.

Acknowledgements

We would like to thank our colleagues at Arrow Therapeutics for their input to this review and to the research programme that led to A-60444.

References

Andries K, Moeremans. Gevers M, Willebrords R, Sommen C, Lacrampe J, Janssens F, Wyde PR. Substituted benzimadazoles with nanomolar activity against respiratory syncytial virus. Antiviral Res 2003; 60: 209–219.

Antonis AFG, Schrijver RS, Daus F, Steverink PJGM, Stockhofe N, Hensen EJ, Langedijk JPM, VanderMost RG. Vaccine-induced immunopathology during bovine respiratory syncytial virus infection: exploring the parameters of pathogenesis. J Virol 2003; 77: 12067–12073.

Barnard DL, Hill CL, Gage T, Matheson JE, Huffman JH, Sidwell RW, Otto MI, Schinazi RF. Potent inhibition of respiratory syncytial virus by polyoxometalates of several structural classes. Antiviral Res 1997; 34: 27–37.

Barnard DL, Huffman JH, Meyerson LR, Sidwell RW. Mode of inhibition of respiratory syncytial virus by a plant flavanoid, SP-303. Chemotherapy 1993; 39: 212–217.

Bitko V, Barik S. Phenotypic silencing of cytoplasmic genes using sequence-specific double-stranded short interfering RNA and its applications in the reverse genetics of wild type negative-strand RNA viruses. BMC Microbiol 2001; 1: 34.

Bitko V, Musiyenko A, Shulyayeva O, Barik S. Inhibition of respiratory viruses by nasally administered siRNA. Nat Med 2005; 11: 50–55.

Bond S, Sanford VA, Lambert JN, Lim CY, Mitchell JP, Draffan AG, Nearn RH. Polycyclic agents for the treatment of respiratory syncytial virus infections. 2005; WO 2005/061516 A1.

Budge PJ, Li Y, Beeler JA, Graham BS. RhoA-derived peptide dimers share mechanistic properties with other polyanionic inhibitors of respiratory syncytial virus (RSV), including disruption of viral attachment and dependence on RSV G. J Virol 2004; 78: 5015–5022.

Calfee DP, Peng AW, Cass LM, Lobo M, Hayden FG. Safety and efficacy of intravenous zanamivir in preventing experimental human influenza A virus infection. Antimicrob Agents Chemother 1999; 43: 1616–1620.

Carter MC, Alber DA, Baxter RC, Bithell SK, Cockerill GS, Dowdell VCL, Henderson EA, Keegan SJ, Kelsey RD, Stables JN, Wilson LJ, Powell KL. Investigation of 1, 4-Benzodiazepine as inhibitors of respiratory syncytial virus. J Med Chem 2006; 49: 2311–2319.

Chiba T, Shigeta S, Numazaki Y. Inhibitory effect of pyridobenzazoles on virus replication *in vitro*. Biol Pharm Bull 1995; 18: 1081–1083.

Cianci C, Genovesi EV, Lamb L, Medina I, Yang Z, Zadjura L, Yang H, D'Arienzo C, Sin N, Yu K-L, Combrink K, Li Z, Colonno R, Meanwell N, Clark J, Krystal M. Oral efficacy of a respiratory syncytial virus inhibitor in rodent models of infection. Antimicrob Agents Chemother 2004a; 48: 2448–2454.

Cianci C, Langley DR, Dischino DD, Sun Y, Yu K-L, Stanley A, Roach J, Li Z, Dalterio R, Colonno R, Meanwell NA, Krystal M. Targeting a binding pocket within the trimer-of-hairpins: small-molecule inhibition of viral fusion. Proc Natl Acad USA 2004b; 101: 15046–15051.

Cianci C, Meanwell N, Krystall M. Antiviral activity and molecular mechanism of an orally active respiratory syncytial virus fusion inhibitor. J Antimicrob Chemother 2005; 55: 289–292.

Cianci C, Yu K-L, Combrink K, Sin N, Pearce B, Wang A, Civiello R, Voss S, Luo G, Kadow K, Genovesi EV, Venables B, Gulgeze H, Trehan A, James J, Lamb L, Medina I, Roach J, Yang Z, Zadjura L, Colonno R, Clark J, Meanwell N, Krystal M. Orally active fusion inhibitor of respiratory syncytial virus. Antimicrob Agents Chemother 2004c; 48: 413–422.

Collins PL, Chanock RM, Murphy BR. Respiratory syncytial virus. In: Fields Virology (Knipe DM, Howley PM, editors). 4th ed. Philadelphia, PA: Lippincott, Williams & Wilkins; 2001; pp. 1433–1485.

Cook PM, Eglin RP, Easton AJ. Pathogenesis of pneumovirus infections in mice: detection of pneumonia virus of mice and human respiratory syncytial virus mRNA in lungs of infected mice by *in situ* hybridization. J Gen Virol 1998; 79: 2411–2417.

De Vicenzo JP, El Saleeby CM, Bush AJ. Respiratory syncytial virus load predicts disease severity in previously healthy infants. J Infect Dis 2005; 191: 1861–1868.

Dent J, Grieve S, Harland D, Alber D, Keegan S, Sanderson B, Lonsdale F, Thompson E, Smith G, Allan G, Powell K. Multi-dose safety and pharmacokinetics of A-60444, a novel compound active against respiratory syncytial virus (RSV). Abstract F438/287 45th ICAAC meeting, Washington, DC; 2005.

Douglas JL, Panis ML, Ho E, Lin K-Y, Krawczyk SH, Grant DM, Cai R, Swaminathan S, Chen X, Cihlar T. Small molecules VP-14637 and JNJ-2408068 inhibit respiratory syncytial virus fusion by similar mechanisms. Antimicrob Agents Chemother 2005; 49: 2460–2466.

Dubovi EJ, Geratz JD, Tidwell RR. Inhibition of respiratory syncytial virus by bis (5-amidino-2-benzimidazolyl) methane. Virology 1980; 103: 502–509.

Eckstein F. Small non-coding RNAs as magic bullets. Trends Biochem Sci 2005; 30: 445–452.

Falsey AR, Formica MA, Treanor JJ, Walsh EE. Comparison of quantitative reverse transcription-PCR to viral culture for assessment of respiratory syncytial virus shedding. J Clin Microbiol 2003; 41: 4160–4165.

Field HJ, Bell SE, Elion GB, Nash AA, Wildy P. Effect of acycloguanosine treatment on acute and latent herpes simplex infections in mice. Antimicrob Agents Chemother 1979; 15: 554–561.

Fytas G, Marakos P, Kolocouris N, Foscolos GB, Pouli N, Vamvakides A, Ikeda S, De Clercq E. 3-cyclopentyl-1-adamantanamines and adamantemethanamines. Antiviral activity evaluation and convulsion studies. Farmacology 1994; 49: 641–647.

Gabrielsen B, Phelan MJ, Barthel-Rosa L, See C, Huggins JW, Kefauver DF, Monath TP, Ussery MA, Chmurny GN, Schubert EM. Synthesis and antiviral evaluation of N-carboxamidine-substituted analogues of 1-beta-D-ribofuranosyl-1,2,4-triazole-3-carboxamidine hydrochloride. J Med Chem 1992; 35: 3231–3238.

Gower TL, Graham BS. Antiviral activity of lovastatin against respiratory syncytial virus *in vivo* and *in vitro*. Antimicrob Agents Chemother 2001; 45: 1231–1237.

Groothius JR, Simoes E, Levin MJ, Hall CB, Long CE, Rodriguez WJ, Arrobio J, Meissner HC, Fulton DR, Welliver RC, Tristram DA, Siber GR, Price GA, Van Raden M, Hemming VG. for the Respiratory Syncytial Virus Immune Globulin Study Group Prophylactic administration of respiratory syncytial virus immune globulin to high-risk infants and young children. New Engl J Med 1993; 329: 1524–1530.

Hall CB. Prevention of infections with respiratory syncytial virus: the hopes and hurdles ahead. Rev Inf Dis 1980; 2: 384–392.

Hancock GE, Tebbey PW. Antiviral compositions which inhibit Paramyxovirus infection. WO 2005/066205 A2; 2005.

Hayden FG, Andries K, Janssen PA. Safety and efficacy of intranasal pirodavir (R77975) in experimental rhinovirus infection. Antimicrob Agents Chemother 1992; 36: 727–732.

Hayden FG, Herrington DT, Coats TL, Kim K, Cooper EC, Villano SA, Liu S, Hudson S, Pevear DC, Collett M, McKinlay M, Pleconaril Respiratory Infection Study Group. (2003) Efficacy and safety of oral pleconaril for treatment of colds due to picornaviruses in adults: results of 2 double-blind, randomized, placebo-controlled trials. Clin Inf Dis 2003; 37: 1523–1532.

Hayden FG, Treanor JJ, Fritz RS, Lobo M, Betts RF, Miller M, Kinnersly N, Mills RG, Ward P, Straus SE. Use of the oral neuraminidase inhibitor oseltamivir in experimental human influenza: randomized controlled trials for prevention and treatment. J Am Med Assoc 1999; 282: 1246–1249.

Herman RC. Synthesis of respiratory syncytial virus RNA in cell-free extracts. J Gen Virol 1989; 70: 755–761.

Hruska JF, Bernstein JM, Gordon Douglas Jr. R, Hall CB. Effects of Ribavirin on respiratory syncytial virus *in vitro*. Antimicrob Agents Chemother 1980; 17: 770–775.

Huang RC, Panin M, Romito RR, Huang YT. Inhibition of replication of human respiratory syncytial virus by 6-diazo-5-oxo-L-norleucine. Antiviral Res 1994; 25: 269–279.

Huntley CC, Weiss WJ, Gazumyan A, Buklan A, Feld B, Hu W, Jones TR, Murphy T, Nikitenko AA, O'Hara B, Prince G, Quartuccio S, Raifeld YE, Wyde P, O'Connell JF. RFI-641 a potent respiratory syncytial virus inhibitor. Antimicrob Agents Chemother 2002; 46: 841–847.

Ikeda S, Neyts J, Verma S, Wickramasinghe A, Mohan P, De Clercq E. *In vitro* and *in vivo* inhibition of ortho- and paramyxovirus infections by a new class of sulfonic acid polymers interacting with virus-cell binding and/or fusion. Antimicrob Agents Chemother 1994; 38: 256–259.

Kapikian AZ, Mitchell RH, Chanock RM, Shvedoff RA, Stewart CE. An epidemiological study of altered clinical reactivity to respiratory syncytial (RS) virus infection in children previously vaccinated with an inactivated RS virus vaccine. Am J Epidemiol 1969; 89: 405–421.

Kimura K, Ishioka K, Hashimoto K, Mori S, Suzutani T, Bowlin TL, Shigeta S. Isolation and characterization of NMSO3-resistant mutants of respiratory syncytial virus. Antiviral Res 2004; 61: 165–171.

Kimura K, Mori S, Tomita K, Ohno K, Takahashi K, Shigeta S, Terada M. Antiviral activity of NMSO3 against respiratory syncytial virus infection *in vitro* and *in vivo*. Antiviral Res 2000; 47: 41–51.

Lackey JW, Kinder DS, Tvermoes NA. Benzimidazole compounds and antiviral uses thereof. WO 02/092575 A1; 2002.

Larder BA, Purifoy DJM, Powell KL, Darby G. Site-specific mutagenesis of AIDS virus reverse transcriptase. Nature 1987; 327: 716–717.

Leaman DW, Longano FJ, Okicki JR, Soike KF, Torrence PF, Silverman RH, Cramer H. Targeted therapy of respiratory syncytial virus in African green monkeys by intranasally administered 2-5A antisense. Virology 2002; 292: 70–77.

Lee FE, Walsh EE, Falsey AR, Betts RF, Treanor JJ. Experimental infection of humans with A2 respiratory syncytial virus. Antiviral Res 2004; 63: 191–196.

Maggon K, Barik S. New drugs and treatment for respiratory syncytial virus. Rev Med Virol 2004; 14: 149–168.

Markland W, McQuaid TJ, Jain J, Kwong AD. Broad-spectrum antiviral activity of the IMP dehydrogenase inhibitor VX-497: a comparison with ribavirin and demonstration of antiviral additivity with alpha interferon. Antimicrob Agents Chemother 2000; 44: 859–866.

Mason SW, Lawetz C, Gaudette Y, Dô F, Scouten E, Legacé L, Simoneau B, Liuzzi M. Polyadenylation-dependent screening assay for respiratory syncytial virus RNA transcriptase activity and identification of an inhibitor. Nucleic Acids Res 2004; 32: 4758–4767.

McKimm-Breschkin J. VP-14637 ViroPharma. Curr Opin Invest Drugs 2000; 1: 425–427.

Nikitenko AA, Raifeld YE, Wang TZ. The discovery of RFI-641 as a potent and selective inhibitor of the respiratory syncytial virus. Bioorg Med Chem Lett 2001; 11: 1041–1044.

Ohki S, Liu JZ, Schaller J, Welliver RC. The compound DATEM inhibits respiratory syncytial virus fusion activity with epithelial cells. Antiviral Res 2003; 58: 115–124.

Pastey MK, Gower TL, Spearman PW, Crowe Jr. JE, Graham BS. A RhoA-derived peptide inhibits syncytium formation induced by respiratory syncytial virus and parainfluenza virus type 3. Nat Med 2000; 6: 35–40.

Perkins SM, Webb DL, Torrance SA, El Saleeby C, Harrison LM, Aitken JA, Patel A, DeVincenzo JP. Comparison of a real-time reverse transcriptase PCR assay and a culture technique for quantitative assessment of viral load in children naturally infected with respiratory syncytial virus. J Clin Microbiol 2005; 43: 2356–2362.

Prince GA, Horswood RL, Berndt J, Suffin SC, Chanock RM. Respiratory syncytial virus infection in inbred mice. Infect Immun 1979; 26: 764–766.

Starpharma web site – www.starpharma.com

Sudo K, Konno K, Watanabe W, Shigeta S, Yokata . Mechanism of selective inhibition of respiratory syncytial virus by a benzodithiin compound (RD3-0028). Microbiol Immunol 2001; 45: 531–537.

Sudo K, Miyazaki Y, Kojima N, Kobayashi M, Suzuki H, Shintani M, Shimizu Y. YM-53403, a unique anti-respiratory syncytial virus agent with a novel mechanism of action. Antiviral Res 2005; 65: 125–131.

Taylor G, Stott EJ, Hughes M, Collins AP. Respiratory syncytial virus infection in mice. Infect Immun 1984; 43: 649–655.

Taylor G, Thomas LH, Furze JM, Cook RS, Wyld SG, Lerch R, Hardy R, Wertz GW. Recombinant vaccinia viruses expressing the F, G or N, but not the M2, protein of bovine respiratory syncytial virus (BRSV) induce resistance to BRSV challenge in the calf and protect against the development of pneumonic lesions. J Gen Virol 1997; 78: 3195–3206.

The Impact-RSV Study Group. Palivizumab, a humanized respiratory syncytial virus monoclonal antibody, reduces hospitalization from respiratory syncytial virus infection in high-risk infants. Pediatrics 1998; 102: 531–537.

Tidwell RR, Geratz JD, Clyde Jr. WA, Rosenthal KU, Dubovi EJ. Suppression of respiratory syncytial virus infection in cotton rats by Bis (5-Amidino-2-Benzimidazolyl) Methane. Antimicrob Agents Chemother 1984; 26: 591–593.

Van den Hoogen BG, Bestebroer TM, Osterhaus AD, Fouchier RA. Analysis of the genomic sequence of a human metapneumovirus. Virology 2002; 295: 119–132.

Watanabe W, Sudo K, Sata R, Kajiyashiki T, Konno K, Shigeta S, Yokota T. Novel anti-respiratory syncytial (RS) viral compounds: benzodithiin derivatives. Biochem Biophys Res Commun 1998; 249: 922–926.

Woolums AR, Anderson ML, Gunther RA, Schelegle ES, LaRochelle DR, Singer RS, Boyle GA, Fribertshauser KE, Gershwin LJ. Am J Veter Res 1999; 60: 473–480.

Wyde PR, Ambrose MW, Meyerson LR, Gibert BE. Antiviral Res 1993; 20(2): 145–154.

Wyde PR, Ambrose MW, Meyer HL, Gilbert BE. Toxicity and antiviral activity of LY253963 against respiratory syncytial and parainfluenza type 3 viruses in tissue culture and in cotton rats. Antiviral Res. 1990a; 14: 237–247.

Wyde PR, Ambrose MW, Meyer HL, Zolinski CL, Gilbert BE. Evaluation of the toxicity and antiviral activity of carbocyclic 3-deazaadenosine against respiratory syncytial and parainfluenza type 3 viruses in tissue culture and in cotton rats. Antiviral Res 1990b; 14: 215–225.

Wyde PR, Chetty SN, Timmerman P, Gilbert BE, Andries K. Short duration aerosols of JNJ 2408068 (R170591) administered prophylactically or therapeutically protect cotton rats from experimental respiratory syncytial virus infection. Antivir Res 2003; 60: 221–231.

Wyde PR, Laquerre S, Chetty SN, Gilbert BE, Nitz TJ, Pevear DC. Antiviral efficacy of VP14637 against respiratory syncytial virus *in vitro* and in cotton rats following delivery by small droplet aerosol. Antivir Res 2005; 68: 18–26.

Wyde PR, Moore DK, Pimentel DM, Blough HA. Evaluation of the antiviral activity of N-(phosphonoacetyl)-L-aspartate against paramyxoviruses in tissue culture and against respiratory syncytial virus in cotton rats. Antiviral Res 1995; 27: 59–69.

Wyde PR, Wilson SZ, Petrella R, Gilbert BE. Efficacy of high dose—short duration ribavirin aerosol in the treatment of respiratory syncytial virus infected cotton rats and influenza B virus infected mice. Antiviral Res 1987; 7: 211–220.

Zhang L, Peeples ME, Boucher RC, Collins PL, Pickles RJ. Respiratory syncytial virus infection of human airway epithelial cells is polarized, specific to ciliated cells and without obvious cytopathology. J Virol 2002; 76: 5654–5666.

Zhang W, Yang H, Kong X, Mohapatra S, Juan-Vergara HS, Hellermann G, Behera S, Singam R, Lockey RF, Mohapatra SS. Inhibition of respiratory syncytial virus infection with intranasal siRNA nanoparticles targeting the viral NS1 gene. Nat Med 2005; 11: 56–62.

Respiratory Syncytial Virus
Patricia Cane (Editor)

DOI 10.1016/S0168-7069(06)14010-0

Pneumonia Virus of Mice

Andrew J. Easton[a], Joseph B. Domachowske[b], Helene F. Rosenberg[c]

[a]*Department of Biological Sciences, University of Warwick, Coventry CV4 7AL, UK*
[b]*Department of Pediatrics, State University of New York Upstate Medical University, 750 East Adams Street, Syracuse, New York 13210, USA*
[c]*Laboratory of Allergic Diseases, National Institute of Allergy and Infectious Diseases, National Institutes of Health, Bethesda, MD 20892, USA*

In 1939, Horsfall and Hahn reported the isolation of a new virus which caused pneumonia in mice (Horsfall and Hahn, 1939, 1940). The virus was obtained by passage of lung suspensions from apparently healthy mice into equally healthy outbred recipient mice. The virus became known as pneumonia virus of mice (PVM). Thirty-five years later, PVM was identified as the first isolated pneumovirus.

Infection of mice is only possible by the intranasal route. In the original studies, the inoculated mice showed considerable lung consolidation and by passage six of the original material, approximately 24% of animals succumbed to a fatal pneumonia. The lung consolidation seen with PVM is distinct from that seen with other viruses such as influenza and observation of the pathology shows that the disease progresses from a bronchiolitis to pneumonia. We now know a great deal about the pathogenesis of PVM infection in inbred strains of mice, as discussed in detail below. The pathology that is seen with PVM is strikingly similar to that observed with severe respiratory syncytial virus (RSV) in humans, suggesting that the PVM/mouse system is an excellent model for the study of pneumovirus infections in a natural host.

The natural history of PVM

From the nature of its original isolation it was clear that PVM was a common infection in laboratory mice. Early serological studies detected PVM-specific antibodies in a wide range of laboratory animals, suggesting that it was widespread (Horsfall and Curnen, 1946; Table 1).

Table 1

Seropositivity for PVM in laboratory animals

Animal	% seropositive (n)
Mice	85.7
Hamster	48.6 (580)
Guinea-pig	66.7 (60)
Cotton rat	22.6 (1458)
Rabbit	13 (210)
Monkey	23.6 (106)
Chimpanzee	33.3 (6)

Source: Horsfall and Curnen (1946).

Later studies confirmed that PVM was prevalent in laboratory rodent colonies, in which it causes a mild or symptom-free infection in inbred strains of mice (Horsfall and Curnen, 1946; Parker et al., 1966; Poiley, 1970; Gannon and Carthew, 1980). Once established, PVM is extremely difficult to eradicate (Cunliffe-Beamer, 1988) and regular screening is now recommended to prevent infection. PVM infection has also been detected among wild rodent species. One study performed to estimate the prevalence of PVM in wild rodents in the UK demonstrated disease in 45% of wood mice and in 30% and 40% of two species of vole, respectively (Kaplan et al., 1980).

Initial analysis of human sera showed that PVM, or a serologically closely related virus, also infected humans (Horsfall and Curnen, 1946). Subsequently, using a more sensitive analysis, Pringle and Eglin (1986) showed that more than 75% of adults were seropositive for PVM, suggesting prior exposure or infection. Age-related studies showed that the anti-PVM-specific neutralising antibodies are acquired early in life, similar to what has been reported for RSV (Pringle and Eglin, 1986). No known clinical disease has been associated with PVM infection, and thus it is not considered to represent a health burden at the current time.

Neutralising antibodies specific for either PVM or RSV present in human sera or by inoculation of animals show no cross reactivity with the other virus. Despite this, as explained below, there is some serological cross reactivity between some of the RSV and PVM proteins, demonstrating their close evolutionary relationship (Gimenez et al., 1984; Ling and Pringle, 1989a). However, unlike RSV, PVM can agglutinate mouse red blood cells (Mills and Dochez, 1944, 1945). Since the virus does not appear to spread beyond the lung it is likely that this characteristic is not relevant to disease but merely reflects the ability of the virus to bind to carbohydrates present on the surface of murine red blood cells.

Characteristics of the PVM virion

Electron microscopic analysis of the PVM virion gave the first evidence that it was a pneumovirus (Compans et al., 1967; Berthiaume et al., 1974). The virion is enveloped and pleiomorphic, with a variety of morphologies ranging from spherical to filamentous. The structure of the virion nucleocapsid distinguishes pneumoviruses from all other paramyxoviruses and presumably reflects the distinct nature of the proteins which constitute the nucleocapsid complex.

The molecular biology of PVM

The complete nucleotide sequence of three isolates of PVM have now been determined (Krempl et al., 2005; Thorpe and Easton, 2005). Initial sequencing studies focused on strain 15, obtained from the original stock of PVM deposited at the American Type Culture Collection (ATCC). This strain was passaged continuously in tissue culture for almost 20 years and animal studies showed that it was non-pathogenic in mice though it replicated efficiently (Cook et al., 1998; see below). Subsequently, an aliquot of strain 15 from ATCC tested directly in mice was shown to have retained pathogenicity (Krempl and Collins, 2004). The likeliest explanation for the difference in pathogenicity of the two stocks is that the extensive passage in tissue culture has moderated the pathogenicity of the virus, although this has not been demonstrated directly (Krempl and Collins, 2004). For ease, the original strain 15 will be referred to as strain 15 (Warwick). Both of these strains have been completely sequenced. Another isolate obtained in the early studies, designated strain J3666, which has been maintained in mouse passage only, and which is highly pathogenic, has also been sequenced (Thorpe and Easton, 2005).

Genome organisation

The genome organisation of PVM closely resembles that of RSV. The genome encodes 10 mRNAs arranged in a linear array along the genome (Fig. 1). The genes are flanked by conserved gene start and gene end sequences. The consensus PVM gene start sequence (AGGAyAArT) shows a high degree of conservation and has feature of those of RSV (GGGGCAATa) and avian pneumovirus (GGGACAAGT) (Collins et al., 1986; Chambers et al., 1990; Yu et al., 1991, 1992a, b, 1995; Li et al., 1992, 1996; Ling et al., 1995; Randhawa et al., 1996a, b). In contrast, the PVM gene end sequence (tAGTtAnnn(An)) is not well conserved between the genes (Chambers et al., 1990).

The similarity of genome organisation of PVM and RSV suggests that the two viruses are likely to share many common features in their replication and gene expression strategies. Most, but not all, PVM genes and the proteins they encode share a high degree of similarity with their homologues in RSV (Barr et al., 1991, 1994; Chambers et al., 1991, 1992; Randhawa et al., 1995; Easton and Chambers, 1997; Ahmadian et al., 1999; Table 2).

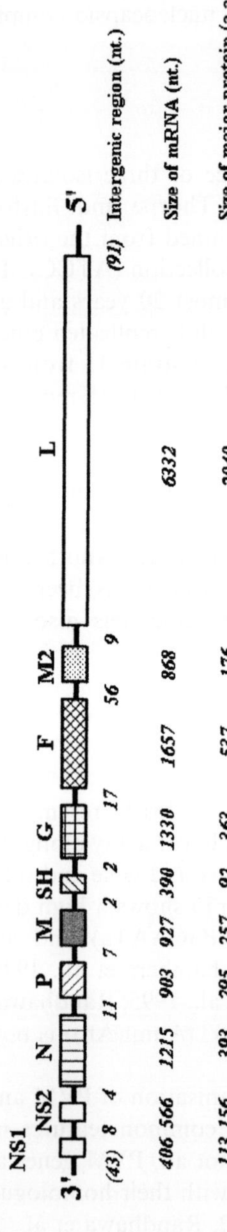

Fig. 1 Organisation of the genome of PVM strain 15 (Warwick). The sizes of the mRNAs, the sizes of the major encoded proteins and the intergenic regions are shown. The sizes of the 3′ terminal (leader) and 5′ terminal (trailer) regions are shown in brackets.

Table 2

Amino acid similarities between human RSV (strain A2) and PVM (strain 15 Warwick) genes and the encoded proteins

	NS1	NS2	N	P	M	SH	G	F	M2-1	L
Amino acid identity	21	28	61	37	42	27	18	40	40	43

PVM proteins

The proteins of the nucleocapsid complex

The nucleocapsid (N) protein of PVM shares the highest degree of similarity with the RSV counterpart of all of the virus proteins (Barr et al., 1991) and is believed to play the same structural role in the formation of the helical nucleocapsid complex in association with the viral RNA genome. The PVM and RSV N proteins show cross reactivity with specific antisera and the central portion of the proteins contain a region of 68 identical residues out of 71 (96% identity). Sequence alignments of the pneumovirus, and all other paramyxovirus, nucleocapsid proteins suggest that they contain a similar arrangement of structural features (Barr et al., 1991). Analysis of the binding of the PVM N protein with the phosphoprotein using a far western approach indicated that both the amino- and carboxy-termini of the N protein were involved in the interaction (Barr and Easton, 1995).

A significant difference between PVM and RSV is seen in the coding capacity of the phosphoprotein (P) gene. The RSV P gene contains a single open-reading frame (ORF) that encodes the P protein (Lambden et al., 1985). A second, minor, protein produced by internal initiation within the RSV P mRNA ORF has also been described (Caravokyri et al., 1992). In contrast, the PVM P gene contains two ORFs(Barr et al., 1994). The first ORF encodes the P protein. The PVM P protein is significantly longer than the RSV homologue and the sequence identity between these proteins is unequally distributed along their lengths (Barr et al., 1994). In particular, the PVM P protein contains a region towards the amino terminus, which does not have a counterpart in the RSV P protein. This region is encoded by the portion of the P gene mRNA which contains the second ORF. The protein product of the second ORF has been detected using P protein-specific antisera raised against peptides predicted from the nucleotide sequence (Barr et al., 1994). The function of this second ORF protein is not yet known. The PVM P gene resembles that of the paramyxovirus Sendai virus in encoding several additional proteins, each translated from AUG initiation codons within the P protein ORF. This process of internal initiation generates a nested set of four additional proteins, with the sequences of each entirely contained within the next largest in the series (Barr et al., 1994; Fig. 2). The functions of the additional P-related proteins are not known. The phosphorylated residues in the PVM P protein have not yet been identified.

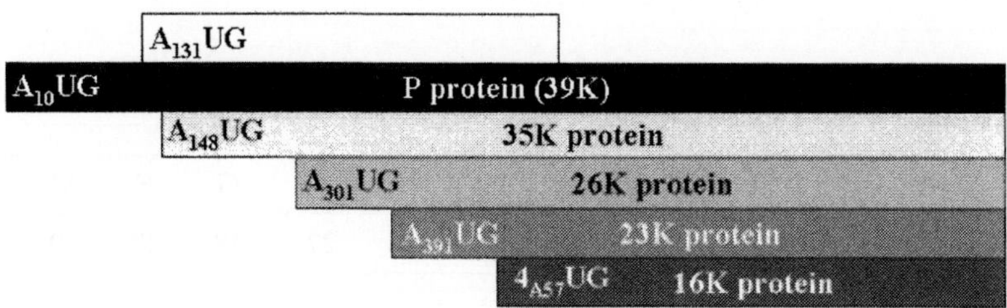

Fig. 2 Organisation of the open-reading frames in the PVM P gene. The positions of the AUG initiation codons in the P gene mRNA are indicated. Adapted from Barr et al. (1994).

Analysis of the interaction between the PVM N and P proteins has shown that the immediate carboxy terminus of the P protein contains the necessary sequences for the interaction to occur, with some potential involvement of the amino terminus (Slack and Easton, 1998). This is similar to the situation with the human and bovine RSV P proteins, suggesting that it is a common feature of pneumoviruses (Garcia-Barreno et al., 1996; Mallipeddi et al., 1996; Hengst and Kiefer, 2000; Khattar et al., 2001).

The L gene of PVM encodes a protein of 2040 amino acids and, by analogy with the L gene of other paramyxoviruses, this is believed to be the catalytic component of the virus RNA polymerase (Thorpe and Easton, 2005). Sequence alignments of the L proteins of PVM and RSV showed that the RSV protein contains a short stretch of amino acids at the amino terminus which is not present in the PVM, or indeed any other paramyxovirus, L protein. The significance of this is not clear. The PVM L protein contains all of the key motifs identified in other L proteins.

Like RSV, PVM contains a gene encoding an M2 protein. The mRNA from this gene contains two ORFs, the first encoding a protein (M2-1) which is highly conserved between the two viruses, and the second encoding a protein (M2-2) which shows essentially no amino acid sequence identity with the protein from the equivalent RSV ORF (Ahmadian et al., 1999). Translation of the second ORF in the RSV M2 gene has been shown to occur by a coupled translation termination/reinitiation process in which a proportion of the ribosomes terminating translation of the first ORF reinitiate translation at the upstream AUG codon at the beginning of the second ORF (Ahmadian et al., 2000). The PVM M2 gene has a similar organisation and the second ORF is accessed using the same process (Gould and Easton, unpublished). By analogy with the RSV homologues, the PVM M2-1 protein is anticipated to act in virus transcription, significantly enhancing the production of full-length mRNA (Grosfeld et al., 1995; Collins et al., 1995, 1996; Yu et al., 1995; Fearns and Collins, 1999). Reverse genetics experiments with PVM-based minigenomes have confirmed that the M2-1 protein acts like the RSV counterpart (Dibben et al., unpublished). The PVM M2-2 protein has been detected in infected cells using monospecific antiserum (Ahmadian et al., 1999). Expression of the RSV M2-2 ORF in reverse genetics experiments resulted in the inhibition of virus gene expression from synthetic genomes (Bermingham and Collins, 1999). Despite the lack of any sequence identity the PVM M2-2 protein also acts like its RSV homologue, inhibiting transcription from the virus genome (O. Dibben et al., unpublished).

The membrane glycoproteins and membrane-associated matrix (M) protein

The PVM G protein shares several structural features with the G protein of RSV. Both proteins contain a large number of serine and threonine residues, representing up to 30% of the total mass (Wertz et al., 1985; Randhawa et al., 1995). Monoclonal antibodies directed against the PVM G protein inhibit the virus haemagglutination activity which is consistent with the role of the G protein as the attachment protein for the virus (Ling and Pringle, 1989b). The G protein is a type II glycoprotein, with the carboxy terminus presented on the external surface of the virion and infected cell. As with the RSV G protein, the PVM protein is extensively modified by addition of both N- and O-linked sugars, which alters the mass from approximately 35,000 for the unmodified protein to approximately 80,000 for the fully processed molecule. The O-linked sugars are the most predominant modification (Ling and Pringle, 1989b). Analysis of the PVM G protein generated in infected cells in the presence of glycosylation inhibitors revealed the presence of two proteins (Ling and Pringle, 1989b). These were not characterised further but suggest that, as for RSV, PVM makes two forms of G protein. In RSV one is membrane-bound and the other, a product of internal initiation in the G protein ORF followed by post-translational proteolytic cleavage, is a secreted form which may play a role in pathogenesis (Roberts et al., 1994; Johnson et al., 1998; Johnson and Graham, 1999).

The sequence analysis of the G genes of the non-pathogenic PVM strain 15 (Warwick) and pathogenic strain J3666 revealed some intriguing differences. The G gene of strain 15 (Warwick) does not have an amino-terminal sequence prior to the putative membrane anchor region. In contrast, the strain J3666 G protein contains a 35-residue sequence prior to the membrane anchor (Randhawa et al., 1995). This represents the most significant genetic difference between the pathogenic and non-pathogenic strains.

Interestingly, both the RSV and PVM G genes contain a short ORF upstream of the major G protein coding ORF (Wertz et al., 1985; Randhawa et al., 1995). This conservation of genetic organisation suggests that the upstream ORF may have a role in the control of expression of the downstream, G protein, ORF.

The pneumovirus fusion (F) proteins are type I glycoproteins and contain an amino-terminal signal sequence which is cleaved during processing of the protein. The proteins contain a small number of potential N-linked glycosylation sites, which are utilised (Collins et al., 1984; Ling and Pringle, 1989b; Chambers et al., 1992). A recent development in studies on the RSV F protein identified a second cleavage site which, when utilised, released a short peptide (Gonzalez-Reyes et al., 2001;

Zimmer et al., 2001, 2002, 2003; Begona Ruiz-Arguello et al., 2002). The peptide, termed virokinin, has significant immunomodulatory properties. Alignment of the PVM and RSV F protein sequences show that the PVM protein lacks this additional cleavage site and also does not contain a sequence equivalent to the virokinin region (Chambers et al., 1992). This raises questions about the precise role of the virokinin in pathogenesis of pneumovirus infections.

PVM encodes a small hydrophobic (SH) protein which is believed to be analogous to that of RSV (Collins and Wertz, 1985; Easton and Chambers, 1997). The PVM protein, with 92 residues is significantly larger than the 64 or 65 residue RSV SH protein. The PVM SH protein contains two hydrophobic domains in contrast to the single domain in the RSV protein. It is not yet known whether the PVM SH protein crosses the membrane twice or whether the protein is anchored by a single hydrophobic domain as is the case with the RSV SH protein. As with RSV, the role of the PVM SH protein during infection is not known. Comparison of the genome sequences of the non-pathogenic strain 15 (Warwick) and pathogenic strain J3666 identified a large amount of variation in the SH gene (Thorpe and Easton, 2005). This may indicate a role in pathogenesis, but this remains to be established.

The matrix (M) protein is an integral protein in the virion, forming a protein layer underneath the virus envelope. It has been proposed that the M protein coordinates the association of the nucleocapsid complex with the cellular membrane containing the virus F, G and SH proteins prior to budding of the virion. The PVM M protein conforms to the structure seen in other matrix proteins and shares a significant degree of sequence identity with the RSV M protein throughout its length (Easton and Chambers, 1997).

The non-structural proteins NS1 and NS2

The NS1 and NS2 genes of RSV have been shown to moderate the host interferon response (Schlender et al., 2000; Bossert & Conzelmann, 2002; Bossert et al., 2003; Valarcher et al., 2003; Spann et al., 2004; Ramaswamy et al., 2006). An initial analysis of the PVM NS genes indicated that they too acted to suppress the interferon response (Bossert et al., 2001). Despite this, the NS1 and NS2 proteins of PVM and RSV show no significant sequence identity (Table 1). Like their RSV counterparts, the sequences of the PVM NS genes show several similarities that suggest that they may have arisen by a gene duplication event after which the genes have diverged. It is tempting to speculate that the conserved function but not sequence may indicate that the genes are 'tailored' for their natural hosts.

Pathogenesis of PVM infection in inbred strains of mice: basic biology

As PVM is a natural pathogen of rodent species, it engages the innate and acquired immune responses of mice in an evolutionarily meaningful fashion. Given the specific nature of the host–pathogen relationship, perhaps it is not surprising that respiratory infection with PVM in mice replicates many of the clinical features of the more severe forms of human RSV infection. (NB: all of the experimental work discussed in this section, except where noted, has been performed with the mouse-passaged, fully virulent PVM J3666 strain.) Intranasal inoculation with as few as 10–60 plaque forming units (pfu) of virus results in robust replication, leading to severe morbidity and mortality, and peak virus titres as high as 10^8 pfu per gram of lung tissue by day 5 post infection and declining rapidly thereafter (Domachowske et al., 2000a, b). This can be compared to the hRSV mouse challenge model, in which inocula of $> 10^6$ pfu are utilised, and limited virus replication is observed in association with minimal clinical symptoms (Taylor et al., 1984; Easton et al., 2004).

Following the course of infection in BALB/c mice using *in situ* hybridisation demonstrated that the virus initially appears in alveolar cells within two days (Cook et al., 1998). From the initial site of infection it spreads to neighbouring cells before appearing in the columnar epithelial cells lining the terminal bronchioles and the adjacent interstitial cells by day 4. It is at this site that the most significant pathological damage is seen (Fig. 3). The infected cells are sloughed off into the bronchiolar lumen. At the same time, additional proteinacous material accumulates in the lumen as is seen in typical bronchiolitis. It is notable that this damage appears before the virus titres reach their peak. The level of cellular damage is at its maximum around day 5 in response to 120 pfu in an inoculum volume of 50 μl. This is the critical time for the infected animals in determining whether they survive or succumb to a fatal pneumonia (Cook et al., 1998). By 8 days after the infection there are only sporadic sites of infection in the lungs of surviving mice. PVM has also been described as a wasting disease (Smith et al., 1984) and in these cases the weight loss is likely to be a secondary phenomenon due to changes in feeding behaviour as a result of respiratory distress.

The immunological response to infection

PVM replication in lung epithelial cells *in vivo* is accompanied by influx of granulocytes (Fig. 4) similar to the situation seen with severe hRSV infection in humans (Garofalo et al., 1992; Harrison et al., 1999; Domachowske et al., 2000b; Bonville et al., 2006a). The chemoattractant macrophage inflammatory protein 1α (MIP-1α), also produced in bronchial epithelial cells (Bonville et al., 2006a), is crucial for granulocyte recruitment in response to PVM infection (Domachowske et al., 2000b; Bonville et al., 2003). Biochemical or genetic elimination of MIP-1α or elimination or blockade of its major receptor, CCR1, results in a profound reduction in the PVM-mediated inflammatory response (Bonville et al., 2003, 2004). MIP-1α has likewise been implicated in eliciting granulocyte influx in response to hRSV infection in human subjects (Harrison et al., 1999) as well as in predicting the severity of disease (Garofalo et al., 2001). Other chemoattractants involved in promoting the inflammatory response to PVM infection include monocyte chemoattractant protein 1 (MCP-1) and MIP-2 (one of the mouse orthologs of interleukin-8 (IL-8)), which are also implicated in hRSV disease in human patients (Fiedler et al., 1996;

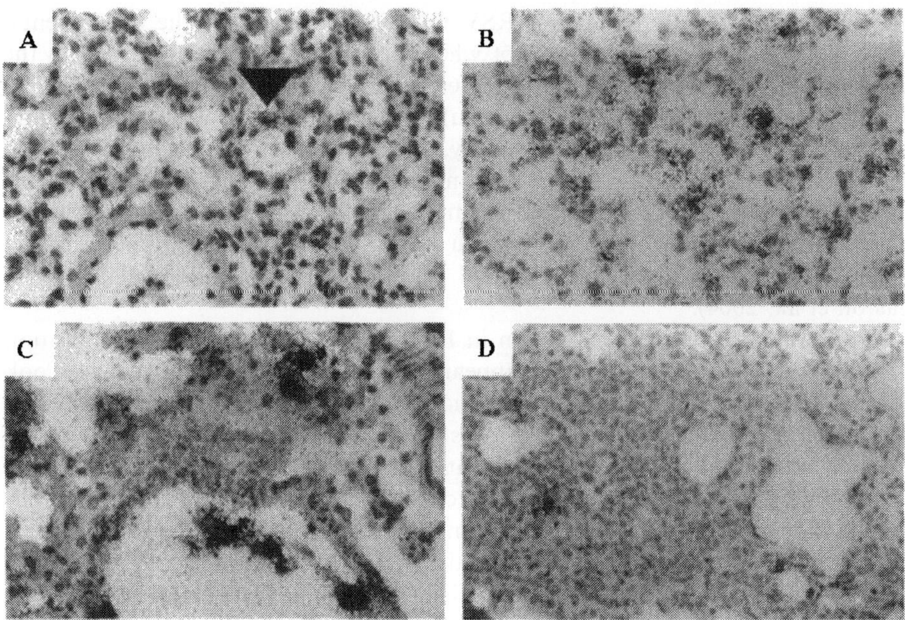

Fig. 3 *In situ* hybridisation showing the progression of PVM infection in mouse lung. Following infection with PVM strain J3666 PVM N gene mRNA was detected by hybridisation with a radioactive probe. Silver grains indicate the regions of infected tissue, indicated by an arrow in panel A. (A) Tissues prepared two days after infection, (B) tissues prepared three days after infection, (C) tissue prepared four days after infection, (D) tissues prepared eight days after infection. Taken with permission from Cook et al. (1998) (for colour version: see colour section on page 329).

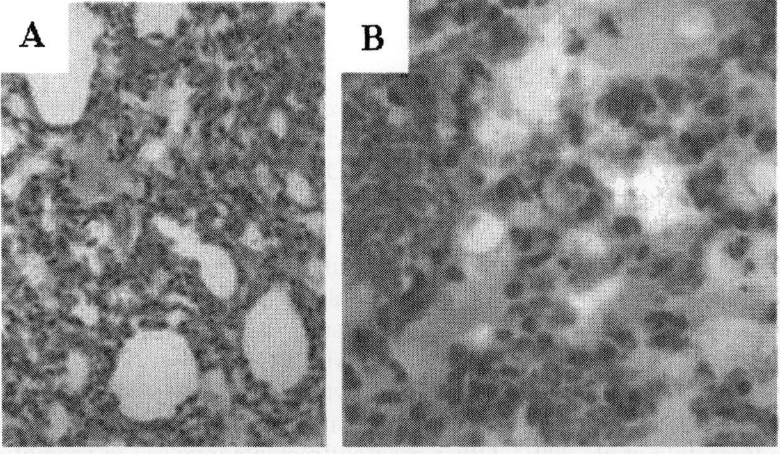

Fig. 4 Inflammation in lung tissue in response to PVM infection. (A) Original magnifications, 20X and (B) 40X. The influx of granulocytes and pulmonary oedema, which can progress to complete compromise of the airways, can be clearly seen. Images courtesy of Dr. John Ellis, Western College of Veterinary Medicine, University of Saskatchewan, Saskatoon, Canada. Reprinted with permission from Rosenberg et al. (2005) (for colour version: see colour section on page 329).

Casola et al., 2000; Hull et al., 2000). Expression patterns of MIP-1α, MCP-1, and MIP-2 correlate with the extent of PVM replication in lung tissue and with objective measures of lung dysfunction and clinical disease (Bonville et al., 2006a).

Antiviral T-cell responses in PVM-infected mice and recurrent pneumovirus infections

Although most of the focus to date has been on granulocyte recruitment, Claassen and colleagues (Claassen et al., 2005) defined three PVM-specific T-cell epitopes (one each on the P, M and F proteins), and have shown that a significant number of CD8+ T cells are recruited to the lungs of PVM-infected BALB/c mice at day 8 post inoculation. Interestingly, only approximately 2% of these CD8+ T cells were cytokine producing and PVM specific; PVM-specific CD8+ T cells were impaired in their ability to produce interferonγ (IFN-γ) and tumour necrosis factor α (TNF-α), suggesting that PVM replication results in their functional inactivation. This is an intriguing finding that the authors relate to the issue of partial immunity and recurrent pneumovirus infections.

Interferon-related responses in PVM-infected mice.

PVM infection in wild type-mice is associated with the transcription of IFN-β and an extensive collection of interferon-response genes (Domachowske et al., 2002). Garvey and colleagues (Garvey et al., 2005) defined the responses of PVM-infected IFNαβR-/- mice, and identified distinct lung pathology associated with preferential expression of eotaxin-2, thymus and activation-regulated chemokine (TARC), and mouse eosinophil-associated ribonuclease 11, and reduced expression of MCP-5, IP-10 and toll-like receptor (TLR3).

Explorations with the PVM infection model: therapeutic directions

PVM infection of mice presents an opportunity to explore potential therapeutic interventions in a natural host–pathogen system with the ease and sophisticated tools that are not readily available for study with the RSV pathogen. The similarity of the pattern of disease and the very close genetic relationship of the two viruses raises the hope that information from the PVM system may open up new possibilities for intervention in RSV infection and disease.

Use of the antiviral agent ribavirin for the treatment of acute pneumovirus infection

Among the more intriguing questions to be approached with the PVM infection model is that of the efficacy (or lack thereof) of the antiviral agent, ribavirin, for the treatment of severe pneumovirus infection. Ribavirin is a nucleoside analogue with a complex mechanism of action (Reyes, 2001; Hong and Cameron, 2002). While remarkably effective at inhibiting virus replication both in tissue culture and *in vivo*, a meta analysis of several crucial studies has supported clinical wisdom, indicating that ribavirin therapy has little impact on therapeutically meaningful outcomes when administered for severe hRSV disease in human infants (Randolph and Wang, 1996).

At the outset, this seems almost counterintuitive—how could a drug that reduces virus replication have so little impact on the outcome of a respiratory virus infection? As a first step, it has been possible to replicate this observation with the PVM infection model. When mice were infected with PVM and treated with ribavirin from day 3 post inoculation, virus replication ceased in response to the ribavirin treatment, while production of the proinflammatory chemokine MIP-1α, and recruitment of granulocytes did not. Ribavirin alone had little effect on measures of morbidity and mortality (Bonville et al., 2003). These results indicate that the inflammatory response is not inextricably linked to virus replication, and, once initiated and left unchecked, inflammation alone can result in morbidity and mortality even when virus replication ceased. Ribavirin alone does nothing to eliminate the inflammatory response to PVM infection in mice, which may explain its limited clinical efficacy in the setting of severe human RSV infection.

The role of glucocorticoids for the treatment of acute pneumovirus infection

A similar situation exists regarding the use of glucocorticoids. Physicians have routinely administered systemic glucocorticoids as broad-spectrum anti-inflammatory therapy for severe hRSV infection, both with and without ribavirin, yet the overall view is that this approach has marginal, if any clinical benefit (Garrison et al., 2000; Black, 2003). Although an evaluation of combination ribavirin–glucocorticoid therapy in the PVM-infected mouse model has not been carried out, the effects of systemic hydrocortisone alone have been evaluated (Domachowske et al., 2001). These studies showed that hydrocortisone administered at either 0.4 or 1.0 mg per mouse per day eliminated recruitment of eosinophils and lymphocytes, but had no effect on the production of proinflammatory chemokines (including MIP-1α) and likewise had no effect on the influx of neutrophils. Interestingly, two independent groups demonstrated that glucocorticoid therapy likewise had no effect on chemokines elicited in response to hRSV infection in human subjects (Thomas et al., 2002; Jafri, 2003). Furthermore, hydrocortisone administration in PVM-infected mice results in the recovery of nearly 10-fold higher virus titres and overall accelerated mortality (mean survival 8.4 ± 0.4 vs. 11.5 ± 1.4 days, $p < 0.05$). The principle to be appreciated is that all inflammatory responses are not the same. Although glucocorticoids have a clear role in reducing allergic inflammation in the lung, here they are clearly unable to reduce the negative impact of the inflammatory response characteristic of pneumovirus infection. Glucocorticoids have been shown to have no effect on the production of MIP-1α (consistent with clinical findings in humans) and the associated influx of neutrophils. A different anti-inflammatory, or immunomodulatory approach might be more effective.

Combined antiviral/immunomodulatory therapy for acute pneumovirus infection

As is clear from both the clinical picture with hRSV and with PVM infected mice, limiting virus replication alone is insufficient to reduce the inflammatory component of severe pneumovirus infection. At the same time, both clinical and experimental experience with systemic glucocorticoids indicates that an approach directed towards the components that elicit neutrophil influx might have a greater overall impact on disease pathogenesis. Towards that end, the responses of PVM-infected mice to treatment with ribavirin in combination with genetic, immunological or biochemical immunomodulatory blockade have been examined (Bonville et al., 2003, 2004). These data showed that it is possible to reduce the mortality of PVM infection if ribavirin is administered to MIP-1α or CCR1 gene-deleted mice, or administered to wild-type mice in conjunction with anti-MIP-1α neutralising antibodies, or with the small-molecule CCR1 inhibitor, met-RANTES (Fig. 5). In a more recent study, similar reductions in morbidity and mortality were observed when ribavirin was combined with the CysLT1 cysteinyl leucotriene receptor antagonist, montelukast (Bonville et al., 2006b). These important new therapeutic directions might ultimately be considered for human phase I trials.

Allergic sensitisation and respiratory virus infection

Respiratory virus infection in early infancy is recognised as among the potential risk factors for the development of childhood asthma, particularly infection with hRSV (Gern, 2004; Jartti et al., 2005). In a recent publication, Barends and colleagues (Barends et al., 2004) used traditional ovalbumin inhalation sensitisation and challenge, with a superimposed virus inoculation, including challenge with influenza, hRSV and PVM. PVM (and hRSV) enhance pulmonary inflammatory responses over and above what would be observed with ovalbumin challenge alone, in association with increased expression of transcripts encoding the Th2 cytokines IL-4, -5, and -13, and increased influx of eosinophils. Although the molecular mechanism remain to be elucidated, the authors present several intriguing hypotheses including structural links related to the PVM and hRSV G proteins, and issues related to chemokine production from infected respiratory epithelial cells.

The role of TLRs in pneumovirus infection in vivo

As noted earlier, Garvey and colleagues (Garvey et al., 2005) reported differential transcription of TLR3 in response to PVM infection in IFNαβR-gene-deleted mice. TLR3 has been characterised as a pathogen-response receptor that detects double-stranded RNA that may (or may not) function in antiviral host defence (Schroder and Bowie, 2005); further exploration of this observation *vis à vis* PVM infection is certainly warranted. More recently, Desmecht and colleagues (Faisca et al., 2006) demonstrated conclusively that TLR4 does not play a role in host defence against PVM infection. TLR4 was originally characterised as a pattern receptor crucial in

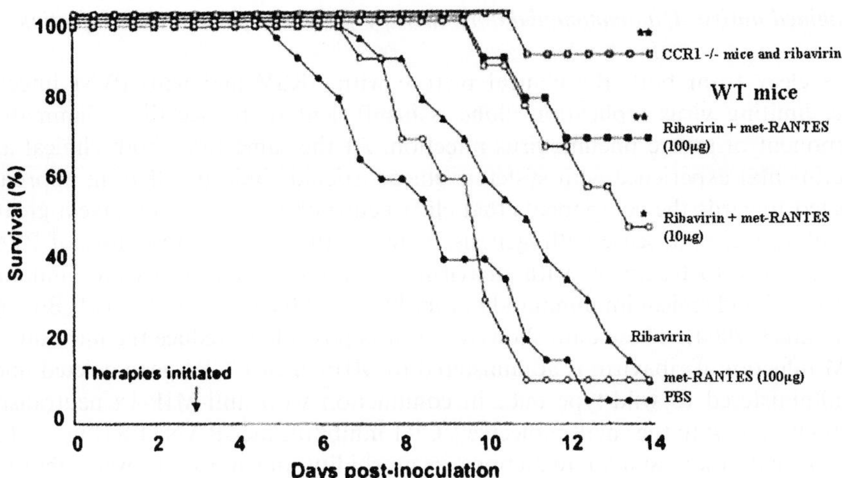

Fig. 5 Improved survival of PVM-infected mice treated with ribavirin and met-RANTES. Significantly improved survival was seen in the +ribavirin +met-RANTES groups (*$p<0.05$) when compared individually to the +met-RANTES alone, +ribavirin alone, or control groups. The combination of ribavirin with the higher met-RANTES dose (100 μg/day) offered additional survival benefit over the ribavirin/met-RANTES (10 μg/day) group (**$p<0.05$), approaching that observed for CCR1-/- mice +ribavirin, representing a theoretical complete receptor blockade. Reprinted with permission from Bonville et al. (2004).

host defence against bacteria, yet several earlier studies suggested that TLR4 also played a role in innate immunity against hRSV. Desmecht and colleagues explored body weight, mortality, respiratory parameters, histopathology and virus titre, and could find no statistically significant differences between TLR4-sufficient and TLR4-gene-deleted mouse strains. These results stand in contrast to earlier findings on TLR4-mediated responses in the hRSV mouse challenge model, which demonstrate higher virus titres in TLR4-gene-deleted mice (Kurt-Jones et al., 2000; Haynes et al., 2001), although the results of these initial studies have since been questioned (Ehl et al., 2004). Human studies suggest that TLR4 mutations are over represented in patients with severe hRSV (Tal et al., 2004), yet overexpression of TLR4 correlates with greater disease severity (Gagro et al., 2004). Desmecht and colleagues conclude appropriately that they cannot rule out the possibility that TLR4 might have some 'RSV –specificity' that cannot be addressed with here; in the absence of this unlikelihood, they have provided conclusive evidence demonstrating that TLR4 has no role to play in host defence against pneumovirus infection *in vivo*.

Explorations of mucosal vaccination using attenuated PVM strain 15

Strain 15 is a tissue culture-passaged variant of the mouse-passaged PVM strain J3666 that has several characterised mutations, most notably in the virion surface

SH gene (Krempl et al., 2005; Thorpe and Easton, 2005). Strain 15 replicates effectively in C57BL/6 mice but causes no clinical symptoms or weight loss and results in seroconversion of intranasally inoculated mice. These mice are then protected from subsequent challenge from lethal PVM (strain J3666) infection. No seroconversion or protection is observed in response to intranasal inoculation of heat-inactivated (non-replicating) strain 15. This live-attenuated vaccine model can be used to explore the efficacy of mucosal vaccination, the role of adjuvants, and the role of various cytokine and signalling pathways via the inclusion of specific gene-deleted mouse strains. The latter has already been explored to some extent, with intriguing results (Ellis et al., 2006).

Basic biological explorations of PVM infection in mice have already provided a great deal of insight into the pathogenesis of pneumovirus infection *in vivo*. In combination with information from animal studies with RSV, these studies will continue to provide us with much additional information, with the added advantage of being able to assess potential therapeutic interventions in a natural situation.

References

Ahmadian G, Chambers P, Easton AJ. Detection and characterisation of proteins encoded by the second ORF of the M2 gene of pneumoviruses. J Gen Virol 1999; 80: 2011–2016.

Ahmadian G, Randhawa JS, Easton AJ. Expression of the ORF-2 protein of the human respiratory syncytial virus M2 gene is initiated by a ribosomal termination-dependent reinitiation mechanism. EMBO J 2000; 19: 2681–2689.

Barends M, de Rond LG, Dormans J, van Oosten M, Boelen A, Neijens HJ, Osterhaus AD, Kimman TG. Respiratory syncytial virus, pneumonia virus of mice, and influenza A virus differently affect respiratory allergy in mice. Clin Exp Allergy 2004; 34: 488.

Barr J, Chambers P, Harriott P, Pringle CR, Easton AJ. Sequence of the phosphoprotein gene of pneumonia virus of mice: expression of multiple proteins from 2 overlapping reading frames. J Virol 1994; 68: 5330–5334.

Barr J, Chambers P, Pringle CR, Easton AJ. Sequence of the major nucleocapsid protein gene of pneumonia virus of mice: sequence comparisons suggest structural homology between nucleocapsid proteins of pneumoviruses, paramyxoviruses, rhabdoviruses and filoviruses. J Gen Virol 1991; 72: 677–685.

Barr J, Easton AJ. Characterisation of the interaction between the nucleoprotein and phosphoprotein of pneumonia virus of mice. Virus Res 1995; 39: 221–235.

Begona Ruiz-Arguello M, Gonzalez-Reyes L, Calder LJ, Palomo C, Martin D, Saiz MJ, Garcia-Berreno B, Skehel JJ, Melero JA. Effect of proteolytic processing at two distinct sites on shape and aggregation of an anchorless fusion protein of human respiratory syncytial virus and fate of the intervening segment. Virology 2002; 298: 317–326.

Bermingham A, Collins PL. The M2-2 protein of human respiratory syncytial virus is a regulatory factor involved in the balance between RNA replication and transcription. Proc Natl Acad Sci USA 1999; 96: 11259–11264.

Berthiaume L, Joncas J, Pavilanis V. Comparative structure, morphogenesis and biological characteristics of the respiratory syncytial (RS) virus and the pneumonia virus of mice (PVM). Arch gesamte Virusforsch 1974; 45: 39–51.

Black CP. Systematic review of the biology and medical management of respiratory syncytial virus infection. Resp Care 2003; 48: 209.

Bonville CA, Bennett NJ, Koehnlein M, Haines DM, Ellis JA, DelVecchio AM, Rosenberg HF, Domachowske JB. Respiratory dysfunction and proinflammatory chemokines in the pneumonia virus of mice (PVM) model of viral bronchiolitis. Virology 2006a; 25(3): 87.

Bonville CA, Easton AJ, Rosenberg HF, Domachowske JB. Altered pathogenesis of severe pneumovirus infection in response to combined antiviral and specific immunomodulatory agents. J Virol 2003; 77: 1237.

Bonville CA, Lau VK, DeLeon JM, Gao J-L, Easton AJ, Rosenberg HF, Domachowske JB. Functional antagonism of chemokine receptor CCR1 reduces mortality in acute pneumovirus infection *in vivo*. J Virol 2004; 78: 7984.

Bonville CA, Rosenberg HF, Domachowske JB. Ribavirin and cysteinyl leukotriene-1 receptor blockade as treatment for severe bronchiolitis. Antiviral Res 2006b; 69: 53.

Bossert B, Conzelmann KK. Respiratory syncytial virus (RSV) nonstructural (NS) proteins as host range determinants: a chimeric bovine RSV with NS genes from human RSV is attenuated in interferon-competent bovine cells. J Virol 2002; 76: 4287–4293.

Bossert B, Easton A, Conzelmann KK. Pneumonia virus of mice non-structural proteins NS1 and NS2 mediate type I IFN resistance. In: Abstracts of Respiratory Syncytial Viruses After 45 Years. Segovia; 2001; 74.

Bossert B, Marozin S, Conzelmann KK. Nonstructural proteins NS1 and NS2 of bovine respiratory syncytial virus block activation of interferon regulatory factor 3. J Virol 2003; 77: 8661–8668.

Caravokyri C, Zajac AJ, Pringle CR. Assignment of mutant tsN19 (complementation group E) of respiratory syncytial virus to the P protein gene. J Gen Virol 1992; 73: 865–873.

Casola A, Garofalo RP, Jamaluddin M, Vlahopoulos S, Brasier AR. Requirement of a novel upstream response element in respiratory syncytial virus-induced IL-8 gene expression. J Immunol 2000; 164: 5944.

Chambers P, Matthews DA, Pringle CR, Easton AJ. The nucleotide sequences of intergenic regions between nine genes of pneumonia virus of mice establish the physical order of these genes in the viral genome. Virus Res 1990; 18: 263–270.

Chambers P, Pringle CR, Easton AJ. Genes 1 and 2 of pneumonia virus of mice encode proteins which have little homology with the 1C and 1B proteins of human respiratory syncytial virus. J Gen Virol 1991; 72: 2545–2549.

Chambers P, Pringle CR, Easton AJ. Sequence analysis of the gene encoding the fusion glycoprotein of pneumonia virus of mice suggests possible conserved secondary structure elements in paramyxovirus fusion glycoproteins. J Gen Virol 1992; 73: 1717–1724.

Claassen EA, van der Kant PA, Rychnavska ZS, van Bleek GM, Easton AJ, van der Most RG. Activation and inactivation of antiviral CD8 T cell responses during murine pneumovirus infection. J Immunol 2005; 175: 6597.

Collins PL, Dickens LE, Buckler-White A, Olmsted RA, Spriggs MK, Camargo E, Coelingh KV. Nucleotide sequences for the gene junctions of human respiratory syncytial virus reveal distinctive features of intergenic structure and gene order. Proc Natl Acad Sci USA 1986; 83: 4594–4598.

Collins PL, Hill MG, Camargo E, Grosfeld H, Chanock RM, Murphy BR. Production of infectious human respiratory syncytial virus from cloned cDNA confirms an essential role for the transcription elongation factor from the 5′ proximal open reading frame of the M2 mRNA in gene expression and provides a capability for vaccine development. Proc Natl Acad Sci USA 1995; 92: 11563–11567.

Collins PL, Hill MG, Cristina J, Grosfeld H. Transcription elongation factor of respiratory syncytial virus, a nonsegmented negative-strand RNA virus. Proc Natl Acad Sci USA 1996; 93: 81–85.

Collins PL, Huang YT, Wertz GW. Nucleotide sequence of the gene encoding the fusion (F) glycoprotein of human respiratory syncytial virus. Proc Natl Acad Sci USA 1984; 81: 7683–7687.

Collins PL, Wertz GW. The 1A protein gene of human respiratory syncytial virus: nucleotide sequence of the mRNA and a related polycistronic transcript. Virology 1985; 141: 283–291.

Compans RW, Harter DH, Choppin PW. Studies of pneumonia virus of mice (PVM) in cell culture. II: Structure and morphogenesis of the virus particle. J Exp Med 1967; 126: 267–277.

Cook PM, Eglin RP, Easton AJ. Pathogenesis of pneumovirus infections in mice: detection of pneumonia virus of mice and human respiratory syncytial virus mRNA in lungs of infected mice by *in situ* hybridisation. J Gen Virol 1998; 79: 2411–2417.

Cunliffe-Beamer TL. Eradication of pneumonia virus of mice (PVM) from mouse colonies. Lab An Sci 1988; 38: 520–521.

Domachowske JB, Bonville CA, Ali-Ahmad D, Dyer KD, Easton AJ, Rosenberg HF. Glucocorticoid administration accelerates mortality of pneumovirus-infected mice. J Infect Dis 2001; 184: 1518.

Domachowske JB, Bonville CA, Dyer KD, Easton AJ, Rosenberg HF. Pulmonary eosinophilia and production of MIP-1α are prominent responses to infection with pneumonia virus of mice. Cell Immunol 2000a; 200: 98.

Domachowske JB, Bonville CA, Easton AJ, Rosenberg HF. Differential expression of proinflammatory cytokine genes *in vivo* in response to pathogenic and nonpathogenic pneumovirus infections. J Infect Dis 2002; 186: 8.

Domachowske JB, Bonville CA, Gao J-L, Murphy PM, Easton AJ, Rosenberg HF. The chemokine macrophage-inflammatory protein-1α and its receptor CCR1 control pulmonary inflammation and antiviral host defense in paramyxovirus infection. J Immunol 2000b; 165: 2677.

Easton AJ, Chambers P. Nucleotide sequence of the genes encoding the matrix and small hydrophobic proteins of pneumonia virus of mice. Virus Res 1997; 48: 27–33.

Easton AJ, Domachowske JB, Rosenberg HF. Animal pneumoviruses: molecular genetics and pathogenesis. J Clin Micro 2004; 17: 390.

Ehl S, Bischoff R, Ostler T, Vallbracht S, Schulte-Monting J, Poltorak A, Freudenberg M. The role of toll-like receptor 4 versus interleukin-12 in immunity to respiratory syncytial virus. Eur J Immunol 2004; 34: 1146.

Ellis JA, Martin BV, Dyer KD, Domachowske JB, Rosenberg HF. Mucosal inoculation with an attenuated mouse pneumovirus protects against lethal challenge. 2006, Personal communication.

Faisca P, Tran Anh DB, Thomas A, Desmecht D. Suppression of pattern-recognition receptor TLR4 sensing does not alter lung responses to pneumovirus infection. Microbes Infect 2006; 8: 621.

Fearns R, Collins PL. Role of the M2-1 transcription antitermination protein of respiratory syncytial virus in sequential transcription. J Virol 1999; 73: 5852–5864.

Fiedler MA, Wernke-Dollries K, Stark JM. Mechanism of RSV-induced IL-8 gene expression in A549 cells before viral replication. Am J Physiol 1996; 271: L963.

Gagro A, Tominac M, Krsulovic-Hresic V, Bace A, Matic M, Drazenovic V, Mlinaric-Galinovic G, Kosor E, Gotovac K, Bolanca I, Batinica S, Rabatic S. Increased toll-like receptor 4 expression in infants with respiratory syncytial virus bronchiolitis. Clin Exp Immunol 2004; 135: 267.

Gannon J, Carthew P. Prevalence of indigenous viruses in laboratory animal colonies in the United Kingdom 1978–1979. Lab Anim 1980; 14: 309–311.

Garcia-Barreno B, Delgado T, Melero JA. Identification of protein regions involved in the interaction of human respiratory syncytial virus phosphoprotein and nucleoprotein: significance for nucleocapsid assembly and formation of cytoplasmic inclusions. J Virol 1996; 70: 801–808.

Garofalo R, Kimpen JL, Welliver RC, Ogra PL. Eosinophil degranulation in the respiratory tract during naturally acquired respiratory syncytial virus infection. J Pediatr 1992; 120: 28.

Garofalo RP, Paii J, Hintz KA, Hill V, Ogra PL, Welliver RC. Macrophage inflammatory protein-1α (not T helper type 2 cytokines) is associated with severe forms of respiratory syncytial virus bronchiolitis. J Infect Dis 2001; 184: 393.

Garrison MM, Christakis DA, Harvey E, Cummings P, Davis RL. Systemic corticosteroids in infant bronchiolitis: a meta-analysis. Pediatrics 2000; 105: E44.

Garvey TL, Dyer KD, Ellis JA, Bonville CA, Foster B, Prussin C, Easton AJ, Domachowske JB, Rosenberg HF. Inflammatory responses to pneumovirus infection in IFNαβR gene-deleted mice. J Immunol 2005; 175: 4735.

Gern JE. Viral respiratory infection and the link to asthma. Pediatr Infect Dis J 2004; 23: S78.

Gimenez HB, Cash P, Melvin WT. Monoclonal antibodies to human respiratory syncytial virus and their use in comparison of different virus isolates. J Gen Virol 1984; 65: 963–971.

Gonzalez-Reyes L, Ruiz-Arguello MB, Garcia-Berreno B, Calder LJ, Lopez JA, Albar JP, Skehel JJ, Wiley DC, Melero JA. Cleavage of the human respiratory syncytial virus fusion protein at two distinct sites is required for activation of membrane fusion. Proc Natl Acad Sci USA 2001; 98: 9859–9864.

Grosfeld H, Hill MG, Collins PL. RNA replication by respiratory syncytial virus (RSV) is directed by the N, P, and L proteins; transcription also occurs under these conditions but requires RSV superinfection for efficient synthesis of full-length mRNA. J Virol 1995; 69: 5677–5686.

Harrison AM, Bonville CA, Rosenberg HF, Domachowske JB. Respiratory syncytical virus-induced chemokine expression in the lower airways: eosinophil recruitment and degranulation. Am J Resp Crit Care Med 1999; 159: 1918.

Haynes LM, Moore DD, Kurt-Jones EA, Finberg RW, Anderson LJ, Tripp RA. Involvement of toll-like receptor 4 in innate immunity to respiratory syncytial virus. J Virol 2001; 75: 10730.

Hengst U, Kiefer P. Domains of human respiratory syncytial virus P protein essential for homodimerisation and for binding to N and NS1 protein. Virus Genes 2000; 20: 221–225.

Hong K, Cameron CE. Pleiotropic mechanisms of ribavirin antiviral activities. Prog Drug Res 2002; 59: 41.

Horsfall FL, Curnen EC. Studies on pneumonia virus of mice (PVM). II. Immunological evidence of latent infection with the virus in numerous mammalian species. J Exp Med 1946; 83: 43–64.

Horsfall FL, Hahn RG. A pneumonia virus of Swiss mice. Proc Soc Exp Biol Med 1939; 40: 684–686.

Horsfall FL, Hahn RG. A latent virus in normal mice capable of producing pneumonia in its natural host. J Exp Med 1940; 71: 391–408.

Hull J, Thomson A, Kwiatkowski D. Association of respiratory syncytial virus bronchiolitis with the interleukin 8 gene region in UK families. Thorax 2000; 55: 1023.

Jafri HS. Treatment of respiratory syncytial virus: antiviral therapies. Pediatr Infect Dis J 2003; 22: S89.

Jartti T, Makela MJ, Vanto T, Ruuskanen O. The link between bronchiolitis and asthma. Infect Dis Clin North Am 2005; 19: 667.

Johnson TR, Graham BS. Secreted respiratory syncytial virus G glycoprotein induces interleukin-5 (IL-5), IL-13, and eosinophilia by an IL-4-independent mechanism. J Virol 1999; 73: 8485–8495.

Johnson TR, Johnson JE, Roberts SR, Wertz GW, Parker RA, Graham BS. Priming with secreted glycoprotein G of respiratory syncytial virus (RSV) augments interleukin-5 production and tissue eosinophilia after RSV challenge. J Virol 1998; 72: 2871–2880.

Kaplan C, Healing TD, Evans N, Healing L, Prior A. Evidence of infection by viruses in small British field rodents. J Hyg Cam 1980; 84: 285–294.

Khattar SK, Yunus AS, Samal SK. Mapping the domains on the phosphoprotein of bovine respiratory syncytial virus required for N–P and P–L interactions using a minigenome system. J Gen Virol 2001; 82: 775–779.

Krempl CD, Collins PL. Reevaluation of the virulence of prototypic strain 15 of pneumonia virus of mice. J Virol 2004; 78: 13362.

Krempl CD, Lamirande EW, Collins PL. Complete sequence of the RNA genome of pneumonia virus of mice (PVM). Virus Genes 2005; 30: 237.

Kurt-Jones EA, Popova L, Kwinn L, Haynes LM, Jones LP, Tripp RA, Walsh EE, Freeman MW, Golenbock DT, Anderson LJ, Finberg RW. Pattern recognition receptors TLR4 and CD14 mediate response to respiratory syncytial virus. Nat Immunol 2000; 1: 398.

Lambden PR. Nucleotide sequence of the respiratory syncytial virus phosphoprotein gene. J Gen Virol 1985; 66: 1607.

Li J, Ling R, Randhawa JS, Shaw K, Davis PJ, Juhasz K, Pringle CR, Easton AJ. Sequence of the nucleocapsid protein gene of subgroup A and B avian pneumoviruses. Virus Res 1996; 41: 185–191.

Ling R, Davis PJ, Yu Q, Wood CM, Pringle CR, Cavanagh D, Easton AJ. Sequence and *in vitro* expression of the phosphoprotein gene of avian pneumovirus. Virus Res 1995; 36: 247–257.

Ling R, Easton AJ, Pringle CR. Sequence analysis of the 22 K, SH and G genes of turkey rhinotracheitis virus and their intergenic regions reveals a gene order different from that of other pneumoviruses. J GenVirol 1992; 73: 1709–1715.

Ling R, Pringle CR. Polypeptides of pneumonia virus of mice. I: Immunological cross-reactions and post-translational modifications. J Gen Virol 1989a; 70: 1427–1440.

Ling R, Pringle CR. Polypeptides of pneumonia virus of mice. II: Characterisation of the glycoproteins. J Gen Virol 1989b; 70: 1441–1452.

Mallipeddi SK, Lupiani B, Samal SK. Mapping the domains on the phosphoprotein of bovine respiratory syncytial virus required for N–P interaction using a two-hybrid system. J Gen Virol 1996; 77: 1019–1023.

Mills KC, Dochez AR. Specific agglutination of murine erythrocytes by a pneumonia virus in mice. Proc Soc Exp Biol 1944; 57: 140–143.

Mills KC, Dochez AR. Further observations on red cell agglutinating agent present in lungs of virus infected mice. Proc Soc Exp Biol 1945; 60: 141–145.

Parker JC, Tennant RW, Ward TG. Prevalence of viruses in mouse colonies. Natl Cancer Inst Mon 1966; 20: 25–36.

Poiley SM. A survey of indiginous mouse viruses in a variety of production and research animal facilities. Lab Anim Care 1970; 20: 643–650.

Pringle CR, Eglin RP. Murine pneumonia virus: seroepidemiological evidence of widespread human infection. J Gen Virol 1986; 67: 975–982.

Ramaswamy M, Shi L, Varga SM, Barik. S, Behlke MA, Look DC. Respiratory syncytial virus nonstructural protein 2 specifically inhibits type I interferon signal transduction. Virology 2006; 344: 328–339.

Randhawa JS, Chambers P, Pringle CR, Easton AJ. Nucleotide sequences of the genes encoding the putative attachment glycoprotein (G) of mouse and tissue culture-passaged strains of pneumonia virus of mice. Virology 1995; 207: 240–245.

Randhawa JS, Pringle CR, Easton AJ. Nucleotide sequence of the matrix protein gene of a subgroup B avian pneumovirus. Virus Genes 1996a; 12: 179–183.

Randhawa JS, Wilson SD, Tolley KP, Cavanagh D, Pringle CR, Easton AJ. Nucleotide sequence of the gene encoding the viral polymerase of avian pneumovirus. J Gen Virol 1996b; 77: 3047–3051.

Randolph AG, Wang EEL. Ribavirin for respiratory syncytiual virus lower respiratory tract infection: a systematic overview. Arch Pediatr Adolesc Med 1996; 150: 942.

Reyes GR. Ribavirin: recent insights into antiviral mechanisms of action. Curr Opin Drug Discov Dev 2001; 4: 651.

Roberts SR, Lichtenstein D, Ball LA, Wertz GW. The membrane-associated and secreted forms of the respiratory syncytial virus attachment glycoprotein G are synthesized from alternative initiation codons. J Virol 1994; 68: 4538–4546.

Rosenberg HF, Bonville CA, Easton AJ, Domachowske JB. The pneumonia virus of mice infection model for severe respiratory syncytial virus infection: identifying novel targets for therapeutic intervention. Pharmacol Therap 2005; 105: 1–6.

Schlender J, Bossert B, Buchholz U, Conzelmann KK. Bovine respiratory syncytial virus nonstructural proteins NS1 and NS2 cooperatively antagonise alpha/beta interferon-induced antiviral response. J Virol 2000; 74: 8234–8242.

Schroder M, Bowie AG. TLR3 in antiviral immunity: key player or bystander? Trends Immunol 2005; 26: 462.

Slack MS, Easton AJ. Characterisation of the interaction of the human respiratory syncytial virus nucleocapsid protein and phosphoprotein using the two-hybrid system. Virus Res 1998; 55: 167.

Smith AL, Carrand VA, Brownstein DG. Response of weanling random bred mice to infection with pneumonia virus of mice (PVM). Lab Anim Sci 1984; 34: 35–37.

Spann KM, Tran KC, Chi B, Rabin RL, Collins PL. Suppression of the induction of alpha, beta, and lambda interferons by the NS1 and NS2 proteins of human respiratory syncytial virus in human epithelial cells and macrophages. J Virol 2004; 78: 4363–4369.

Tal G, Mandelberg A, Dalal I, Cesar K, Somekh E, Tal A, Oron A, Itskovich S, Ballin A, Houri S, Beigelman A, Lider O, Rechavi G, Amariglio N. Association between common toll-like receptor 4 mutations and severe respiratory syncytial virus disease. J Infect Dis 2004; 189: 2057.

Taylor G, Stott EJ, Hughes M, Collins AP. Respiratory syncytial virus infection in mice. Infect Immun 1984; 43: 649.

Thomas LH, Sharland M, Friedland JS. Steroids fail to down-regulate respiratory syncytial virus-induced IL-8 secretion in infants. Pediatr Res 2002; 52: 368.

Thorpe LC, Easton AJ. Genome sequence of the non-pathogenic strain 15 of pneumonia virus of mice and comparison with the genome of the pathogenic strain J3666. J Gen Virol 2005; 86: 159.

Valarcher JF, Furze J, Wyld S, Cook R, Conzelmann KK, Taylor G. Role of alpha/beta interferons in the attenuation and immunogenicity of recombinant bovine respiratory syncytial viruses lacking NS proteins. J Virol 2003; 77: 8426.

Wertz GW, Collins PL, Huang Y, Gruber C, Levine S, Ball LA. Nucleotide sequence of the G protein gene of human respiratory syncytial virus reveals an unusual type of viral membrane protein. Proc Natl Acad Sci USA 1985; 82: 4075–4079.

Yu Q, Davis PJ, Barrett T, Binns MM, Boursnell ME, Cavanagh D. Deduced amino acid sequence of the fusion glycoprotein of turkey rhinotracheitis virus has greater identity with that of human respiratory syncytial virus, a pneumovirus, than that of paramyxoviruses and morbilliviruses. J Gen Virol 1991; 72: 75–81.

Yu Q, Davis PJ, Brown TD, Cavanagh D. Sequence and *in vitro* expression of the M2 gene of turkey rhinotracheitis pneumovirus. J Gen Virol 1992a; 73: 1355–1363.

Yu Q, Davis PJ, Li J, Cavanagh D. Cloning and sequencing of the matrix protein (M) gene of turkey rhinotracheitis virus reveal a gene order different from that of respiratory syncytial virus. Virology 1992b; 186: 426–434.

Yu Q, Hardy RW, Wertz GW. Functional cDNA clones of the human respiratory syncytial (RS) virus N, P, and L proteins support replication of RS virus genomic RNA analogs and define minimal *trans*-acting requirements for RNA replication. J Virol 1995; 69: 2412–2419.

Zimmer G, Budz L, Herrler G. Proteolytic activation of respiratory syncytial virus fusion protein. Cleavage at two furin consensus sequences. J Biol Chem 2001; 276: 31642–31650.

Zimmer G, Conzelmann KK, Herrler G. Cleavage at the furin consensus sequence RAR/KR(109) and presence of the intervening peptide of the respiratory syncytial virus fusion protein are dispensable for virus replication in cell culture. J Virol 2002; 76: 9218–9224.

Zimmer G, Rohn M, McGregor GP, Schemann M, Conzelmann KK, Herrler G. Virokinin, a bioactive peptide of the tachykinin family, is released from the fusion protein of bovine respiratory syncytial virus. J Biol Chem 2003; 278: 46854–46861.

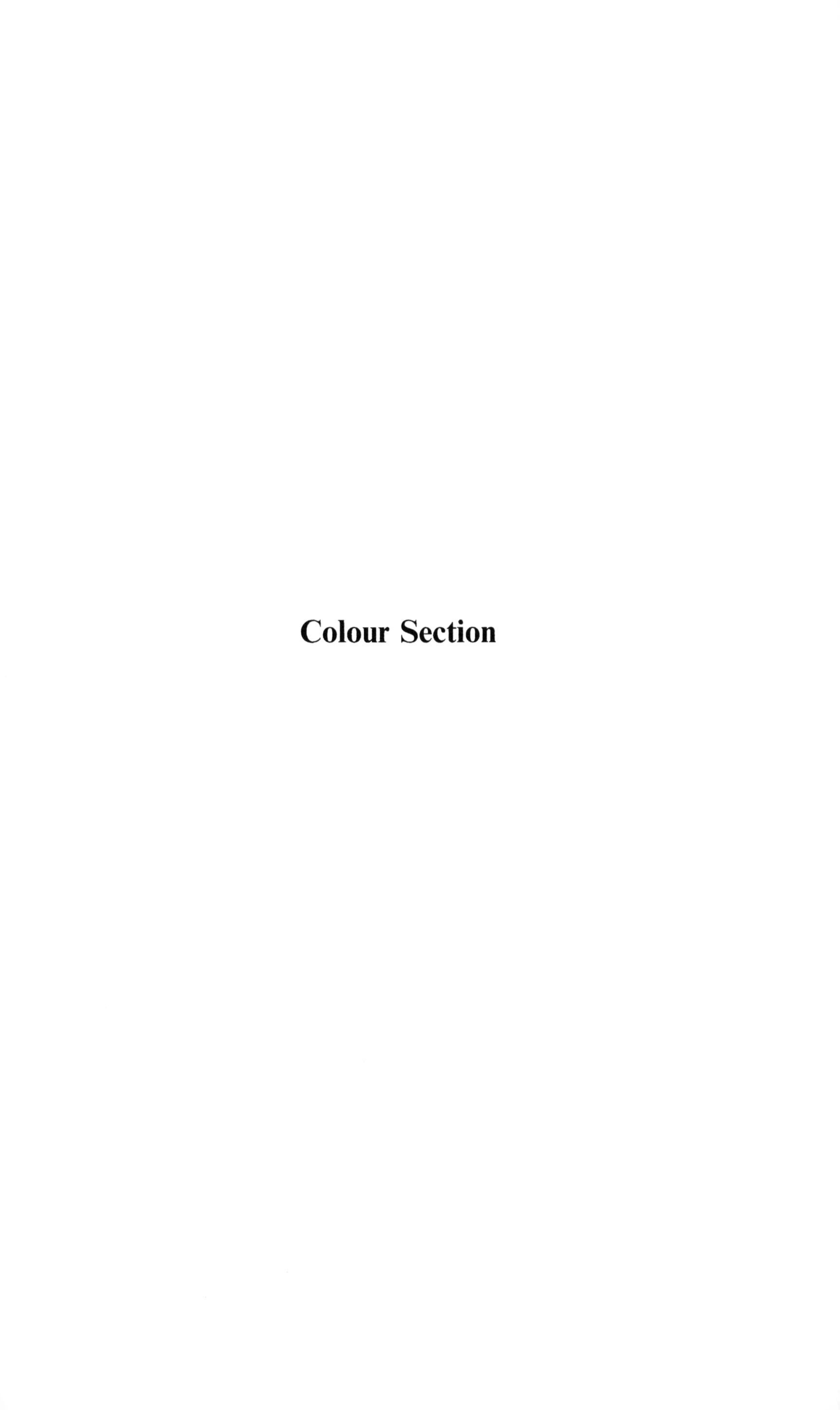

Colour Section

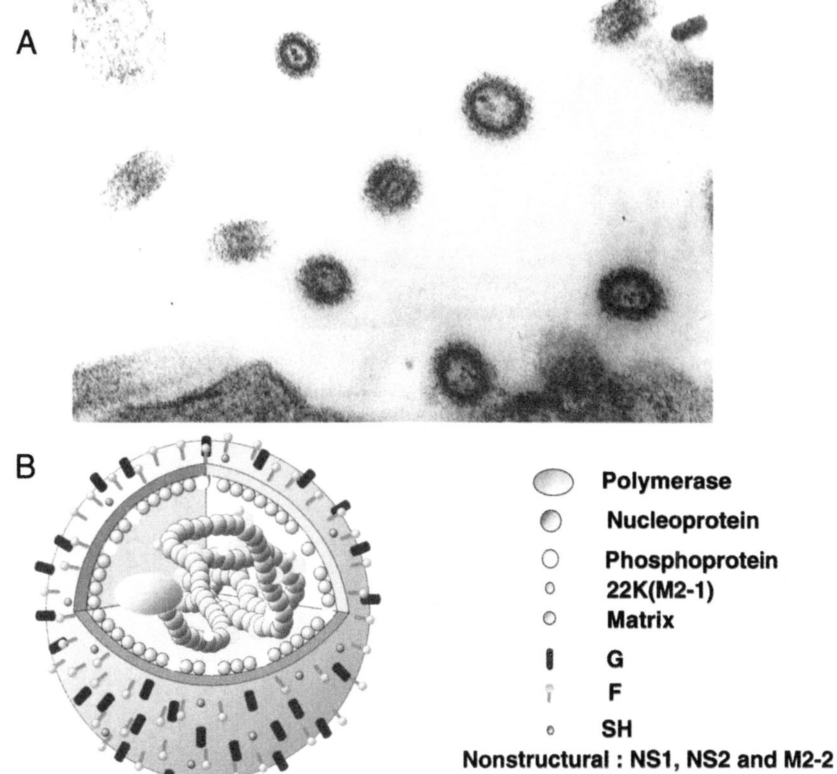

Plate 1 Electron microscopy (A) and scheme (B) of the HRSV virion. The structural (colour-coded) and non-structural proteins are listed in part B of the figure.

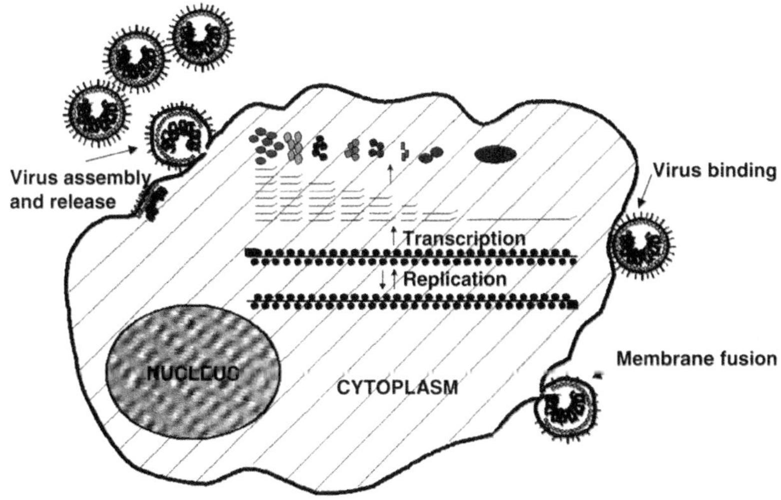

Plate 2 Diagram of the HRSV infectious cycle.

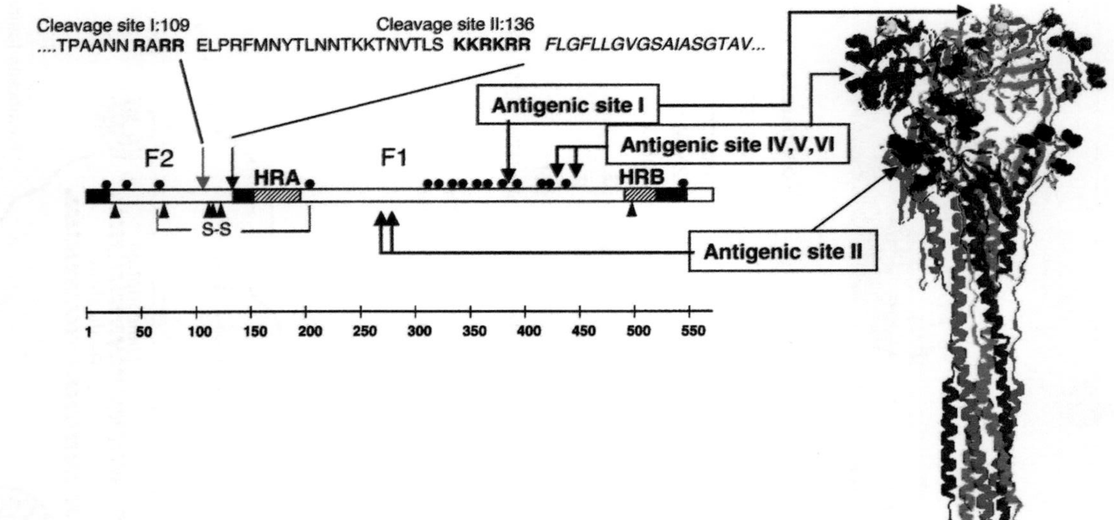

Plate 3 Scheme of the F protein of HRSV. The F0 precursor is depicted as a grey rectangle of 574 amino acids in length. The hydrophobic regions are shown in black and the heptad repeat sequences (HRA and HRB) in shaded rectangles, respectively. The two cleavage sites that yield the F1 and F2 chains are indicated by vertical arrows (red and blue). A partial amino acid sequence of the F protein, including cleavage sites I and II (with the furin recognition sequences shown in boldface) and the fusion peptide (italics), is shown above the protein diagram. Also shown are the N-glycosylation sites (▲), the cysteine residues (●) and the disulfide bond (–S–S–) between the F2 and F1 chains. A 3-D model of the HRSV F glycoprotein, based on the structure determined for the uncleaved parainfluenza type 3 F ectodomain (Yin et al., 2005), is shown at right. Residues that are changed in escape mutants selected with monoclonal antibodies, whose epitopes map in the different antigenic sites of the F molecule, are indicated in the protein diagram and in the 3-D model.

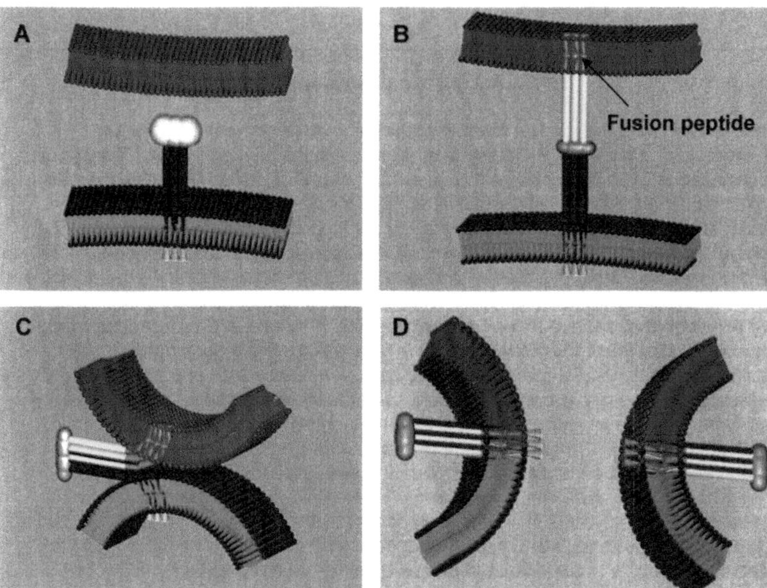

Plate 4 Model of the viral and cell membrane fusion mediated by the HRSV glycoprotein. (A) Only an F protein trimer is shown inserted into the viral lipid bilayer (green) and in the proximity of the cell membrane (red). (B) After activation of the F protein, the fusion peptide is exposed and consequently it is inserted into the target cell membrane. (C) Refolding of the F protein intermediate brings the viral and cell membranes into close proximity. (D) Lipid mixing of the two membranes forms the fusion pore that probably requires the concerted action of several F molecules.

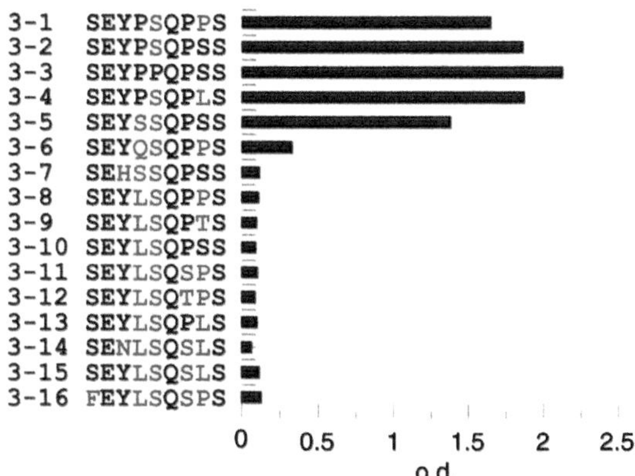

Plate 5 Reaction in an enzyme-linked immunoassay (x-axis) of a baby RSV convalescent serum with peptides based on natural variants of residues 283-291 of the G protein of group A isolates (y-axis). Peptide 3-3 represents the sequence of the infecting virus. The crucial change that abrogated antibody recognition in this case was change of residue 4, proline, to leucine. Change of this residue to serine appeared to have no effect unless residue 3, tyrosine, was also changed to histidine (peptide 3-7) while change of the residue to glutamine reduced but did not eliminate antibody binding. Adapted from Cane (1997).

Single nucleotide polymorphisms

Each person carries 2 copies of each chromosome, apart from the X and Y chromosome in males. Chromosomes are made tightly bundled DNA. The genetic information in DNA is carried by 4 bases, A, T, C and G. When a cell divides, DNA is replicated. Each of the 3 billion bases of DNA is faithfully copied and new chromosomes are made. Very rarely an error occurs, and one base is incorrectly copied. If this happens in a germ-line cell, this base change can be passed on to the next generation Base changes which have only deleterious effects will be rapidly lost from the population and never reach a measurably frequency. Base changes which are either neutral or have some beneficial effects can increase in frequency. Once they occur in at least 1% of the population they called single nucleotide polymorphisms or SNPs (pronounced "snips"). The frequency of a particular SNP depends on how long ago they arose and whether there has been any positive selection of the gene region in which they are located. Eventually most neutral SNPs will drift to 'fixation' - the point when they replace the previous base in all chromosomes in a population. SNPs occur every 100 to 300 bases along the 3-billion-base human genome. Two of every three SNPs involve the replacement of cytosine (C) with thymine (T). SNPs can occur in both coding (gene) and non-coding regions of the genome. Many SNPs have no effect on cell function, but others could predispose people to disease or influence their response to a drug.

Nearly all SNPs are bi-allelic. This means that there are 2 possible bases that can be present at the position of the SNP in the DNA sequence. The 2 different bases are called alleles. Individuals in the population will either carry 2 copies of one allele (homozygotes) or carry one copy of each (heterozygotes). The combination of the 2 alleles together is referred to as a person's genotype. The distribution of genotypes can be predicted according to the frequencies of the alleles – this is called the Hardy Weinberg distribution. The frequency of homozygotes is equal to the square of their allele frequencies and the frequency of heterozygotes is equal to the twice the product of the 2 allele frequencies – this is represented by the equation: $p^2 + 2pq + q^2 = 1$ where p and q are the common and rare allele frequencies respectively. It is expected that all SNP genotypes will conform to this distribution in both cases and controls. Significant deviation away from Hardy Weinberg frequencies can be an indication that the genotyping method is inaccurate.

Person 1
........**AGCTAATCCGCTGGTA**.......
........**AGCTAATCCGCTGGTA**.......

Person 2
........**AGCTAATCCGCTGGTA**.......
........**AGCTAATTCGCTGGTA**.......

Person 3
........**AGCTAATTCGCTGGTA**.......
........**AGCTAATTCGCTGGTA**.......

DNA sequences of 2 copies of each chromosome in each of 3 individuals are shown. Individual 1 is a CC homozygote, individual 2 is a CT heterozygote and individual 3 is TT homozygote.

Plate 6 Single-nucleotide polymorphisms.

Case control study

In a case control study, cases are selected by a given phenotypic characteristic, for example blood culture proven pneumococcal septicaemia. At least an equal number of carefully matched controls are identified. Allele frequencies are then compared between the two groups. For relatively rare diseases (affecting less than 10% of the population), odds ratio gives the best estimate of true relative risk within the population.

Affected D+ Control D-

	D+	D-
Blue allele	16	10
Red allele	8	14

Odds ratio (OR) = (16/8) / (10/14) = 2.8

Note in the example that the OR is the same whether it is calculated as the odds of being affected if carrying the blue variant, or the odds of carrying the blue variant if affected. It estimates the true population risk of being affected if carrying the allele of interest. The probability (p value) is calculated by Chi square or Fishers exact test. In this example, p= 0.08

Family-based study

The family based design can be easily understood by considering the hypothetical family in (a). One of the parents is heterozygous for the marker of interest and carries a blue and a red allele. The other parent is homozygous for the red allele and therefore not informative. When we look at whether the red or blue allele is transmitted from the heterozygote parent to the ten offspring, as expected, five offspring have the red allele and five have the blue allele. If it turns out that the blue allele predisposes to the infection being studied, then more offspring carrying the blue allele will be affected (in this example three blue versus one red). If we now select families on the basis of having an affected offspring, we notice that, because we are now selecting for those offspring who are more likely to carry the blue allele, there is an apparent excess of transmission of this allele from heterozygote parents to their offspring. In the example shown in (b), instead of the 50% transmission expected if there were no effect, we observe the blue allele being transmitted on 6 out of 10 occasions (transmission of 60%). This distortion of expected transmission forms the bases of the transmission disequilibrium test (TDT) used in most family based designs. The probability of this being a non-random variation (p value) is calculated using Chi square, with 50% transmission giving the 'expected' values.

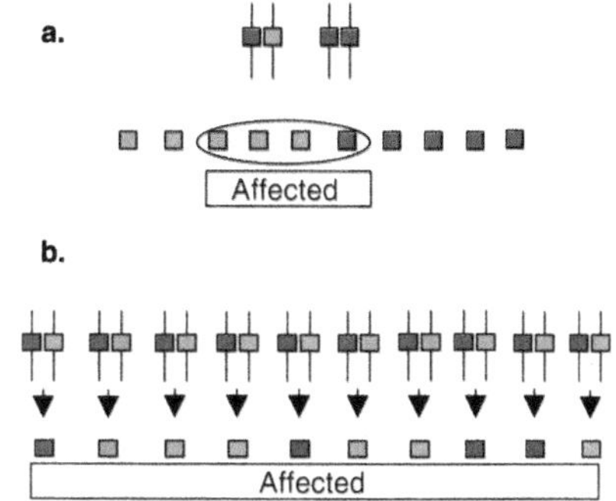

Adapted from Hull, J Genetic susceptibility to infection. in Infection and Immunity, Eds Friedland and Lightstone, publ: Martin Dunitz 2003.

Plate 7 Case–control study.

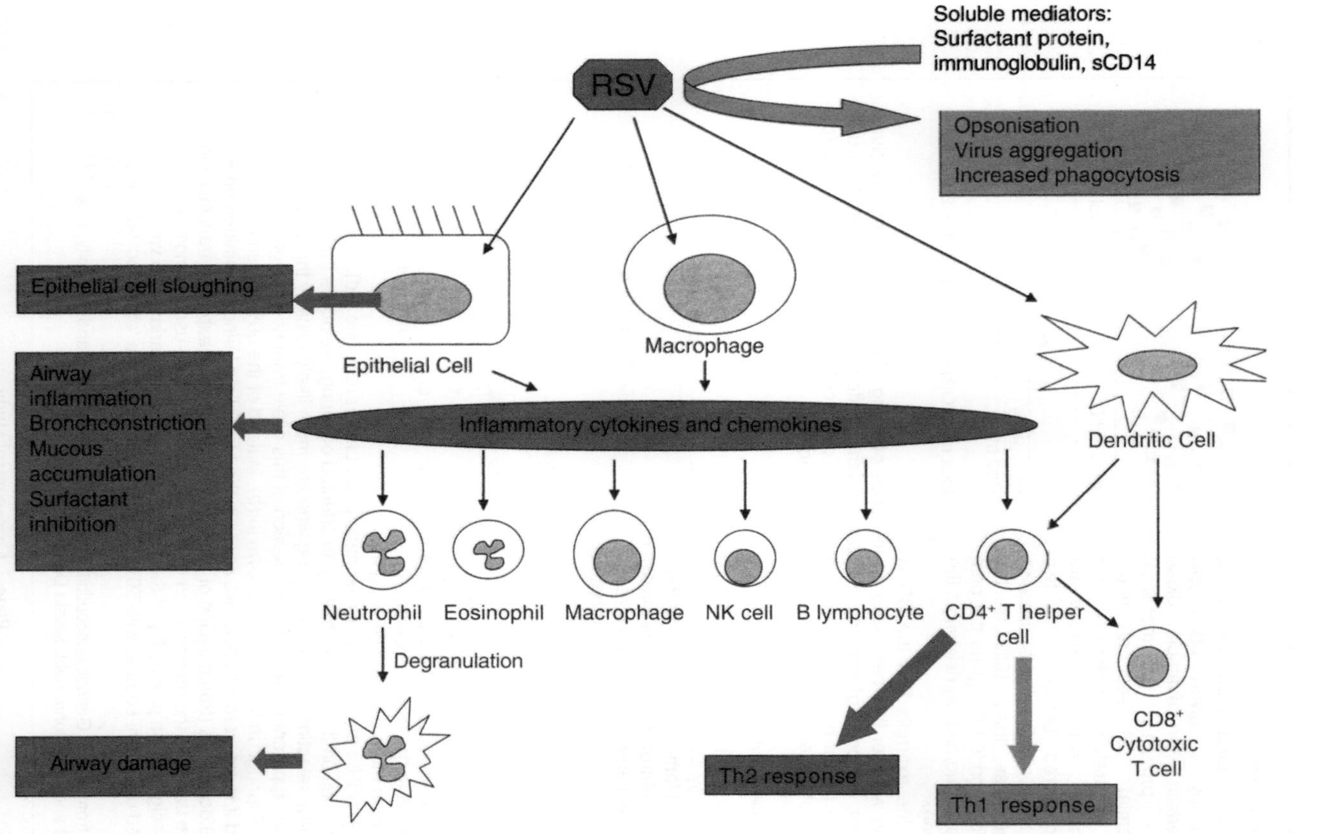

Plate 8 Pathogenesis of RSV bronchiolitis. RSV first infects ciliated epithelial cells of the respiratory tract. Inflammatory cytokines and chemokines, secreted by infected epithelial cells and macrophages, attract inflammatory cells and cause inflammation and bronchoconstriction in the airway. The predominant inflammatory cells in the airway are neutrophils and alveolar macrophages. Dendritic cells are the main antigen-presenting cells that stimulate T-lymphocyte function. Neutrophil survival is prolonged and IL-9 secretion promotes mucus production. CD4+ T-helper lymphocytes may be skewed to produce proinflammatory (Th2) cytokines. The combination of epithelial cell sloughing, mucus plugging and airway inflammation leads to the clinical presentation of acute bronchiolitis.

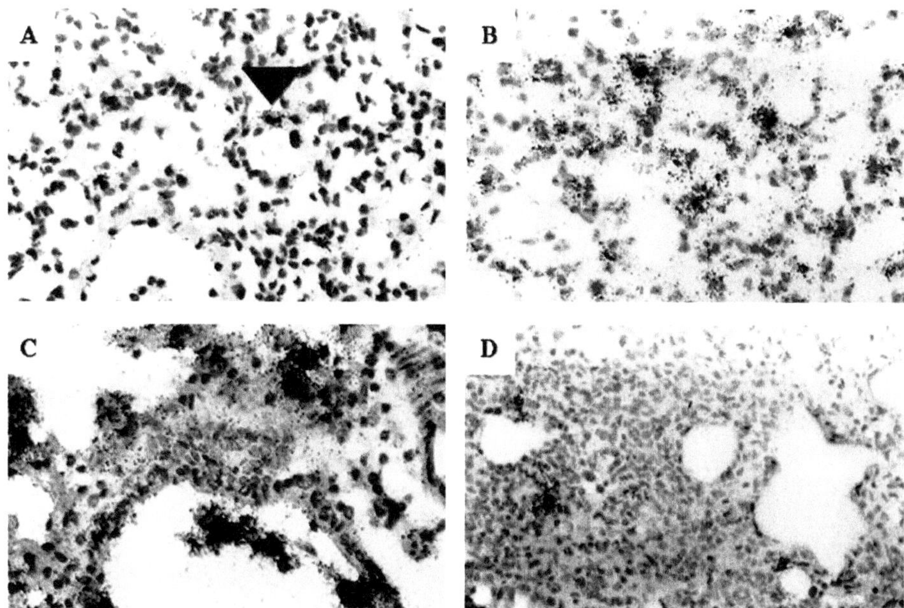

Plate 9 *In situ* hybridisation showing the progression of PVM infection in mouse lung. Following infection with PVM strain J3666 PVM N gene mRNA was detected by hybridisation with a radioactive probe. Silver grains indicate the regions of infected tissue, indicated by an arrow in panel A. (A) Tissues prepared two days after infection, (B) tissues prepared three days after infection, (C) tissue prepared four days after infection, (D) tissues prepared eight days after infection. Taken with permission from Cook et al. (1998).

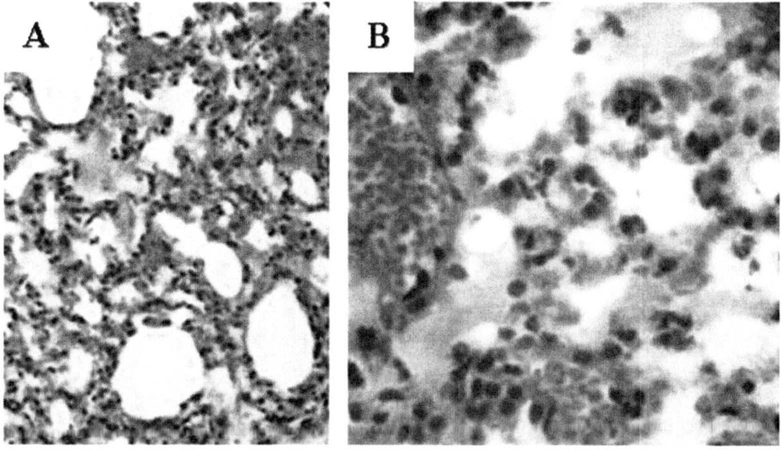

Plate 10 Inflammation in lung tissue in response to PVM infection. (A) Original magnifications, 20X and (B) 40X. The influx of granulocytes and pulmonary oedema, which can progress to complete compromise of the airways, can be clearly seen. Images courtesy of Dr. John Ellis, Western College of Veterinary Medicine, University of Saskatchewan, Saskatoon, Canada. Reprinted with permission from Rosenberg et al. (2005).

List of Contributors

Dagmar Alber
Arrow Therapeutics Ltd.
7 Trinity Street, Borough
London SE1 1DA, UK

Stephen P. Brearey
Division of Child Health
School of Reproductive and Developmental Medicine
University of Liverpool
Alder Hey Children's Hospital
Liverpool L12 2AP, UK

Patricia Cane
Health Protection Agency, Porton Down
Salisbury SP4 0JG, UK

Peter L. Collins
Laboratory of Infectious Diseases
National Institute of Allergy and Infectious Diseases
Building 50, Room 6503, 50 South Dr. MSC 8007
National Institutes of Health
Bethesda, MD 20892-8007, USA

Joseph B. Domachowske
Department of Pediatrics
State University of New York
Upstate Medical University
750 East Adams Street
Syracuse, NY 13210, USA

Andrew J. Easton
Department of Biological Sciences
University of Warwick
Coventry CV4 7AL, UK

Ann R. Falsey
Department of Medicine
Rochester General Hospital
1425 Portland Avenue
Rochester, NY 14621, USA

Jeremy Hull
Department of Paediatrics
John Radcliffe Hospital
Oxford University
Oxford, UK

José A. Melero
Centro Nacional de Microbiología
Instituto de Salud Carlos III
Majadahonda, 28220 Madrid, Spain

Yoshihiko Murata
Department of Medicine
Rochester General Hospital
1425 Portland Avenue
Rochester, NY 14621, USA

Brian R. Murphy
Laboratory of Infectious Diseases
National Institute of Allergy and Infectious Diseases
50 South Dr. MSC 8007
National Institutes of Health
Bethesda, MD 20892-8007, USA

D. James Nokes
Centre for Geographic Medicine Research – Coast (CGMRC)
Kenya Medical Research Institute (KEMRI)/Wellcome Trust
Reasearch Programme
Kilifi, Kenya and
Department of Biological Sciences
University of Warwick
Coventry CV4 7AL, UK

Kenneth L. Powell
Arrow Therapeutics Ltd.
7 Trinity Street, Borough
London SE1 1DA, UK

Helene F. Rosenberg
Laboratory of Allergic Diseases
National Institute of Allergy and Infectious Diseases
National Institutes of Health
Bethesda, MD 20892-8007, USA

Rosalind L. Smyth
Division of Child Health
School of Reproductive and Developmental Medicine
University of Liverpool
Alder Hey Children's Hospital
Liverpool L12 2AP, UK

Geraldine Taylor
Institute for Animal Health
Compton Laboratory
Compton, Newbury RG20 7NN, UK

Index

Printed and bound by CPI Group (UK) Ltd, Croydon, CR0 4YY
08/05/2025
01865007-0004